NORTH CAROLINA
STATE BOARD OF COMMUNITY
LIBRARIES
SOUTHEASTERN COMMUNITY COLLEGE

Keep on Running

Keep on Running

The Science of Training and Performance

Eric Newsholme

Department of Biochemistry, University of Oxford
and Merton College, Oxford, UK

Tony Leech

Gresham's School, Holt, Norfolk, UK

Glenda Duester

Department of Biochemistry, University of Oxford, UK

JOHN WILEY & SONS

Chichester · New York · Brisbane · Toronto · Singapore

Other Wiley Editorial Offices

John Wiley & Sons, Inc., 605 Third Avenue,
New York, NY 10158-0012 USA

Jacaranda Wiley Ltd, G.P.O. Box 859, Brisbane,
Queensland 4001, Australia

John Wiley & Sons (SEA) Pte Ltd, 37 Jala Pemimpin #05-04,
Block B, Union Industrial Building, Singapore 2057

John Wiley & Sons (Canada) Ltd, 22 Worcester Road,
Rexdale, Ontario M9W 1L1, Canada

Library of Congress Cataloguing-in-Publication Data

Newsholme, E. A.
    Keep on running: the science of training and performance / Eric
Newsholme, Tony Leech, Glenda Duester.
      p. cm
    Includes bibliographical references (p.) and index.
    ISBN 0 471 94313 4 (cloth)   ISBN 0 471 94314 2 (pbk)
    1. Running–Training. 2. Running–Physiological aspects.
I. Leech, A. R. II. Duester, Glenda. III. Title.
GV1061.5,N49   1993
796.42–dc20   93.49630
                                                         CIP

British Library Cataloguing in Publication Data

A catalogue record for this book is available from the British Library

ISBN 0 471 94313 4 (cloth)
ISBN 0 471 94314 2 (paper)

Typeset in 10/12pt Century Schoolbook by
Acorn Bookwork, Salisbury, Wilts
Printed and bound in Great Britain by Redwood Books, Trowbridge,
Wiltshire

Contents

Authors

Eric Newsholme, M.A., Ph.D., D.Sc., is a Reader in Cellular Nutrition, at the Department of Biochemistry, University of Oxford, UK. He is an experienced marathon runner, having participated in 37 marathons. Dr Newsholme is co-author of *Regulation in Metabolism* (Wiley 1973), *Biochemistry for the Medical Sciences* (Wiley 1983), *The Runner* (Fitness Press, USA, 1983) and numerous research papers.

Tony Leech, M.A., D.Phil., is a biology teacher at Gresham's School, Holt, UK. He is co-author of *Biochemistry for Medical Sciences* (Wiley 1983) and *The Runner* (Fitness Press, USA, 1983).

Glenda Duester, B.A., M.Sc., is a research assistant in biochemistry at the University of Oxford, UK. She is a club marathon and half-marathon runner.

Bruce Tulloh, Ph.D., was the gold medal winner at 5000 metres in the European Championships (1962). He is a biology master at Marlborough College, Wiltshire, UK and is currently coaching editor of *Runner's World*.

The foreword was kindly written by **Professor P.-O. Åstrand**, Emeritus Professor, Karolinska Institute, Stockholm and author with K. Rodahl of the classic *Textbook of Work Physiology*. He is a world authority on physical education and physiology and since he started in the field in 1946 is now a father figure of science in athletic performance.

Foreword

No other tissue in the human body can vary its metabolic rate so dramatically as skeletal muscle. In fact, active muscles can increase their oxidative processes to more than 50 times the resting level. Such an enormous variation in metabolic rate necessarily creates problems for muscle cells because, while consumption of oxygen and fuel (substrates) increases 50-fold, the rate of removal of produced heat, carbon dioxide, water and "waste products" must be similarly increased. To maintain the chemical and physical equilibrium within the body, there must be a tremendous increase in the exchange of molecules between the inside and outside of the muscle cells. When muscles are thrown into vigorous activity, the ability to maintain the internal equilibrium at a level permitting continuous exercise is entirely dependent on those organs that service the muscles. This dependence is especially true in the case of respiration and circulation, but certainly food intake, digestion and handling of substrates, kidney function, temperature regulation, water balance regulation and the effect of various hormones are also affected by variations in the metabolic rate caused by more or less intensive physical activity.

There is a definite tendency for new scientific frontiers like microbiology, genetics, immunology, developmental biology and neuroscience to dominate both in the award of research grants and in the teaching of medicine, medical science, biochemistry and biology. However, such emphasis on subject specialities by enthusiasts is not without risk. Other sectors of biology and medicine that may in the future become more important run the risk of being neglected. These risks have been emphasized by the American and British Physiological Societies. It is very important that physiologists and biologists convert the lifeless pieces of molecular and cellular biology into living systems.

In my opinion, "exercise physiology" is from these viewpoints particularly important because an exercise situation in various environments provides unique opportunities to study how different functions of the body are regulated and integrated. As stated above, most functions and structures in the body are in one way or another affected by acute and chronic (i.e. training) exercises. Therefore, exercise physiology is to a high degree an integrated science that has as its goal the identification of the mechanisms of overall bodily function and its regulation. It is therefore regrettable therefore, that so few pages in standard textbooks in biochemistry and physiology for medical students are devoted to discussions of the effects of physical activity on different structures and functions.

Newsholme, Leech and Duester have written an excellent and highly needed example of a text that illustrates the importance of a broad, holistic approach when analysing human structures and functions. Walking and running are activities developed millions of years ago during evolution of the hominid family. We have been hunters and gatherers, i.e. nomadic people, during more than 99% of our existence as hominids! Therefore "service systems" securing an optimal internal environment, function and performance during walking and running were developed, modified and adapted. It is very logical to choose running when discussing human biochemistry and physiology because it is a situation in which cells and organs are following the Three Musketeer principle in their functional strategies: "All for one and one for all!" Running can stress the body and mind to its limit and it is important and fascinating to analyse limiting factors, risks of overload, prevention of such risks and treatment of the consequences of overload. These aspects of human athletic achievement have high priorities in this volume.

The text is highly educational and it will serve professional teachers in physiology and medicine. At the same time, the authors have successfully presented and discussed complicated scientific events in a fluent and didactic style so that it can be enjoyed and understood by athletes and general readers with no formal background in biochemistry and physiology. The only prerequisite is curiosity about the function of the human body and this curiosity should have a high priority.

Per-Olof Åstrand

Preface

Most people have a greater understanding of how their car works than how their body works, although this is less likely to be true for athletes, who, in the process of pushing their bodies to the limit, acquire much information about themselves. Many runners will have had little in the way of scientific education and need to work hard if they are to assimilate all the biochemical, nutritional, physiological and psychological information that is now available. The reward for this effort, however, is now considerable, with the real possibility of using the information to improve performance. But even if this were not so, knowledge of what is going on 'under the bonnet' can add greatly to the pleasure of running even for those of us who will gain no medals.

This book has been written for athletes, at any stage of their career, for coaches, for physicians and for anyone who wishes to understand more about the scientific basis of running. It is also intended to help students of sports science, especially those without a strong background in science. For the most part we have emphasized ideas rather than details and, where possible, have presented biochemistry without the equations and physiology without the mathematics.

Understandably the athlete has a muscle-centred view of his or her body and it is with muscles that we begin in Chapter 2. Human muscles can no more defy the laws of physics than can the internal combustion engine so to continue working they require a source of energy. How this is stored, made available and can limit performance in different events is described in the following chapters. To be used, these fuels and the oxygen needed for their combustion must reach the muscles, and an understanding of the body's supply lines, described in Chapter 7, has always been an important aspect of sports science. Although female participation in all track and road events is now accepted, the history of women's running is short and in Chapter 8 we consider some of the few ways in which female runners are different.

The modern holistic approach to training acknowledges that the body as a whole must be trained and that this includes the mind. Although our understanding of the scientific basis of behaviour lags far behind our physiological knowledge, the scientific approach is maintained in Chapter 10. In contrast, much more is known about the connection between diet and human energy metabolism and in Chapter 11 we explore these links, seeking to correct misconceptions and show how the athlete's dietary needs are somewhat different from those of the average person. It is an unfortunate fact that most athletes will have to endure some spell of injury during their career and in Chapter 12 we attempt to explain the nature of common injuries. Whereas dietary manipulations are an accepted part of race preparation, the use of drugs is not and in the final chapter of Part I we present some of the reasons for this.

Above all, we hope to have not lost sight of the practical application of science to running and in Part II offer specific advice, beginning with a set of training schedules for a whole range of distances which can be modified to suit individual requirements. Readers may be surprised to find recipes in a book on scientific principles but any runner trying to cope with the special demands of intense training schedules, and the problem of finding time to prepare satisfactory 'athletic meals', should find them very useful. Part II also contains advice on many other aspects of race preparation, from learning to relax to choosing a bra.

It is, of course, not possible to write a book of this kind without a great deal of help from others. Much of this has been garnered from the written page—that repository of shared knowledge characteristic of scientific endeavour. Many of our sources have been listed as 'Further Reading' but there are inevitably many other pieces of published work which we have made use of, consciously and unconsciously. We are particularly grateful to Craig Sharp and to Priscilla Clarkson, who commented so generously and helpfully on the manuscript and helped us to avoid at least some of the more embarrassing errors. Help with particular parts of the book was provided by C. Pond, Open University, T.F.R.G. Braun, Merton College and J.A.N. Railton, Oxford University Committee for Sport. We would also like to thank the typists who have been involved with the preparation of this book, particularly Judith Kirby and Shirley Greenslade. We thank Brian Taylor, librarian of the Department of Biochemistry, University of Oxford, for his help in obtaining books and journals to aid our access to the information, so that we had more time for preparation of the book. We also thank Stanley Greenberg, honorary statistician to the British Athletic Federation and BBC TV Athletic Statistican for provision of information on current British, Olympic and World records for track and field athletic events and the marathon.

Finally we thank our families for their patience and support during the long periods of writing and preparation of the book.

Part I

Running Principles

Chapter 1

Running In

And it is right that in your Congress here you should study the 'making of a champion', *if I may borrow the title of the monumental book written here at Laval University. It is right that you should study the making of a champion, but it is also right that you should fulfil another and a greater task. Two centuries ago, the French Revolution gave us the concept of the rights of man. A century later, a great French statesman, Baron Pierre de Coubertin, added another right to those demanded by Jean-Jacques Rousseau and Robespierre; he added the right to play, to physical education, to unity of mind and body, to education in the Hellenic Gymnasium and in the playing fields. Baron de Coubertin not only created the Olympic Games, the magnificent assembly of the great élite, he propounded, first and lively to all mankind, the policy of sport for all.*

From a speech by Philip Noel-Baker, Director General of UNESCO, at the opening ceremony of an International Congress of Physical Activity Sciences in 1976 in Quebec City, prior to the Olympic Games in Montreal. Philip Noel-Baker won the silver medal in the 1500 m event at the Antwerp Olympic Games in 1920.

For many animals the ability to survive depends on ability to run, either from danger or to capture food; and human beings have most certainly survived for they are not only good runners but also versatile ones. This ability is still to be seen in modern times although we rarely have to run for survival. In the 1988 Olympic Games Carl Lewis won the gold medal in the 100 m, running at 43 km/h, and Gelindo Bordin won the marathon (42.195 km) in 2 h 10 min 32 s. In 1989 Tony Rafferty covered 1000 miles on the track in 14 days 11 h 59 min. These athletes were running not for survival but for pleasure—the pleasure of competing and the pleasure of winning. Many more men and women gain pleasure from maintaining their bodies in an optimal state of fitness, indeed the running 'high' has been likened to a state of drug-induced euphoria. Such pleasures are not new; two and a half thousand years ago professional Greek athletes, with their professional coaches, competed in organized competition for rich rewards.

Competition implies training—techniques and behaviour practised to improve performance. For, in contrast to machines, which begin to

Box 1.1   The Real Olympic Games

The first Olympic Games were held in 776 BC, although athletic competition had become popular in Greece long before that date. By AD 93 Games were held in 300 places, with four—Delphi (Pythian Games), Corinth (Isthmian Games), Nemea and, of course, Olympia—staging the most prestigious events (Figure 1.1). In their general nature they were probably similar to present-day Highland Games but the events were quite different and included:

- Boxing.
- Wrestling (including *pankration*, a form of all-in wrestling).
- Pentathlon (long jump, javelin, discus, foot racing and wrestling).
- Running events (the *stade* (hence stadium) of 200 m; the *diaulos* of 400 m and the longest race, the *dolichos*, of about 5 km) (Figure 1.2).

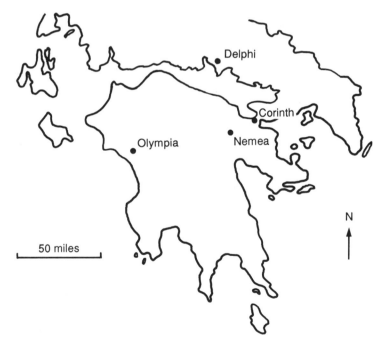

Figure 1.1. Map of Greece showing locations of the major Games in the Ancient Greek sporting calendar

continued

continued

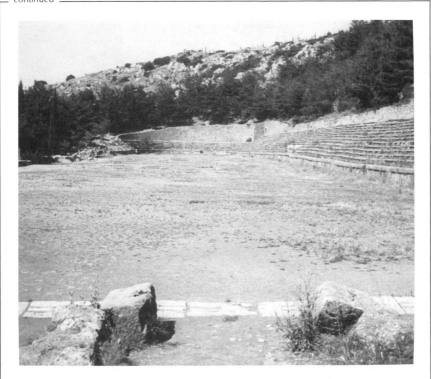

Figure 1.2. The athletic stadium at Delphi, Greece. Photograph kindly provided by the Ashmolean Museum, Oxford

Despite its Ancient Greek origin, the first marathon in the Olympic Games was run in Baron de Coubertin's resurrected Games of 1896 in Athens.

It is intriguing to see how many of the practices which we associate with modern athletics were common in this classical period. Take financial reward, for example. At first there was no prize money; winners were honoured with wreaths and laurels and only the wealthy could afford to travel to the Games, which existed primarily for the benefit of local people. However, when military conquests increased the wealth of the nation, prize money was offered and, by the second century BC, this had become generous enough to produce professional or 'career' athletes. All the available evidence suggests that, for these athletes in Ancient Greece, winning—not just participating— was the important thing!

continued

continued

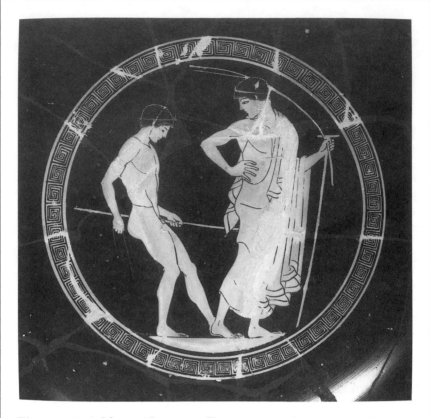

Figure 1.3. Athlete with trainer. Trainers were always depicted clothed and with a forked stick. Photograph kindly provided by the Ashmolean Museum, Oxford

The change from amateur to professional status was gradual but total. With it came specialization, so that athletes rarely won prizes in more than one event, and the combined event—the pentathlon—was relegated to a low status from which it has hardly recovered. The professional athlete's whole day was taken up by exercise, eating and sleeping—a lifestyle deplored by some writers of the time and no doubt by some of the population in general since athletes would have lacked the skills necessary for war and did little to benefit society as a whole. Euripides put the case against the athlete in his last play, *Autolycus*, in which he writes 'Of all the countless evils throughout

continued

continued

> Hellas (Greece) none is worse than the race of athletes ... slaves of their belly and their jaws they know not how to live well.'
>
> In the early years of Greek athletics, from about the sixth to the fourth centuries BC, it was considered that the daily toil of the farmer—lifting heavy weights, pulling a plough, grinding corn and, best of all, catching horses by running them down—provided adequate training. But with the professional approach came specific training (Figure 1.3) and by the end of the fourth century BC, training programmes, often involving a 4-day cycle, were in use:
>
> - Day 1   Preparation—short, brisk exercises.
> - Day 2   Concentration—all-out effort to exhaustion.
> - Day 3   Relaxation —rest and recovery.
> - Day 4   Moderation—technical exercises to prepare for special events.
>
> There is even evidence from paintings on vases that runners were paced by others on horseback—equivalent to the current practice of pacing by car.

wear out from the moment they are first used, human bodies actually improve with use. By imposing on ourselves patterns of activity and controlled stresses, we can improve our strength, endurance and co-ordination, but what every athlete would dearly like to know (and perhaps prevent his or her rivals from knowing) is what methods and duration of training are most effective. Since different events demand different qualities, the first principle of training must have been, if you want your body to do something well, make it do it again and again and again. Experience, however, has shown that this is not the most effective approach, so that, for example, a sprinter might gain more benefit from an hour of circuits or weight-training than from a day of sprinting. Through accumulated experience, athletes and coaches have devised methods which work. But are they the best possible?

TRAINING: A HISTORICAL PERSPECTIVE

Even in Ancient Greece the professional trainer was an important person. Often they had themselves been champions, like Iccus of

Tarentam (Taras) who won the pentathlon at Olympia some time during the fifth century BC. He is said to have been the first to write a book on training but, unfortunately, it has not survived. (The chances of any copies of *this* book being around in the year AD 4400 are pretty remote, too!).

Trainers knew that diet was important and ensured that the athlete's whole day was taken up by eating, sleeping and training. They also appreciated the importance of psychology in winning races, identifying the 'ideal' athlete as one able to face hard work, possessing a healthy appetite and who was rarely ill (and recovered quickly if he was). The importance of 'warming-up' was understood and a series of exercises, including running on the spot, was carried out before each event. There was also controversy. In his *De Ante Gymnastica*, Philostratus (third century AD) defended athletes against Euripides' diatribe but blamed trainers who indiscriminately applied hard-and-fast rules about diet and training techniques without regard to age or individual requirements. Have we heard this criticism elsewhere and more recently?

Reading the records of the nineteenth century is a pleasant pastime for today's runners (Table 1.1). If, a hundred years ago, you could have run 10 000 m in 30 min you would have been a world champion and hero; today's (November 1994) record for men stands at 26:52.23. But a record of that era which even today demands respect was set by Walter George, who ran the mile, in 4 min 12¾ s in 1886. During his running career, which spanned twenty years, Walter George set British records for all distances from the half-mile to 10 miles. His training methods influenced British athletes up to the Second World War and included the following features:

- Training was frequent—twice a day during the running season.
- Training was not excessively strenuous.
- Training was specific; if he wished to run at a pace of 65 s laps, that was the speed he trained at.
- Rest before races.

His general advice was 'run every day but do not run fast. Steady, long runs—anything up to 2 miles, with occasional shorter bursts of a quarter or half a mile and a few sprints, will soon make one fit.'

This would have seemed demanding at the time but by present-day standards it is very limited. Walter George may have been able to maintain a high level of fitness without the need for really hard training. During the winter, for example, he would not train at all

Table 1.1. Times for various track events and the marathon for male runners in some of the Olympic Games since 1896

Event	Times (h:min:s)					
	1896	1908	1924	1936	1960	1988
100 m	12.0	10.8	10.6	10.3	10.32	9.92
400 m	54.2	50.0	47.6	46.66	45.07	43.87
800 m	2:11.0	1:52.8	1:52.5	1:52.9	1:46.48	1:43.45
1 500 m	4:33.2	4:03.4	3:53.6	3:47.8	3:35.6	3:35.96
5 000 m	–	14:36.6[a]	14:31.2	14:22.2	13:43.4	13:11.70
10 000 m	–	31:20.8[a]	30:23.2	30:15.4	28:32.18	27:46.70
Marathon	2:58:50.0[b]	2:55:18.4[c]	2:41:22.6	2:29:19.2	2:15:16.2	2:10:32.00

[a] Olympic Games of 1912.
[b] Marathon distance 40 km.
[c] Marathon distance of 42.195 km for the first time.

except for his favourite 'hundred up', which consisted of running on the spot, lifting his knees to his waist 100 times. The training benefit must have been minimal.

Several generations of British runners religiously followed George's regime and some aspects were taken to extremes. George's concept of 'rest-preparation' has much to commend it but it was extended to justify training on alternate days only, and then only lightly. Sydney Wooderson, for example, who held the world records for the mile and half mile in the 1930s, did little more than short intervals, half or three-quarter miles, at race speed, in preparation for international events. The prevalent attitude towards energy expenditure, or rather its conservation, is well illustrated by Sir Adolphe Abrahams, brother of the 1924 Olympic sprint victor Harold Abrahams, who commented: 'We would even walk around gingerly the day before a race, putting our feet gently on the ground to avoid any undue effort.'

With the increasing international competition which developed between the world wars, something more than natural ability was needed. The extra factor was proper training and it was recognized that this played a large part in the increasing success of Germans and Scandinavians in international events. In particular, the Finns dominated the distance events, taking five gold medals in the 5000 m, 10 000 m and steeplechase races at the Olympic Games between 1920 and 1936. Their training regime was hard—much harder than that of the contemporary British athletes. The victorious Finns were farmers and foresters used to spending many hours each day on foot or on skis. The Finnish runners, Hannes Kolehmainen, Paavo Nurmi, Ville Ritola and others, became known as the 'Flying Finns' and set the standards which others followed. In the Stockholm Olympic Games of 1912, Kolehmainen, who was only 22 years old, won three gold medals: in the 10 000 m (31 min 20.8 s), in the 5000 m (in world record time of 14 min 36.6 s, which was 25 s faster than anyone had run this distance before) and in the 8000 m cross-country race. Eight years later, he won the Olympic marathon in the remarkable time in 1920 of 2:32.36. Kolehmainen was no simple peasant; he read and studied the training methods employed by other leading athletes and added to these his own 'year-round' conditioning programme.

More recently, Paavo Nurmi further developed intensive training techniques. From 1920 to 1924 he trained twice a day doing 6–7.5 miles with some sprints in the morning and, in the afternoon, a 2.5–4.5 mile run with a fast pace over the last mile. The afternoon session was finished with four or five 80–100 m sprints. During his running career he progressively increased the intensity of his training and as he prepared for the 1924 Paris Olympic Games included an extra late-morning session in which he ran four or five 80–120 m sprints, a timed 400–1000 m run, and followed this with 3000–4000 m at an even pace but with a fast last lap. In addition to the training, he would warm up 30 min before a race, wear a sweat-suit before and after races, use a stop-watch to learn to run at an even pace and was massaged before and after races.

The next major development, bringing us into more modern times, was interval training, first introduced by a German cardiologist for the benefit of his cardiac patients! It was the German coach, Woldemar Gerschler, who first used interval training systematically for top-class track athletes.

THE SCIENTIFIC APPROACH

It is unlikely, in the era before records were kept, that performances approached those of modern-day athletes, despite the claims of legend. It was said of the seventeenth-century Welsh runner Guto Nythbran that he was so fleet of foot that he could catch a hare on the mountain or that he could run down to the village and back before the kettle came to boil. Unfortunately for legends, science requires precise and quantitative information so that any claims can be tested and checked.

Box 1.2 Beating the clock

The Great Court of Trinity College is the largest quadrangle in Cambridge. On the first stroke of the midday chime on 7th June 1927, Lord Burghley (Figure 1.4), an undergraduate of Magdalene College, sprinted away from the Hall steps with the aim of running right round the perimeter of the court before the clock finished striking. In his own words: 'Ran round Trinity Great Court on the flags while the clock struck twelve, doing it just before the one but last stroke, time 42½ seconds. Witnesses: Tuckit, Allan, Howland and others.' The claim that Lord Burghley achieved this feat in full evening dress, patent leather shoes and that he ran at midnight is apocryphal; he was actually wearing running shorts and running shoes. The event was highlighted in the film *Chariots of Fire*, which publicized the

continued

continued

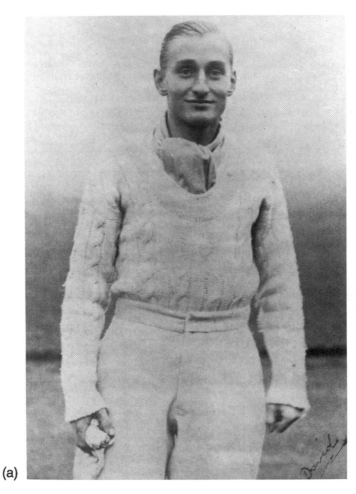

(a)

Figure 1.4. (a) Lord Burghley at Fenners in 1925. Lord Burghley represented England in the 400 m hurdles in the Olympic Games of 1924 and won the event in the 1928 Games. He died in 1981. Photograph reproduced by kind permission of the Masters and Fellows, Magdalene College, Cambridge

continued

continued

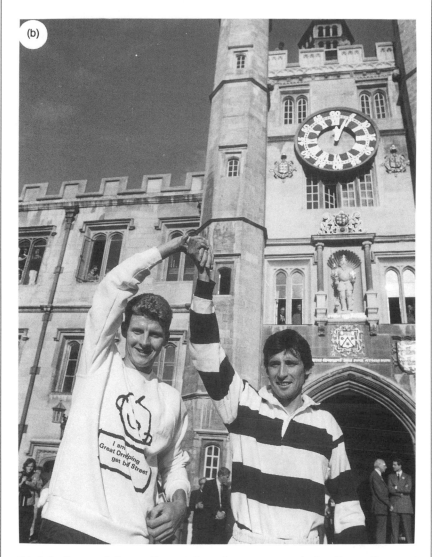

(b) Seb Coe and Steve Cram after the run around the Great Court of Trinity College, Cambridge, in 1988, and in front of the famous clock. Photograph reproduced by kind permission of the *Cambridge Evening News*

continued

continued

endeavour and is now not infrequently attempted by undergraduates at Trinity but usually at midnight and following a formal dinner.

On 29th October 1988, the run was re-enacted as a charity event with Sebastian Coe and Steve Cram taking up the challenge. Coe took 46 s to complete the circuit and Cram was 0.3 s slower. Cheers from the crowd made it difficult to tell whether they literally 'beat the clock' but a video recording confirmed that they did not. It is intriguing to speculate, therefore, on whether Lord Burghley really was the fastest runner. If he was then it would have been a remarkable achievement for the Olympic record for the 400 m was 3.7 s higher in 1924 than 1988. There must be doubts; for one thing the time taken for the clock to complete its 32 chimes varies: according to the state of winding, currently from 42.5 to 45 s. Conceivably this range could have been greater in 1927. Also how Lord Burghley's time of 42.5 s was measured is not clear. The other doubt concerns corners and the precise distance run. Like Lord Burghley, Coe and Cram started at the Hall steps, two thirds of the way along the western straight of the court, thereby including all four corners in the race. Lord Burghley stuck to the flags but whether he strode across the corners is not recorded: if the corners are cut so that the athlete runs on the cobbles at the corners, the distance is minimally 320 m; the full distance on the flags, upon which Lord Burghley claims to have run, is 341.6 m.

From Thorne, C.J.R. (1989). Trinity Great Court Run: the facts. *Trackstats*, **27**, 12–22.

How old was the hare? How far away was the village? How big was the fire under the kettle? Even timed records from previous centuries would not be accepted by modern-day officials. Take for example that of Tom Prince, the butcher from Newport who in 1774 ran, it was reported, 12 miles in 'ten minutes under the hour'. At 50 min for 19 320 m this compares more than favourably with the current (July 1994) record for the 20 000 m of 57 min 18.4 s. However, since he ran from one village to another, it is likely that his start and finish were recorded on two *different* church clocks—a timing procedure that science would never accept.

Until recently, science has done little for track athletes except provide accurate chronometers. In contrast, sportsmen who depend on equipment have, for some time, felt the impact of technology; balls bounce higher, vaulting poles are more springy and archery bows stronger. Although track athletes have benefited from improved shoe design and track surfaces, their performance depends almost entirely on their own bodies. Only recently has scientific understanding of human performance reached the stage where it can effectively influence training schedules, but we predict that the scientific approach will become increasingly useful to the athlete and the coach who understand science and who know how to apply its findings.

So, what do we mean by the scientific approach? We do not mean the use of high-tech gadgets and we do not mean discarding techniques which come 'naturally'. Science is about *understanding* things that are natural. When phenomena are understood they can be better manipulated to achieve a specific end. Science begins with observation and careful measurement. In biology there is often so much variation between individuals that many measurements have to be taken to ensure that any difference is not just the result of natural variation but is the result of, for example, a particular training programme or a particular diet. From such data, plausible explanations are constructed. Then comes the crucial part, the distinctive features of science: these explanations are tested, usually by experiment. Situations are contrived in which the outcome of treatment or an element of a training programme depends on the validity of the original explanation. The explanation is tried and tested, with the jury consisting of other scientists who will demand high standards of reliability and reproducibility before accepting the explanation. If the original explanation is not supported by the evidence, it will be modified or even rejected and new explanations put forward and these, in turn, will also be tested.

The more fundamental a newly discovered piece of knowledge, the more useful it is, because it can be used to explain a wider range of observations. Science depends on communication so that others can use these pieces of knowledge to construct more explanations—and so it continues, building up an ever-increasing framework of tested knowledge about our world. The application of this knowledge, although not without its detrimental aspects, has contributed immeasurably to the well-being of the human race. There is no reason why it should not also contribute, perhaps dramatically, to athletic performance.

When Mike Boit, the great Kenyan 3.49 miler, returned after winning his first Olympic medal, they said to him:

'So, you must be very fast.'

'Yes, quite fast.'

'Can you catch an antelope?'

'No, I don't think so.'

'Then you cannot be very fast. We have men here who can catch an antelope.'

As working biologists we know that science is not a magic potion that will turn any man or woman into an 'antelope catcher'. But, if properly applied, it should be capable of improving antelope-catching ability—or, at the very least, of telling us exactly how fast an athlete needs to run to catch the antelope.

To be useful, any introduction of science into the understanding of scientific performance or athletic training must involve us understanding:

- How our bodies work under normal conditions.
- How this working changes at maximum performance.
- Which processes limit our performance.
- How these limitations can be reduced.

At the same time we must *avoid* two pitfalls:

- The assumption that all individuals will respond in the same way to a particular training method (although, in time, the scientific approach should enable us to explain such variations and so tailor the training programmes more effectively to the individual).
- The rejection of training methods which, as yet, lack a scientific basis but which experience shows do work.

In 1989 the Finnish Society of Sports Medicine celebrated their fiftieth anniversary by hosting the 'Paavo Nurmi Congress: Advanced European Courses on Sports Medicine' and in the subsequent publication from the Finnish Society of Sports Medicine (edited by Martti Kvist and published in 1989), Tero Viljanen of Turku provided the following account of Paavo Nurmi, providing an insight into the reasons for Nurmi's remarkable athletic performances and highlighting his use of biological scientific knowledge as early as the first part of this century (Figure 1.5).

Paavo Nurmi was born in the City of Turku in Finland on 13th June 1887. The 'King of Runners' or the 'Flying Finn', as he was known, won a total of nine Olympic gold medals and three silver medals. He set sixty world records. He owned at the same time all world records in distances from 1500 to 20 000 metres. Nurmi died on 2nd October 1973.

Paavo Nurmi was superman of his age. He seldom lost a competition. He never did lose any cross-country race during his long top-athlete

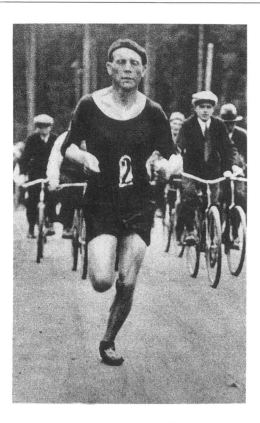

Figure 1.5. Paavo Nurmi, one of the 'Flying Finns', on the road from Heinä-joki to Viborg running his first and only marathon, in which he achieved a time of 2 h 22 min 03 s, for a 40 km marathon. Nurmi was preparing for the 1932 Olympic Games in Los Angeles but was not allowed to run because of doubts concerning his amateur status. Nurmi won more Olympic gold medals than any other athlete. Reproduced by kind permission of Yhtyneet Kuvalehdet Oy

career. His first record is dated in 1908 and the last competition happened in 1934, which means a 26-year long athlete career. Today he is one of the greatest legends ever seen on the fields of sports.

The kind of sports career Nurmi created cannot be explained by one or two factors. It is necessary to think about many kinds of factors needed for his successful top-athlete career.

Nurmi made his final decision to become a runner in the year of the Stockholm Olympic Games, 1912. This is the first important point; the aims were clear to him and the personal decisions firm enough to achieve them. His training was progressive and he continually observed the functioning of his body. He learned to know himself very well. He was trying and searching new training methods. Already in the early twenties he understood the very important relation between training, rest and good results. This phenomenon is still a big mystical problem to many present-day athletes. He followed his training programme exactly, but flexibly. His famous stop-watch was one of his best assistants—in training and competitions—showing him how to go on. He was able to conduct his exercises and competitions through a sound knowledge of his body. And the body learned to obey his will. His training included warming up and cooling down, but also gymnastics. He used to have massage and sauna regularly. His training was many-sided and occasionally also involved cross-country running in woods. Nurmi trained in the right way physiologically.

Nurmi's living habits were modest. He went to sleep early and did not smoke or drink spirits. He tried also vegetarian food, but he soon rejected this trial as not suitable to him. Everything served in a natural way the achievement of his aims. Finally the warm and religious spirit in his parents' home cannot be forgotten.

Nurmi was an extremely talented runner and a clever man. He had very strong willpower. All this together made it possible for him to become a self-made, legendary runner, well known all over the world.

The self-created and effective running style was like a crown on the head of the King of Runners.

Chapter 2

Muscles and Movement

Around 2600 years before the birth of Christ, human muscle power (in the form of some 4000 men working for 20 years) manoeuvred over 2 000 000 stone blocks, each weighing about two and a half tons, to construct the Great Pyramid for King Khufu at Giza. The enterprise depended on the ability of muscle to contract, the ability of men to work together and the application of science.

Over four and a half thousand years later, athletic success depends on the same factors: muscle contraction, cooperation between athlete and coach and, increasingly, the harnessing of scientific understanding to get the very best from those muscles.

But what is muscle? At its simplest, a muscle is a device which can be made to shorten, i.e. contract, and so pull closer together whatever its ends are attached to—usually bones. Hold your upper arm firmly with the opposite hand and bend the arm at the elbow with the palm facing upwards, as though you are doing a biceps curl with weights. You should be able to feel your biceps muscle as it contracts (and so bulges) to raise you forearm and relaxes when the forearm is lowered. In order to find out exactly how muscle works, the special tools of science must be brought to bear. Microscopes help, although ordinary ones tell us little more than that muscles are composed of many fine fibres arranged side by side. Contraction depends on the organization within the fibre, and to see this the much more powerful electron microscope is needed, with its magnification of up to a million times. This tool reveals the way that some of the protein molecules are arranged in the fibres and what happens to them when the muscle contracts (Figure 2.1).

The energy needed to power these contractions comes from chemical reactions which are the province of the biochemist who must, in comparison, work 'blind', for most of the molecules involved are too small to be seen by any microscope. By applying chemical methods of separation, identification and even modification of these molecules, a remarkably detailed picture emerges of just how a muscle works.

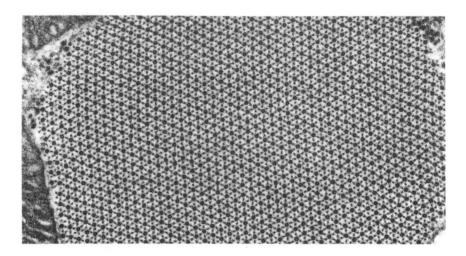

Figure 2.1. Insect flight muscle in cross-section, as seen magnified 112 000 times by an electron microscope. Each of the dots is an end-on view of a small cluster of molecules which form a filament. Contraction is caused by the thick filaments (large dots) and the thin filaments (small dots) sliding over each other. Electron micrograph kindly provided by Professor D. S. Smith, Oxford University

The picture is one of very small changes adding together to produce ever larger changes. Shape-changing molecules cause miniature rods to slide over each other; the sliding of thousands of rods, end to end, shortens whole fibres; the shortening of fibres, side by side, sums to generate the force of an entire muscle, and muscles contracting in perfect synchrony win gold medals.

GETTING MOVING

Muscles are attached to bones by tendons—tough, strong strands of connective tissue which transmit force from muscle to bone. Bones which need to be moved are connected at joints and held in place by ligaments. The contraction of a muscle therefore results in one bone moving relative to another. But contraction alone does not result in locomotion; it must be repeated at frequent intervals, which means that a muscle must extend as well as contract. Since muscles are incapable of returning to their original length through their own devices, they must be extended by some external force. Usually, this

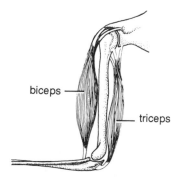

Figure 2.2. To deliver a punch, the arm is first flexed by contraction of the biceps brachii muscle (the 'biceps') and relaxation of the triceps brachii muscle (the 'triceps'). The arm is then rapidly extended by contraction of the triceps and relaxation of the biceps. Several other muscles are involved in flexion of the elbow

force is provided by other muscles which, because they pull in an opposite direction, are known as antagonistic muscles. This arrangement is seen in the muscles which move the forearm (Figure 2.2) but, even for such an apparently simple movement, many additional muscles are involved, contracting and relaxing to produce the smooth movement that we take for granted. And we do too readily take it all for granted, even when the whole structure—the bones, the muscles, the tendons and the ligaments—is drastically stressed during each training session. Knowledge of what actually happens as we run may convince us to treat our muscles and skeleton with respect, to avoid overtraining and to appreciate the problems that can arise as we train harder and harder (Chapter 12).

MUSCLES FOR RUNNING

The body contains approximately six hundred muscles (Figure 2.3). Almost all of these muscles play some part when we run but it is the numerous muscles of the leg which provide most of the power. Movements about three main joints—the hip, the knee and the ankle—are combined to produce each stride. By focusing on each joint in turn, and considering the role of each of the major muscles, we begin to form a picture of the complex patterns of contraction and relaxation involved in human locomotion (Figure 2.4).

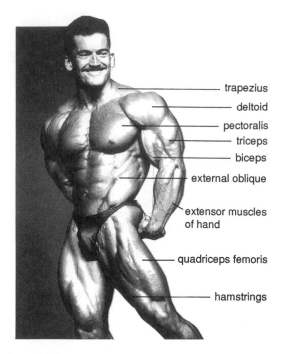

Figure 2.3. A body-builder, Lee Labrado, puts his muscles on view. Photograph © ALLSPORT/Bill Bobbins

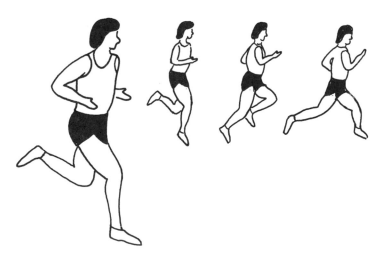

Figure 2.4. Positions of the legs in running. After Alexander (1992)

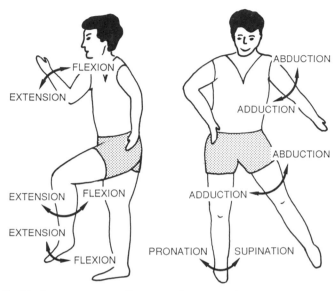

Figure 2.5. Limb movements. Some authors use the terms dorsiflexion and plantarflexion to replace the terms extension and flexion, respectively, at the ankle, and inversion and eversion (of the plantar surface) in place of supination and pronation

The hip joint is formed from the ball-shaped head of the femur and the socket on the outside of the pelvic girdle. This arrangement permits movement of the whole leg forwards, backwards and sideways (Figure 2.5). Three gluteal muscles stretch from the back of the pelvic girdle to the femur (Figure 2.6). The largest of these is the gluteus maximus, which forms the bulk of the buttocks and, when it contracts, pulls the femur back in line with the trunk (retraction). This backward drive of the leg is particularly important when running uphill, as indicated by the tender buttocks of the athlete who has just started hill-training in earnest. The other two buttock muscles help to support the trunk while the weight is on one leg.

A second set of muscles, known as the iliopsoas, draws the femur up and so opposes the movement produced by the gluteus. The iliopsoas and gluteus are therefore antagonistic muscles. The iliopsoas consists of the iliacus muscle, which runs from the top of the femur to the upper part of the pelvis, and the psoas muscle, which connects the top of the femur to the lumbar vertebrae (Figure 2.7). The iliopsoas is stressed, and so trained, by sit-ups.

The remaining hip muscles are those of the groin. Their contraction pulls the leg towards the midline but also, because of the way they are

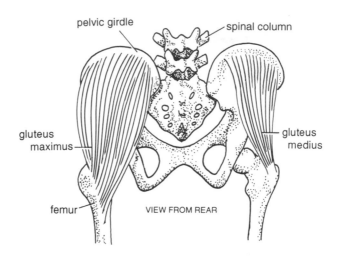

Figure 2.6. Muscles of the buttock. A third buttock muscle, the gluteus minimus, is situated under the gluteus medius

attached to the femur, rotates it outwards. This occurs during each stride in running but these adductor muscles are maximally stressed and sometimes damaged, in the twisting and swerving associated with sports like soccer and rugby. All the adductor muscles are attached at one end to the pelvis but at distances successively further down the leg as we go from the pectineus, through the adductor longus to the gracilis muscle, which is actually inserted in the head of the tibia— the lower leg bone. Longest of all, in fact the longest muscle in the body, is the sartorius muscle, which is involved in the rotation of both knee and hip.

Coming down now to the knee the picture is, at least superficially, simpler because the knee is a hinge joint and therefore is only capable of significant movement in a single plane. In fact, the elaborate organization of ligaments in the knee makes some twisting possible. The main flexor muscles of the knee, which contract as a stride is taken, are the hamstrings, which form the back of the thigh (Figure 2.8). All of the muscles which constitute the hamstrings are attached to the bones of the lower leg just below the knee. The upper ends of the semimembranosus, semitendinosus and one branch of the biceps femoris muscle are attached at the pelvis via long tendons which can be felt through the skin, and it is these that have given rise to the popular name hamstrings. The second 'head' of the biceps femoris attaches itself to the femur via a tendon.

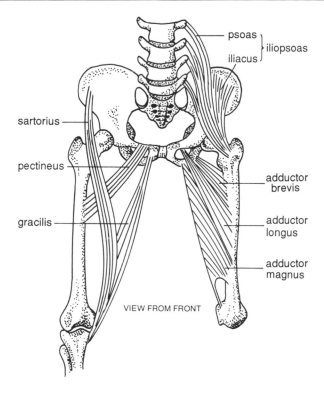

Figure 2.7. Muscles of the thigh. The iliopsoas complex lifts the leg as a stride is taken. The groin (adductor) muscles not only pull the leg inwards but also rotate it. Note that the lower ends of the gracilis and sartorius muscles are inserted (i.e. attached to the bone) below the knee and so contribute to movements at that joint

The group of muscles at the front of the thigh, which is antagonistic to the hamstrings, is known as the quadriceps. Literally this name means 'four-headed' and refers to the upper insertions; in fact the quadriceps is composed of four separate muscles. Of these, three vastus muscles are attached near the head of the femur and the rectus femoris is attached to the pelvis. All these muscles are inserted, via tendons, into the kneecap, which is connected to the tibia by the patellar ligament. When the quadriceps contracts the leg is extended.

We still have to explain how the ankle moves. This is another hinge joint and is extended by contraction of both soleus and gastrocnemius muscles, which form the calf. Since the gastrocnemius is attached to the femur, its contraction also flexes the knee. Both of the calf muscles are attached to the heel bone by the Achilles tendon—the longest

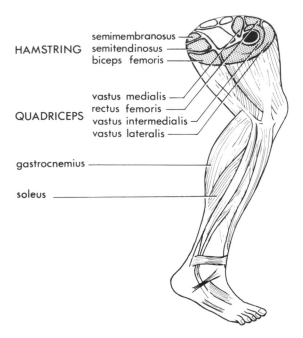

HAMSTRING
- semimembranosus
- semitendinosus
- biceps femoris

QUADRICEPS
- vastus medialis
- rectus femoris
- vastus intermedialis
- vastus lateralis

gastrocnemius

soleus

Figure 2.8. Muscles of the leg

tendon in the body. Antagonism to these calf muscles is partly provided by gravity pulling the weight of the body downwards but a series of muscles in the upper part of the foot also serve as flexors for the ankle. The foot also plays an important part in running and is discussed, along with foot injuries, in Part II(E).

Most of the energy expended while running at constant pace on the flat involves these major muscles, but a whole host of additional muscles play important roles in smoothing the runner's movements and extending the repertoire of leg movements. As the exhausted runner makes the final sprint to the tape, these minor muscles probably contribute a larger proportion of the energy expended, so their training, through such varied exercises as speed-running, fartlek (running at different speeds for different periods of time as dictated by mood rather than the coach or the stop-watch), grass-running, hill-running and circuit training, is important to the athlete.

Although a muscle is pre-eminently a contractile tissue, i.e. one which shortens as a result of chemical energy expenditure, it does not always operate in this way in the body. Try pushing against a wall. The wall doesn't move, so neither do your arm muscles, despite your very obvious expenditure of energy. Your muscles are contracting isometrically (or statically). The force developed per unit of energy expended is in fact greatest for these isometric contractions, so that muscles work most efficiently when their change in length is small— i.e. when they shorten very little or not at all. There is, however, a cost. Isometric contraction compresses arterioles within the muscle, so reducing blood supply. This increases dependence on anaerobic metabolism but at the same time decreases the rate of removal of its harmful by-products, which is why isometric contractions are uncomfortable and cannot be sustained. A further problem is that static exercise stimulates the heart more effectively than dynamic exercise (probably as a consequence of the impaired circulation) and can increase blood pressure dramatically—something that should be remembered by those pushing vehicles which have failed to start.

Isometric contractions occur when the force of contraction exactly equals the force preventing movement. In some cases the latter is actually greater, so that the muscle is extended despite expenditure of chemical energy. Such contractions are termed eccentric (in contrast to normal concentric contractions). During running, eccentric contraction occurs in the quadriceps on landing since the muscle is insufficiently strong to oppose the force generated by the descending body mass. The effect is greatly magnified when running downhill and may cause muscle damage and subsequent soreness and stiffness. Indeed, it is well established that such eccentric contractions do cause more damage than the usual contractions.

CONTROLLING THE CONTRACTIONS

With so many muscles involved in the apparently simple act of running (and the outline presented above *is* greatly simplified), their coordination is essential. Muscles must be instructed not only when to contract but by how much to contract and, just as importantly, when not to contract (Figure 2.9). A small error in the timing of contraction of a sprinter's hamstring muscle could result in its being torn by its powerful antagonist—the quadriceps—leaving the sprinter nursing a pulled hamstring for weeks.

The brain and spinal cord, together constituting the central nervous system, are responsible for this control, communicating with the muscles via peripheral nerves. Each of these nerves is a bundle of nerve fibres or neurones, some of which, the motor neurones, carry signals from the central nervous system to the muscles, while others, the

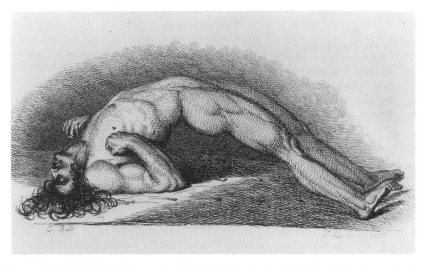

Figure 2.9. This soldier, wounded in 1809 at the Battle of Corunna during the Peninsular War in Spain, is suffering from the simultaneous contraction of *all* his muscles. His wounds have become infected with the tetanus bacterium, which produces a toxin that releases the inhibition of antagonistic muscles so that they also contract. From Bell, C. (1824). *The Anatomy and Philosophy of Expression*. John Murray, London

Box 2.1   When muscles don't get the message

Franklin D. Roosevelt, President of the USA from 1936 to 1945, had to use a wheelchair because he was paralysed below the waist. Not that there was anything wrong with his leg muscles but in 1921 he had contracted poliomyelitis and the virus responsible damaged his motor nerves, which could no longer carry impulses. When denied stimulation, muscles cannot contract and, instead, they undergo a kind of training in reverse—they waste away. However, the wasting only occurs in those muscles which do not receive electrical stimulation (Figure 2.10).

Paralysis can also occur when both nerve and muscle are in working order but are not in communication. Nerves and muscles interface at the neuromuscular junction, and South American Indians have long exploited its properties. When an impulse reaches the neuromuscular junction it releases a minute amount of a chemical called acetylcholine. With a delay of only a millisecond or so, this acetylcholine

continued

— continued —

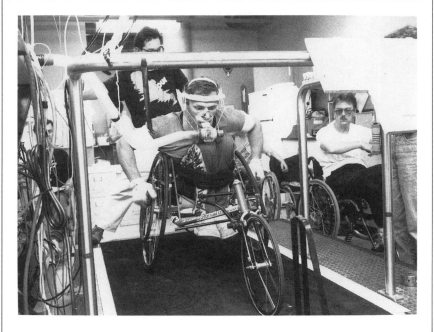

Figure 2.10. A wheelchair athlete undergoing performance testing on a treadmill at the Rehabilitation Research Centre, Cumberland College of Health Sciences, Widcombe, NSW, Australia. Photograph kindly provided by Associate Professor Gregory Gass

triggers the membrane of the muscle fibre into producing another electrical impulse which spreads through the fibre and stimulates contraction. The Indian hunter applies the sap of the Wurali tree (*Chondrodendron tomentosum* and other species) to his blowpipe darts. This sap, known as curare, contains *d*-tubocararine, which powerfully blocks this stimulation of the muscle fibre membrane by acetylcholine. When the dart strikes its animal target the drug passes rapidly into the bloodstream and then to the neuromuscular junctions, causing paralysis. If the animal is in a tree it lets go and falls to the ground. Paralysis of the respiratory muscles results in the death of the animal but it remains suitable for human consumption because cooking destroys the *d*-tubocurarine. For a while, *d*-tubocurarine was used clinically as a muscle relaxant but its use has been superseded by synthetic drugs which, nevertheless, act in a similar way.

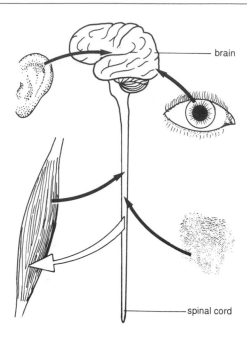

Figure 2.11. Together, the brain and spinal cord constitute the central nervous system, which receives information from receptors all over, and within, the body. In response, signals are sent out to muscles and glands to initiate the appropriate response

sensory neurones, bring information in. The central nervous system integrates and coordinates, matching responses to information received from the environment and from within the body (Figure 2.11). But the brain is no mere biological telephone exchange; the 6 000 000 000 neurones which constitute it add on such higher functions as memory, judgement, intelligence and consciousness.

The signals transmitted by neurones consist of electrical impulses, tiny changes in electrical potential which pass along the fibres at speeds of up to 100 m/s—faster than any sprinter. Since every impulse is identical (a potential change of around one-tenth of a volt lasting for less than 1/200 s) it is the frequency—the number of impulses per second—which conveys the information.

Limb movements are initiated in a part of the forebrain known as the motor cortex, where different regions correspond broadly to different parts of the body. From here, electrical signals pass down the spinal cord (except those to facial muscles which leave the brain

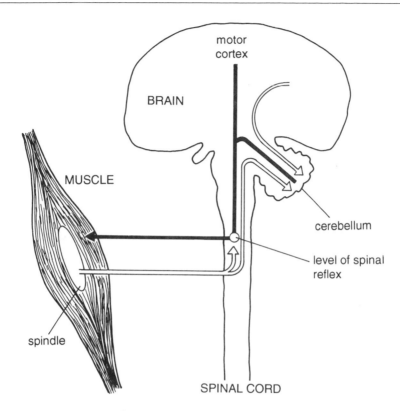

Figure 2.12. Outline of nervous control of muscle contraction. Black arrows
   represent motor pathways; white arrows represent sensory pathways

directly via the cranial nerves) and through motor neurones in the
appropriate peripheral nerve to the muscles (Figure 2.12). A single
impulse would cause the muscle to 'twitch', i.e. to undergo a single,
small contraction—not very useful for running. However, as the frequency of impulses rises, so the fibres in the muscle begin to sustain
a smooth contraction, or tetanus, which is much more useful (Figure
2.13). Furthermore, over a limited frequency range, say 20–45
impulses per second, the tension produced varies with the frequency.

Frequency changes are one way in which muscle tension can be
varied, but a more important way is by switching in additional motor
units. Since there are many fewer motor neurones than muscle fibres
in a muscle, each neurone must innervate many fibres, all of which
will therefore contract at the same time. Such a set of fibres, and the
neurone which controls it, form a motor unit (Figure 2.14). In muscles

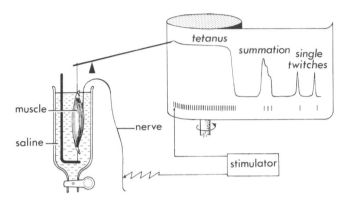

Figure 2.13. Under the right conditions, muscles are able to contract even after removal from an animal. Here, the nerve to an isolated muscle is being stimulated via the motor nerve at different frequencies and the resulting contractions recorded on a moving chart

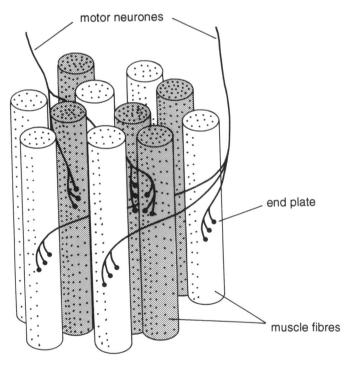

Figure 2.14. Part of two motor units. In reality the fibres would be more closely packed

where fine control of tension is important, motor units have few fibres—just 10 or so, for example, in the rectus muscles which move the eyeball in its socket. Motor units in the gastrocnemius, by contrast, typically contain a couple of thousand fibres. Consider your biceps as you lift a pen from the desk; sufficient force is generated by a few motor units. Now lift a heavy book and many more motor units will be recruited. Motor units overlap so that adjacent fibres may be innervated by different neurones. Furthermore, the contractile properties (e.g. speed of contraction, maximum force, fatigue resistance) of motor units vary, so that by controlling the firing pattern of motor neurones, different tensions and rates of movement can be smoothly achieved.

You go to pick up a suitcase you thought was full but is actually empty. Because the brain carries a 'memory' of the weights of objects, based on previous experience, more motor units are stimulated than are needed, so the suitcase is jerked upwards but, very quickly, the brain re-evaluates the situation and the vigour of the movement is moderated. This implies that the brain is being informed about the loads on the relevant muscles and their rates of contraction; indeed it receives this information via sensory nerves that run from every muscle into the central nervous system.

Much of the feedback control of movement is handled at the level of the spinal cord, where the right connections between neurones ensure that appropriate responses occur. Such reflex actions require no conscious intervention and are executed very rapidly, making them particularly suitable for controlling the basic patterns of movement. One such element is the stretch reflex, which serves to maintain a muscle at constant length despite changes in tension. Embedded between muscle fibres are sensory structures known as spindles, so that if a muscle is stretched the spindle, too, is extended and responds by sending impulses back to the spinal cord via sensory neurones (Figure 2.12). These result in stimulation of motor neurones so that tension rises and muscle length is restored. Such negative feedback is particularly important in postural muscles; without it we would collapse on the floor every time we tried to stand. It is also the basis for that classic demonstration of a reflex action, the knee-jerk response, when a light blow just below the bent knee results in the involuntary extension of the lower limb. Striking the patellar ligament suddenly extends the quadriceps muscle and the resulting small increase in length is detected by spindles within, which 'report' to the central nervous system. The response is a signal for contraction of the quadriceps. The functional significance of this is not clear but it may be that a stumble would produce a similar extension which would be corrected by the contraction. In a reflex action, a given stimulus always elicits the same response; this is both the strength and the weakness of the reflex as a controlling element in locomotion.

One further property of muscle spindles deserves comment. In order to maintain optimal sensitivity of the spindle over a wide range of muscle lengths, the tension within the spindle, and hence the 'resting' signal, can be adjusted by contraction of muscle fibres *within* it. The spindle thus becomes independent of the state of contraction of the muscle of which it is a part, so that it responds only to *changes* in length.

Spinal reflexes also play a large part in ensuring that antagonistic pairs of muscles never contract simultaneously, but signals passing up and down nerve tracks in the spinal cord keep the brain 'informed' and allow it to influence events. The cerebellum—a region of the hind-brain—is of particular importance in 'fine tuning' our movements. It sets the sensitivity of reflexes and controls levels of tension to produce the smooth coordinated movements of the dozens of muscles involved in taking a single stride. The cerebellum receives input not only from muscle spindles but also from visual, auditory and balance centres. Through its action, muscle tone is established and becomes affected by emotional state.

On top of all this complexity comes the safety override. Situated in the tendons (and also occurring in ligaments) Golgi tendon organs respond to changes in tension created either as a result of muscle shortening or due to a suddenly imposed external force. If such forces approach in magnitude those which would cause physical damage, connections are made in the spinal cord which result in the relaxation of the appropriate muscle and reduction of the tension to a safer level. And this safety factor is not redundant since muscles are sufficiently powerful that, if they contract at the wrong time, tendons and liga-ments can be damaged and bones can be broken!

TAKING A MICROSCOPE TO MUSCLE

If cooked meat is pulled apart, its fibrous nature becomes apparent. The fibres in muscle vary in length from about 1 to 60 mm and in thickness from about 10 to 100 micrometres (μm; i.e. from 0.01 to 0.1 mm). For comparison, a human hair is approximately 50 μm thick.

Each muscle is composed of many fibres—long thin cells, packaged into bundles of about one thousand each to form fasciculi (Figure 2.15). Each fasciculus is surrounded by connective tissue, to which each fibre

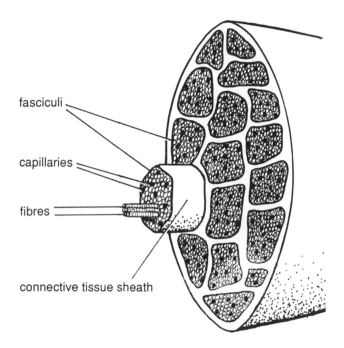

fasciculi

capillaries

fibres

connective tissue sheath

Figure 2.15. Arrangement of fibres and capillaries within a muscle

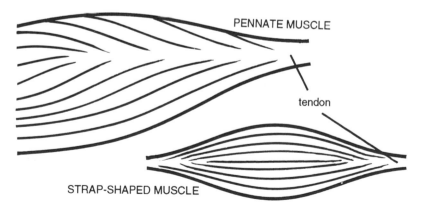

PENNATE MUSCLE

tendon

STRAP-SHAPED MUSCLE

Figure 2.16. Arrangement of fibre bundles in muscles

is attached and which in turn also links the fasciculi. The arrangement of these fasciculi varies from muscle to muscle. In strap-shaped muscles such as the psoas, the fasciculi run parallel to the long axis of the muscle—an arrangement which allows rapid and extensive shortening. Other muscles, such as the gluteus and indeed most human limb muscles, show a pennate arrangement of fasciculi in which the fibres are shorter and orientated at an angle to the contractile axis (Figure 2.16). Such pennate muscles are more powerful on a weight-for-weight basis because more fibres are contracting in parallel but, since each fibre is shorter, they contract over a shorter distance and more slowly. Since more work is obtained from a given amount of chemical energy when percentage length change is least, pennate muscles are inherently more efficient.

In a strap-shaped muscle there is little connective tissue within the muscle mass; most is concentrated in tendons at the end. Such muscles produce the tenderest meat; fillet steak is the psoas muscle of a cow. Pennate muscles contain more connective tissue and form the cheaper cuts at the butcher's.

To see any useful detail within the fibre it is necessary to view a very, very thin slice of the muscle in an electron microscope. Each fibre is enclosed in a membrane, composed of fat-like molecules and proteins, which isolate its contents from the outside. Inside the cell the most prominent feature is the contractile apparatus (the machinery that actually causes the muscle to contract), which occupies some 60–70% of the total volume and consists of myofibrils. A molecular telescoping system enables these myofibrils to shorten and so cause the whole fibre, and in turn the whole muscle, to contract.

Within the fibre, but outside the myofibrils, are other structures which make contraction possible (Figure 2.19). Mitochondria provide

Box 2.2   Moving molecules

Like the internal combustion engine, the working of the muscle engine is wonderfully simple in principle. Complexity comes with the need to maintain fuel supply, remove waste products and regulate power output. The fundamental units of contraction are the rod-like myofibrils which run the length of each fibre. Within these myofibrils are

———————— continued ⏘

continued

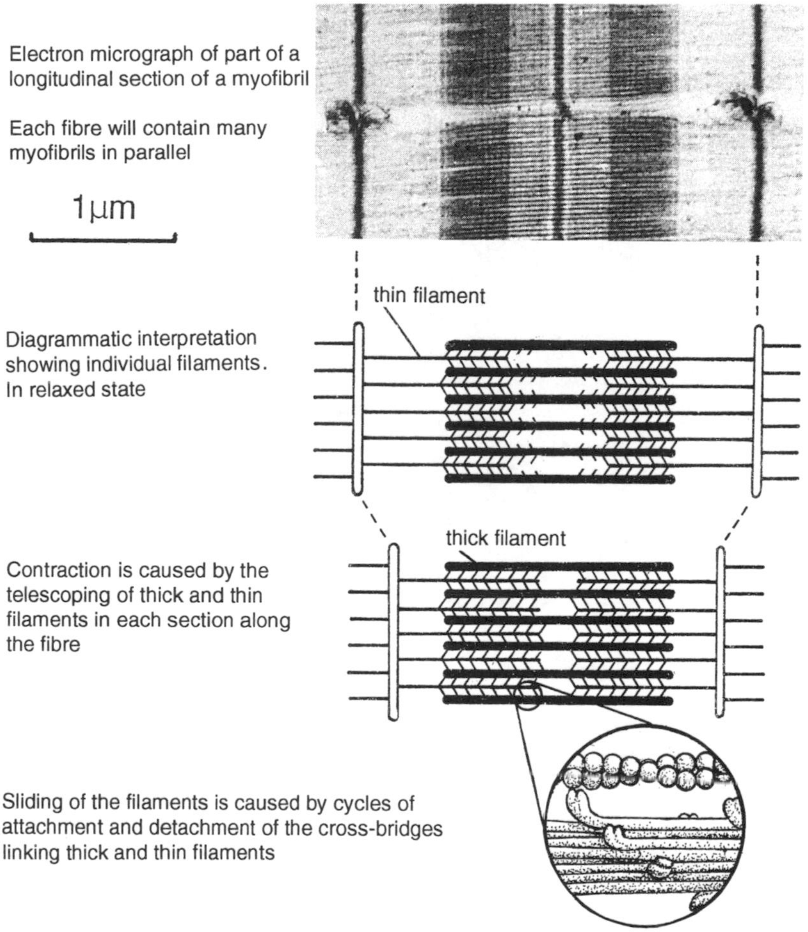

Electron micrograph of part of a
longitudinal section of a myofibril

Each fibre will contain many
myofibrils in parallel

1 μm

Diagrammatic interpretation
showing individual filaments.
In relaxed state

thin filament

thick filament

Contraction is caused by the
telescoping of thick and thin
filaments in each section along
the fibre

Sliding of the filaments is caused by cycles of
attachment and detachment of the cross-bridges
linking thick and thin filaments

Figure 2.17. The sliding-filament mechanism of muscle contraction. Electron micrograph kindly provided by Professor D. S. Smith, Oxford University

sets of overlapping thick and thin filaments (Figure 2.17) arranged in such a way that adjacent sets of filaments slide over each other. When this happens the myofibril (and hence the fibre and the muscle) shortens. What causes this sliding? The filaments are linked by cross-bridges, each a flexible connection between the protein molecules that form the filaments. These cross-bridges are not static but constantly attach and detach. Chemical energy in the form of ATP (see

continued

continued

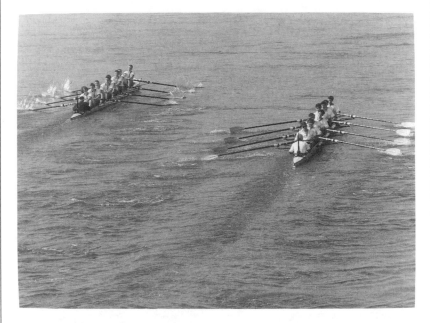

Figure 2.18. A rowing eight. The making and breaking of cross-bridges pull filaments past each other to produce movement in a similar manner to the oars of a rowing crew which make and break contact with the water in order to move the boat. In this photograph for one boat the oars are in the water (attached) while for the other the oars are out of the water (detached). Photograph kindly provided by Eadden Lilly Photography, Cambridge

pp. 63), made available by the oxidation of fuels, causes the cross-bridges to change shape so that re-attachment occurs further along the filament. In this way the thin filaments are pulled over the thick. A rowing eight propels the boat through water in much the same way (Figure 2.18). Think of the boat as the thick filament and the water as the thin filament; the oars form the cross-bridges and the crew provide the energy. As the oars dip into the water (attachment) their shape changes and the boat is drawn along. The oars are then lifted from the water (detachment) and the stroke repeated. Any oarsman will tell you that the process requires energy—as indeed does its molecular counterpart.

the energy needed for contraction by organizing chemical reactions between stored fuels and oxygen. Some mitochondria are present just below the plasma membrane, where they have immediate access to oxygen entering the cell. These mitochondria are sausage-shaped and are just a few micrometres long, but mitochondria closer to the myofibrils may consist of a branching tubular network rather than existing as isolated components. Anaerobic energy-releasing reactions, which do not involve oxygen, take place in the spaces between the myofibrils and are especially important in muscles which maintain a high power output for short periods.

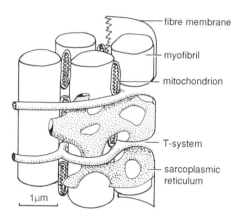

Figure 2.19. Diagrammatic three-dimensional view of part of a single muscle fibre. An electron microscope is needed to observe such detail

Most of the remainder of the fibre is filled with a much-convoluted system of internal membranes known as the sarcoplasmic reticulum. This membrane system encloses a space within the fibre, inside which the concentration of calcium ions is about 10 000 times greater than outside. This calcium is of vital importance; it provides a chemical link between the nerve and the contractile machinery. When a nerve impulse reaches a muscle fibre, it causes the release of some of this calcium into the vicinity of the myofibril and provides the chemical signal which causes the myofibrils to contract. As long as the impulses arrive at the muscle above a certain frequency, calcium remains around the myofibrils and contraction is maintained. A fall in frequency results in calcium being pumped back into the sarcoplasmic

FUEL (fat droplets)   OXYGEN SUPPLY (tracheole)

ENGINE (myofibril)

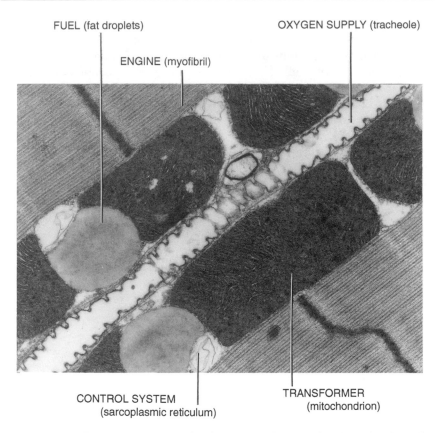

CONTROL SYSTEM   TRANSFORMER
(sarcoplasmic reticulum)   (mitochondrion)

Figure 2.20. Electron micrograph of insect flight muscle, showing the relationship between structure and function. Electron micrograph kindly provided by Mrs Barbara Luke, Oxford University

reticulum faster than it moves out, so the calcium concentration around the myofibril falls and contraction ceases (Figure 2.20).

STRENGTH, SPEED AND ENDURANCE

The thicker the muscle, the more myofibrils it contains and the stronger it is. In other words, the force that a muscle can develop is proportional to the cross-sectional area of the muscle. Sprinters, shot-putters, discus and javelin throwers know this and appreciate the importance of the type of training that 'builds' muscle, i.e. increases the number of myofibrils. In contrast, the performance of long-distance runners is limited by the supply of oxygen, the accumulation of end-products or, in some cases, the availability of fuels. For these athletes, muscle *strength*, and hence size, is much less important (Figure 2.21).

The muscles of sprinters and long-distance runners differ not only in size but in colour. Since there are very few opportunities for the

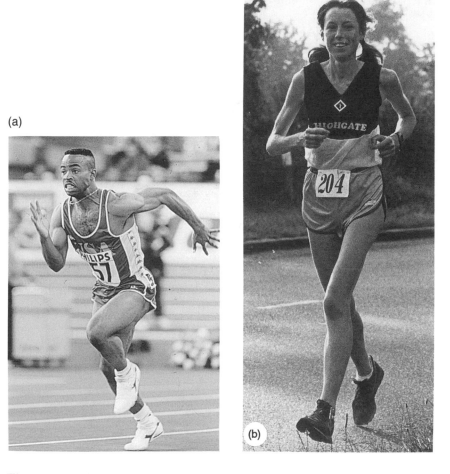

(a)

(b)

Figure 2.21. The contrasting physiques of (a) sprinter (André Cason winning the 100 m sprint at the World Indoor Championships, Seville, 1991, photograph © ALLSPORT/Gray Mortimore) and (b) ultra-distance runner Lyn Fitzgerald who has run the world best times for 50 miles (6:34.47) (October 1982), 100 miles (15:44.20) (July 1983) and the world best distance in 24 hours (133 miles 939 yards) (May 1982)

direct examination of human muscles, these differences are best observed in the sprinters and endurance athletes of the animal world. A biology laboratory is not needed; all the evidence can be seen in the kitchen. Compare the breast muscle of a chicken with that of a duck or pigeon. The chicken is the sprinter, using its wings only for escaping from predators, and the breast muscle (or pectoral muscle) that operates the wings is very pale. In contrast, the pigeon or duck can fly long distances and its breast muscle is dark red. The terms *white muscle* and *red muscle* have been used to describe the two different types of skeletal muscle exemplified by these birds, in which the difference in colour is a consequence of differences in the mechanisms of aerobic and anaerobic energy generation. For escape mechanisms, such as sprinting, large amounts of energy have to be generated very quickly but only for a short time. This is best achieved anaerobically. In contrast, for sustained exercise, less energy is required but it must be generated continuously over a long period of time. As will be seen in Chapter 4, this is best achieved by the oxidation of fuels by oxygen—a process which involves substances called cytochromes which are responsible for the dark red colour.

Different muscles within the same animal have different functions, so they too often have different colours. The darker meat of the chicken leg indicates that it is more of an endurance muscle (hens walk about all day) than a sprint muscle. The difference is even more apparent in many fish. Next time you have a trout for dinner observe that, while the bulk of the muscle is pale, a much darker thin strip runs along each flank, just under the skin (Figure 2.22). Ingenious experiments have revealed that only this dark (or red) muscle is used during normal swimming. The white muscle, although more than 90% of the total, is

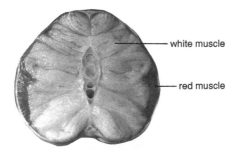

white muscle

red muscle

Figure 2.22. Cross-section of a dogfish showing the large amount of white (anaerobic) muscle and the much smaller bands of red (aerobic) muscle along the flanks of the fish

Box 2.3 A question of fibre type

Fibre composition not only varies from muscle to muscle; it also varies from individual to individual. This is one reason why some of us are better sprinters and others are better endurance athletes.

Only a small piece of muscle is needed to determine the percentage of the different fibre types, and this is taken with a biopsy needle (Figure 2.23). The skin above the muscle is anaesthetized and a small

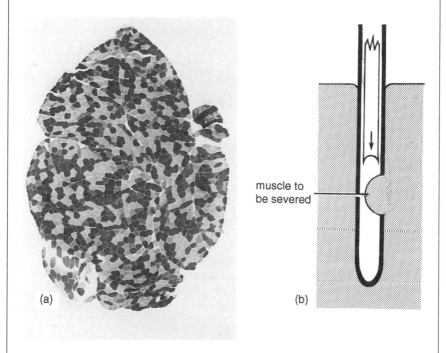

(a)

muscle to be severed

(b)

Figure 2.23. The mosaic (a) is a magnified transverse section of human quadriceps muscle stained to reveal the different fibre types. Fast-twitch glycolytic fibres have stained most strongly and slow-twitch fibres least. For fibre-typing studies and other investigations, small samples of muscle can be removed from human volunteers using a biopsy needle (b). The device is pushed through a small cut made in the skin (using local anaesthetic) and into the muscle. Micrograph kindly provided by Dr C. A. Maunder-Sewry and Prof. V. Dubowitz, University of London

continued

continued

incision made. Through this and into the muscle is inserted the biopsy needle—a hollow needle with a small 'window' in one side. As the needle is inserted, muscle bulges into this 'window' and is severed by a sharp-edged plunger. After withdrawal the muscle sample is thinly sliced, treated with a series of chemicals that stain the fibres and then the thin slices are viewed in cross-section. The fibres stain differently according to their type, and the different fibres can then be counted and the proportion of each calculated. Although the procedure is relatively painless, élite athletes are understandably reluctant to have their muscles interfered with in this way. Nevertheless the available data do show very large differences among individual athletes (Table 2.1).

What an athlete needs to know is whether these percentages can be changed by training. The answer is a qualified 'yes' (Table 2.2). First, fast-twitch glycolytic and fast-twitch oxidative can be 'interchanged' by training; endurance exercise training converts the former into the latter and strength training does the opposite. This explains why the percentage of fast-twitch glycolytic fibres in the muscle of long-distance runners is very small. There is some evidence that a *small* proportion of slow-twitch fibres may be converted into fast-twitch fibres by sprint training (Table 2.2) and a *small* proportion of fast-twitch might be converted into slow twitch by endurance training. These findings suggest that for the marathon runner, sprint training (intervals of less than 100 m and power training with weights) should not be done and, in particular, sprinters should never engage in

Table 2.1. Percentage fibre composition of gastrocnemius muscles in élite athletes (mean values are given; individual variation is large)

Athlete	Percentage of fibres	
	Slow-twitch	Fast-twitch
Sprinter	24	76
Middle-distance runner	52	48
Marathon runner	79	21
Cross-country skier	80	20

Data from Costill, D.L., Daniels, J., Evans, W. *et al.* (1976). Skeletal muscle enzymes and fiber composition in male and female track athletes. *J. Appl. Physiol.*, **40**, 149–154.

continued

─ *continued* ───────

Table 2.2. Percentage of different fibres in muscle (vastus lateralis) from distance runners, endurance trained or sprint trained

Condition of athlete	Percentage		
	Slow-twitch fibres	Fast-twitch oxidative fibres	Fast-twitch glycolytic fibres
Distance runner, hard endurance training for 18 weeks	69	20	11
Same distance runner trained for sprinting for 11 weeks	52	8	40[a]

[a]This includes a small percentage of a new type of fibre which may be 'halfway' between fast-twitch oxidative and fast-twitch glycolytic.
Data from Jansson, E., Sjodin, B. and Tesch, P. (1978). Changes in muscle fibre type distribution in man after physical training. *Acta Physiol. Scand.*, **104**, 235–237.

endurance exercise. Total inactivity can result in a decrease in the number of slow-twitch fibres, probably because they have changed to fast-twitch fibres—a problem for athletes when a limb has to be immobilized due, for example, to the fracture of a bone.

only used when the fish 'sprints' to catch prey, escapes from a predator or when it is caught on an angler's hook. In the latter case, the angler experiences not only the power of the white muscle but also its susceptibility to fatigue, allowing the fish to be landed with ease. This fatigue has the same cause as that in the Olympic 400 m champion and is discussed in Chapter 6.

Human muscles vary in the same way but the distinction is less apparent since all muscles contain both 'red' and 'white' fibres. In fact, it has proved useful to distinguish at least *three* types of fibre in mammalian muscles: slow-twitch, fast-twitch oxidative and fast-twitch glycolytic (Table 2.3). Slow-twitch fibres are most abundant in red muscles; they generate their power aerobically, contract relatively slowly and are fatigue resistant. Fast-twitch glycolytic fibres are most abundant in white muscles, where they generate power anaerobically,

Table 2.3.   Characteristics of human muscle fibre types

Characteristics	Slow-twitch fibres	Fast-twitch oxidative fibres	Fast-twitch glycolytic fibres
Blood supply	Good	Good/moderate	Poor
Short-term fatigue	Resistant	Resistant	Susceptible
Anaerobic capacity	Moderate	Moderate	Good
Major fuels stored	Glycogen and fat	Glycogen and some fat	Glycogen
Contraction velocity	Slow	Fast	Fast
Fibre diameter	Small	Intermediate	Large
Motor unit size	Small	Intermediate	Large
Size of motor neurone fibre	Small	Intermediate	Large

From Saltin, B., Henriksson, J., Nygaard, E. *et al.* (1977). Fibre types and metabolic potentials of skeletal muscles in sedentary man and endurance runners. *Ann. NY Acad. Sci.*, **301**, 3–29.

contract rapidly but are easily fatigued. Fast-twitch oxidative fibres are somewhat intermediate in properties; they contract rapidly but have both aerobic and anaerobic capacities. Within a single motor unit all fibres are of the same type.

Just as we all vary in characteristics such as eye colour, height and shape of nose, so too do we differ in the proportion of the different fibre-types in our muscles (Box 2.3). If you have a preponderance of fast-twitch glycolytic fibres there is no chance of your winning an Olympic gold medal in the marathon; nor will you be a top-class sprinter if you are well-endowed with slow-twitch oxidative fibres (Table 2.1). And as with other characteristics, such as eye colour, fibre composition is largely inherited. Top athletes should be aware of how important it was to have chosen their parents carefully! There is some evidence that training can make a small difference to fibre proportions (Table 2.2), but its major effect is on what happens inside and outside the fibres.

DIFFERENT MUSCLES FOR DIFFERENT TASKS

The kind of muscle of greatest interest to athletes, and the one so far exclusively referred to, is *skeletal* muscle. As its name suggests, that is the muscle which is attached to bones and causes their movement. Skeletal muscle has long fibres which under an ordinary microscope appear transversely striated (Figure 2.24). In general, such muscle has a high power output and can contract rapidly, but not all tasks require these characteristics.

Another type of muscle, which is literally of vital importance to us all, is quite different. Although its fibres are also striated, they are short and branched (Figure 2.24). Their contraction is more gentle than that of skeletal muscle and occurs without any conscious control. Unlike skeletal muscle, this muscle continues to contract and relax rhythmically even when deprived of all its nerves. It is, of course, cardiac muscle, from which the heart is formed. Cardiac muscle is the endurance muscle *par excellence*, contracting and relaxing non-stop approximately 2 500 000 000 times in a lifetime.

We are much less aware, although equally dependent on, our smooth muscles. These are composed of elongated cells rather than fibres and show no sign of cross-striations (Figure 2.24). The power output of smooth muscles is lower than that of skeletal and cardiac muscle, but smooth muscles are responsible for the usually gentle, involuntary

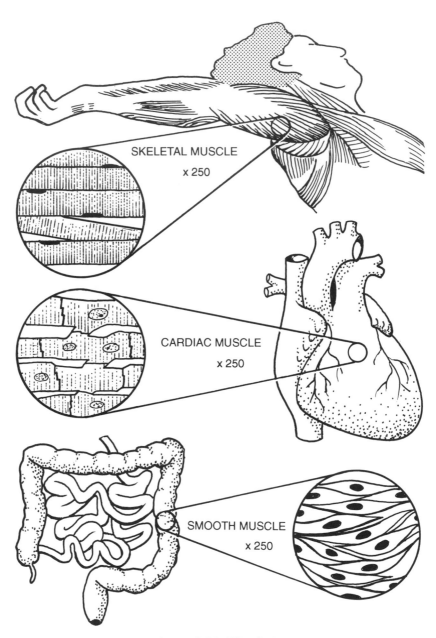

Figure 2.24. Muscle types

movements about which we know little unless they go wrong. These movements including the squeezing of food through the intestine, the changing of the iris diameter in response to variations in light intensity and, of particular importance to athletes, the control of blood flow through small arteries and veins.

Chapter 3

Energy Matters

A marathon runner is totally exhausted after running 26 miles in about 2½ h; so is a sprinter after running 400 m in 45 s (Figure 3.1). Although the sprinter will be able to perform almost as well within an hour, the marathon runner usually requires several days' recovery before another long race can be run. Both athletes might claim they have 'run out of energy' but they have not, for their hearts continue to pump, their breathing muscles work and their brains function; plenty of energy is still available.

The confusion arises because the everyday use of the term 'energy' means different things to different people. When we say we 'have no energy' what we actually mean is that we have plenty of energy (stored in chemical form as fuels) but lack the ability (or will) to use it fast enough to support the desired level of activity. The rate of energy utilization is what athletics is all about but to make any sense of this we have first to be comfortable with the concept of energy itself.

Energy is, in fact, an irritatingly difficult term to define in a useful way. Physicists come straight to the point and define it as the 'capacity to do useful work', which is fine if you understand precisely what is meant by 'useful work'. For an athlete, useful work means overcoming, rapidly and effectively, the forces that prevent movement, including gravity, air resistance and friction.

HOW MUCH ENERGY?

It is not always easy to measure energy precisely but, if a few approximations are accepted, it is not all that difficult. If you are reading this book in a suitable place you could try right now. First, you will need to know the mass (weight) of your body, at least approximately. Now climb some stairs and estimate the total height you have raised yourself. You should also time your climb, for that information will be of use later. If you live in a bungalow, step on and off a chair 20 times and use the total height 'climbed', i.e. 20 times the height of the chair. Now plug your data into the equations in Figure 3.2 to find out how much energy you have used moving against the pull of gravity. Bear in mind that the value you get will not be the *actual* energy you expended but a smaller value because some additional energy will have been used to overcome internal friction in your body, which is

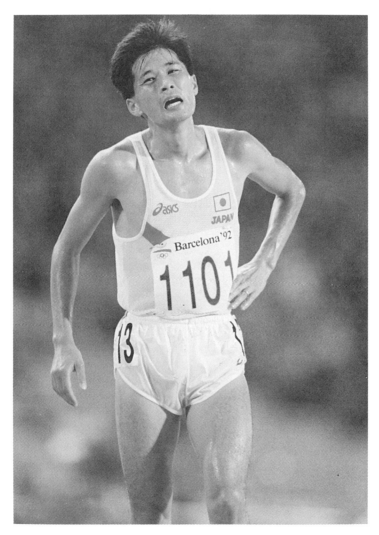

Figure 3.1. Exhausted runner. A Japanese runner after completing a 10 000 m heat in the Barcelona Olympics. Photograph © ALLSPORT/Mike Powell

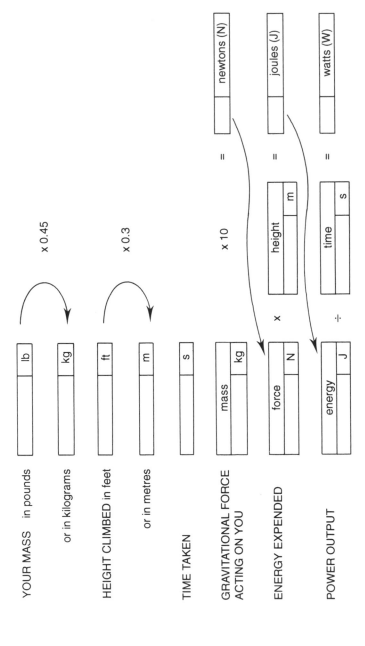

Figure 3.2. Measuring energy output—the amateur way

not easy to measure. Energy is measured in joules (J), which is now the most widely used unit for all forms of energy. Formerly energy was measured in calories, with one calorie equal to 4.18 J.

It will be obvious that if you ran up the stairs, rather than walked, more effort would be needed, although the total energy used would be exactly the same. Time must come into the calculation and the *rate* at which you expended energy (i.e. the amount in a specified period of time) is your *power output*. The importance of power output is apparent from the fact that all of us have enough energy to run a marathon but only a select few can achieve a high enough power output in our leg muscles, for a sufficient length of time, to support a 2 h 10 min marathon! Divide the number of joules you used climbing the stairs

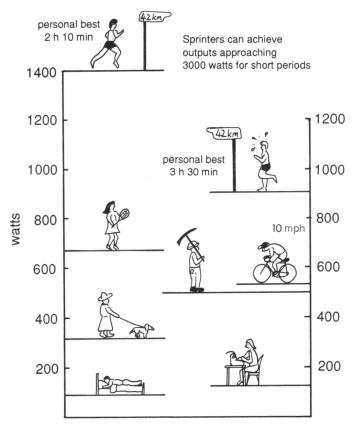

Figure 3.3. Power output during various activities. Power is the rate at which energy is expended or work is done. One watt is one joule per second

by the number of seconds it took you to reach the top to give your power output in watts (W).

A non-élite marathon runner (say, 3 h 30 min personal best) will have a power output of about 900 W during the race—almost the same as a small electric heater (Figure 3.3) An élite marathon runner will achieve about 1400 W and a first-class sprinter expends energy at the rate of about 3000 W.

ENERGY IN ALL ITS GUISES

One consequence of running is that we feel hot. Heat is another form of energy—not one used by the athlete but produced during all forms of exercise. In fact, so much heat is sometimes produced that it can interfere with performance and, in extreme cases, result in death. Of course, on a cold day this heat is used to maintain the body temperature; we feel cold at the start of the run but once into the activity we soon warm up and may have to shed some clothes to prevent overheating, despite the low ambient temperature. From where is all this heat coming? The answer is from *chemical* energy which we obtain from food. Food is a complex mixture of chemical compounds—carbohydrates, fats and proteins—which release their energy when they are broken down to smaller molecules. A variety of energy-releasing reactions occur in muscle and one of the most important is that between sugar (glucose) and oxygen. The products of this reaction—carbon dioxide and water—contain less energy than the reactants, so some is released. Equations are the chemist's shorthand for describing what happens in a chemical reaction, with reactants (starting materials) on the left and products on the right:

$$\text{glycose + oxygen} \longrightarrow \text{carbon dioxide + water}$$

Whether this reaction takes place by burning in a fire or in a more controlled way in a muscle, the amount of energy released from a fixed amount of glucose is *always* the same (16 000 J per gram of glucose). The difference is that on the fire all the energy is released as heat (except, perhaps, for a very small amount as light), but in the muscle some of the energy is converted into movement, i.e. into kinetic energy.

With this information you can work out how much sugar you would have to eat to replace the energy lost climbing those stairs. Simply divide the energy you used into 16 000 and you get the answer in grams. You may be surprised at how little this is. Since you will have

Table 3.1. Approximate energy expenditure in some exercise activities

Activity	Energy used (kJ)	Number of large loaves of bread to provide this energy
Soccer game (90 min)	6000–8000	1
Marathon race (42.2 km)	12 000	1¼
Six months training for the marathon	400 000	52

Note that kilojoules (kJ) equal to 1000 joules are used.
From Ekblom, B. (1992). Energy expenditure during exercise. In *Obesity*, pp. 136–144 (eds Bjorntorp, P. and Brodoff, B.N.). Lippincott, Philadelphia.

probably used less than half a gram, do not reward yourself with a whole bar of chocolate. To replace the energy used running a marathon, you would have to eat one and a quarter large loaves of bread (Table 3.1).

Calculations of this kind have to be carried out by anyone engaged in 'weight-watching' because any chemical energy, i.e. food, consumed in excess of that required will be stored as reserve fuel—mostly fat. It is important therefore, if body weight is to be maintained, that intake does not exceed demand. Measuring your intake is easy enough, if rather tedious, with the help of food composition tables, but measuring energy expended is more difficult.

The do-it-yourself method described in Figure 3.2 is not widely applicable so exercise physiologists have used the principle of calorimetry. In so-called direct calorimetry, heat production is measured by imprisoning the subject, together with facilities for exercise, in an extremely well-insulated chamber. Energy expended is calculated from the thermal capacity of the contents of the chamber (including the subject) and the rise in temperature, which is likely to be exceedingly small. Very few laboratories in the world are equipped with human calorimeters.

More widely used is the principle of indirect calorimetry—so indirect in fact that heat is not measured at all. What is measured is oxygen uptake and carbon dioxide production. By making certain assumptions it is possible to determine what fuel (fat or carbohydrate) and how much is being used in a specific exercise. One litre of oxygen is equivalent to 21 kJ of energy when glucose is oxidized. (If you are using oxygen at a rate of 4.1 l/min, which is an average value for élite marathon runners, you are expending energy at a rate of 1435 watts). An advantage of this method is that the subject does not have to be totally enclosed provided that respiratory gases can be collected. It

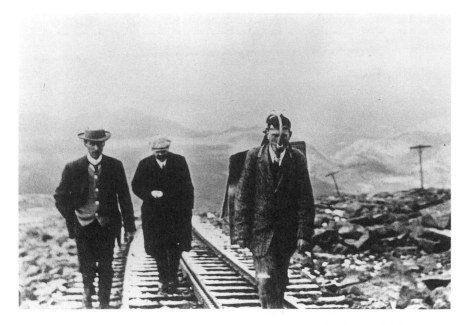

Figure 3.4. C. G. Douglas, the inventor of the Douglas bag, which enables oxygen uptake during exercise to be measured. Professor Douglas is exercising at the high-altitude research station, Pikes Peak, Colorado. J. S. Haldane is timing the walk and E. C. Schneider is observing. Photograph kindly provided by the University Laboratory of Physiology, Oxford University

must be said, however, that running a marathon while wearing a mask and with a Douglas bag strapped to your back is unlikely to improve your personal best (Figure 3.4).

The latest means of assessing how much fuel has been used in a particular situation involves the use of heavy isotopes and some clever thinking (Box 3.1).

For many practical purposes, energy expenditure is not measured but estimated. A typical man is judged to expend around 10 500 kJ per day and a typical woman about 10% less, due to her smaller lean body mass (mainly muscle). Note that human energy expenditure is normally reported in kilojoules (kJ), each equal to 1000 J. Energy expenditure also depends on body size, with larger people having to expend more. But the main cause of difference in energy expenditure between individuals is the amount of exercise they take; a Tour de France cyclist can burn up 40 000 kJ on a tough day in the saddle.

These energy calculations are only possible because energy can neither be created nor destroyed; what disappears in one form must

Box 3.1   Heavy isotopes—the truth drug

The chemical properties of an element (e.g. carbon, oxygen or iron) depend on the electrons surrounding the nucleus of each atom. For some elements, variations in the structure of this nucleus can occur to form isotopes, some of which occur naturally and others are formed in nuclear reactions. Although isotopes of the same element are *chemically* identical, their physical properties do vary and this makes it possible to use isotopes to trace the fate of atoms in organisms and biochemical reactions. An unnatural isotope is introduced and its physical properties used to find where in the organism, or in what chemical compound, it ends up. Isotopes which emit radiation (radioisotopes) are particularly useful, for this radioactivity is quite easy to detect and measure. On the other hand, *heavy* isotopes are not radioactive but their greater atomic mass can be detected and measured, with a little more difficulty, using a mass spectrometer. Oxygen does not have a convenient radioisotope but its heavy isotope, ^{18}O, has an atomic mass of 18 rather than the normal 16. Similarly, heavy hydrogen (^2H, deuterium) atoms have a mass of 2 compared with normal hydrogen, which has an atomic mass of 1.

To put all this to use to measure total energy expenditure requires a glass of $^2H_2{}^{18}O$ (quite harmless), a mass spectrometer (quite expensive) and some ingenious reasoning. The $^2H_2{}^{18}O$ consumed will mix with all the other water in the body and then it will appear slowly in the urine. Samples of urine can be collected and the amount of ^2H and ^{18}O in the water measured. Any respiration which occurs will form normal H_2O (from stored fuels and inhaled oxygen) and slow down the appearance of $^2H_2{}^{18}O$ in the urine. But CO_2 is also produced by oxidative processes in the body, so that there will be a greater dilution of ^{18}O in the H_2O compared to the dilution of ^2H. This difference between dilution of ^{18}O and ^2H is therefore a measure of the rate of CO_2 formation, i.e. oxidation. Thus, the difference between the rates of excretion of ^2H and ^{18}O in the urine over a period of days can be related precisely to the rate of oxidation of fuels, i.e. to energy expenditure. Since these measurements require only the collection of urine samples (e.g. one sample per day), they do not affect performance in any way and have been used, for example, to study energy expenditure during the Tour de France cycle race and indeed in women during pregnancy.

continued

— *continued* —

But why call it a truth drug? It is notoriously difficult to measure accurately the amount of food energy consumed by human beings. If volunteers are asked to keep a diary of all they eat each day, they tend to under-report the amount consumed. If the measurement is done by an independent observer, the quantity of food consumed may be less than normal—the observer effect. However, if body weight does not change, the amount of food energy consumed must equal the amount expended and is measured accurately by this isotopic method. Over a period of several days, it tells the truth about how much food energy has been consumed.

The problem with this method for the athlete, coach or physiologist is that it is not accurate over short periods and should only be used for measuring energy expenditure over at least 3 days. It will not estimate energy expenditure in the 800 m or even the marathon, but it is useful (*very* useful, since no equipment needs to be used by the athlete) for long-term events such as the Tour de France race. It can, also be used to provide a measure of the energy expenditure during several days of training. In one study on élite female endurance runners it was calculated that running 10 miles per day increased daily energy expenditure by 4200 kJ.

reappear in another—a universally true fact which has been dignified with the title of the *first law of thermodynamics* (Figure 3.5). We can now take a closer look at the energy released from the combustion of glucose as you climbed those stairs earlier in the chapter. Energy cannot be destroyed so where has it gone? Some was converted into kinetic energy—your movement—and then into potential energy— the energy due to your position further from the centre of the earth as you climbed the stairs. It was this potential energy that you actually calculated. At each conversion, chemical to kinetic, kinetic to potential, a proportion of the energy is inevitably released as heat which, after warming you, is passed to your environment. Finally, when you come downstairs your potential energy was transformed into heat so, ultimately, virtually all the chemical energy we consume ends up as heat—just as happens when glucose is burned on the fire. The difference is that we have made use of some of the chemical energy, to climb up (and down) the stairs.

Now we have met energy in four of its guises: chemical, heat, kinetic and potential. Two others—light and electricity—are important for living organisms. Light is the sole source of energy for green plants, which convert it into chemical energy through the process of photosynthesis. A few organisms, like fireflies, can actually produce light, converting chemical energy directly to light energy. Differences in electrical potential, again generated by expenditure of chemical energy, are used to convey information along nerves. Much greater potentials can be generated by some fish which use shocks, in excess of 200 volts, to stun prey and to deter predators.

An important factor in the energetics of running is the energy which is stored elastically, like that in a stretched rubber band. Much of the

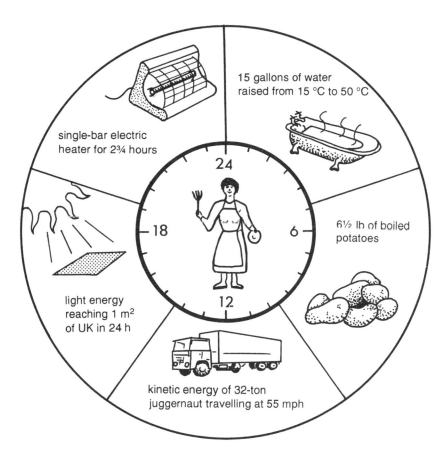

Figure 3.5. Each item in the sectors shown contains or expends approximately 10 000 kJ, the average daily energy expenditure of a normally active woman

energy cost of running on the flat is expended against the pull of gravity since at each step the body is raised. Not all of this energy is lost, however. Just as a pogo-stick transforms potential energy into kinetic energy for the next bounce (Fig. 3.6) so elastic components of the leg allow some of the energy used to raise the body's centre of gravity to be recovered for the next stride (Box 3.2).

Of all the various forms of energy, chemical energy has an especially important role because of the ease with which it can be stored, whether as food in a freezer, oil in a tank, or glycogen (a polymer of glucose, see pp. 72–73) stored in your muscles. Provided a suitable reaction can take place, the energy in such fuels can be made available in other

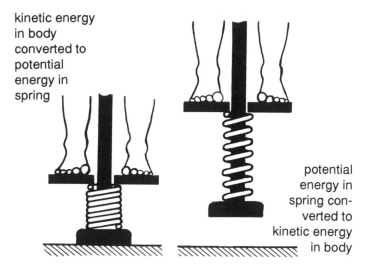

kinetic energy in body converted to potential energy in spring

potential energy in spring converted to kinetic energy in body

Figure 3.6. Pogo stick. Running uses the principle of the pogo stick and this principle may be particularly important in élite track athletes. And just as the precise length and tension in the springs of the pogo stick are important for optimal propulsion, so it is for the athlete. Muscles must maintain the correct length and tension to absorb and release as much energy as possible in elastic recoil. Indeed it has been shown that a certain amount of muscle tightness, presumably to maintain tendon length, is important for efficient energy expenditure in man during jogging. From Gleim, G.W., Stacherfeld, N. S. and Nicholas, J. A. (1990). The influence of flexibility on the economy of walking and jogging. *J. Orthop. Res.*, **8**, 814–823

Box 3.2   Kangaroos have it

A simple analysis of the mechanics of running reveals it to be a strange means of locomotion. In each stride, one leg accelerates while not bearing a load and then decelerates as it hits the ground to bear the load. This mechanism would appear to be equivalent to putting the foot alternatively on the accelerator and then the brake while driving a car—but the runner is more like a bouncing ball in which kinetic energy is retained in the elastic stretch of the ball and is released again in the recoil.

The Achilles tendon (Figure 3.7) is the main spring, stretching by about 6% of its length (1.5 cm) and returning over 90% of its stored energy to the next stride. Flattening of the arch of the foot also returns energy but somewhat less efficiently.

Kangaroos have really made the pogo-stick principle work for them (Figure 3.8) and it appears that élite athletes are much more kangaroo-like than the average population. It has been calculated that tendon elasticity raises the efficiency of conversion of chemical energy into mechanical energy from 25% to 40% or *more*. The good news is that tendon elasticity can be improved by training but the bad news is that as we age this energy recycling property of the muscle and tendons is progressively lost, and so the pace must slow!

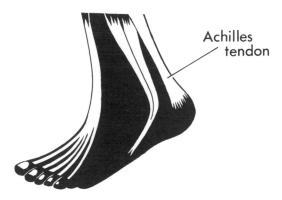

Figure 3.7. Tendons in human foot

continued

— continued

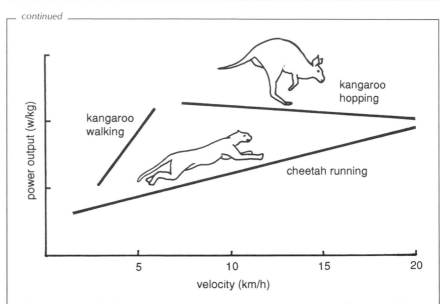

Figure 3.8. In the hopping kangaroo the combination of long Achilles tendon and powerful quadriceps muscle means that faster locomotion does not use more energy! As the kangaroo lands, the tendon is stretched and the muscle contracts almost isometrically (or even eccentrically), its most efficient mode. Note that the cheetah is even more economical than the kangaroo, possibly because of its flexible back and length of stride, Goldspink, G. (1977). Energy cost of locomotion. In *Mechanics and Energetics of Animal Locomotion* pp. 153–167 (Eds. R. McN. Alexander and G. Goldspink) Chapman and Hall, London. The cost of running is determined primarily by the cost of supporting body weight and by the time that the foot is on the ground (which governs the time course of force application) (Kram and Taylor, 1990).

Running economy is a major factor in determining athletic performance at the highest levels. Given 10 runners with $\dot{V}O_{2\,max}$ values between, for example, 78 and 85 ml oxygen per kilogram body weight per minute, it would not be possible to predict from these tests the winner in a 10 km race. Once the athletes are in the top class, running economy—an economical gait and good, very good, springs—are just as important as the precise value of their $\dot{V}O_{2\,max}$!

So if springs are important, what do our muscles do? Contraction of

— continued

continued

the muscles of the leg will get limbs moving, will maintain the optimal length of the Achilles tendon to absorb as much energy in elastic stretch as possible and stabilize the joints so that there is no loss of energy caused by a poor gait. However, springs are only effective on a firm surface. A bouncing ball does not bounce very well in a field of mud, nor do élite track athletes. Super-elastic tendons provide little benefit in cross-country races run under wet and muddy conditions. Steve Ovett illustrated this point memorably in his autobiography when he described his performance as a schoolboy in the English Cross-Country Championships at Blackburn in 1970.

> The race was a disaster. It was pouring with rain all day and by the time my event started the course was churned into a quagmire and at one point looked like a river. I am a fluid runner and this was a course for sloggers . . . It was desperately tough and when I got back to the changing rooms in the school, there was my father, Pop and my Uncle looking like characters out of *The Grapes of Wrath*, soaking wet and bitterly disappointed . . . I think I finished twenty-seventh!!

forms. The most common reaction is oxidation—a process which uses oxygen and produces carbon dioxide and water. In the internal combustion engine, oxidation of the fuel converts the chemical energy first to heat energy then, via expansion of gases, to kinetic energy. Living organisms, by contrast, convert their fuels directly to kinetic, electrical and even light energy, but a proportion of the chemical energy is always lost as heat. What makes all this possible has been the evolution of a relatively simple, but remarkable, chemical called adenosine triphosphate, or ATP for short.

ATP: BIOLOGICAL ENERGY INTERMEDIATE

Adenosine triphosphate can undergo a chemical reaction with water in which it is split to form a molecule of adenosine *di*phosphate (ADP) and one of phosphate. Although cells contain much water, this reaction does not happen spontaneously. It needs a catalyst—something that speeds up a chemical reaction without itself becoming changed. In cells, enzymes perform this function and have the advantage that their catalytic activity can be regulated but, in the chemistry laboratory, simple acids or alkalis are more likely to be used as catalysts. If a little ATP is sprinkled into a test-tube containing dilute acid or alkali, the mixture becomes warm. Energy is being released as heat. None of this is remarkable; chemists are aware of many kinds of molecules which release heat energy when they react with water (i.e. undergo hydrolysis). What is remarkable is that, in the right circumstances, the energy released appears not as heat but as *movement*. The right circumstances occur in a muscle fibre, where the minute amount of energy released when a single ATP molecule is hydrolysed is enough to bend a cross-bridge linking the thick and thin filaments within the myofibril of the muscle (see Box 2.2). If a sufficient number of cross-bridges bend, the filaments slide over each other and, if enough filaments slide, the muscle contracts. Each time a sprinter takes a stride, something like 10 000 000 000 000 000 000 molecules of ATP are converted into ADP with the transfer of energy to the cross-bridges. On a more tangible basis this would mean that a marathon runner would get through 75 kg of ATP during the race. Clearly the marathon runner cannot possibly carry this amount of ATP—most marathon runners weigh less than this anyway. In fact ATP is not stored and as little as 100 g may be present in the whole of the athlete's body. This paradox is resolved when it is appreciated that as soon as any of this ATP is used, more is made from ADP and phosphate. This synthesis needs energy, which is provided by breakdown of the fuels themselves (see Chapter 4). Think of ATP as a ball at the top of a slope. As it rolls down it can do work but, in so doing, it becomes changed into ADP—the ball at the bottom of the slope. For more work to be carried out the ball must be raised back to the top of the slope—an energy-*requiring* process. In other words, for the chemical energy in fuels to be used, it must first be converted into chemical energy in ATP. This conversion, involving oxidation of fuels such as glucose and fat, is known as cellular respiration and occurs in all living organisms, from bacteria to human beings.

The advantage of this arrangement is simplicity. A large number of different energy-yielding reactions all generate the *same* intermediate, namely ATP. Moreover, all muscles, from the flight muscle of an aphid to the calf muscle of man, are powered by the same chemical reactions. In fact, so are *all* the other energy-requiring processes in living organisms, including the transport of molecules across cell membranes, the generation of electricity in nerve cells, the production of light in bioluminescent organisms and the synthesis of complex molecules in all cells. ATP is the universal energy intermediate in biology. Its simultaneous production in energy-yielding reactions and its utilization in energy-requiring processes constitute what is called the ADP/ATP cycle (Figure 3.9). The central importance of this cycle to athletes has been recognized by the International Committee of the Biochemistry of Exercise, who have adopted it as their logo (Figure 3.10).

But what is ATP? If you are a chemist, the answer might be 'a nucleotide in which adenine is linked via ribose to a triphosphate

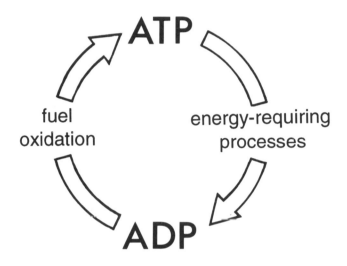

Figure 3.9. ATP/ADP cycle

group'. If you are not a chemist, the description might be 'a white powder which is in solution in biological tissues but can be readily made by chemists in the laboratory' (Figure 3.11). For the athlete, what ATP *is* is unimportant, while what it *does* is vitally important. Much the same can be said about currency. Dollar bills or banknotes are merely pieces of paper printed with designs and symbols. A member of a primitive human society would find no value in a £5 note or a dollar bill save that of burning it to provide a little heat. We, however, can put banknotes to good use.

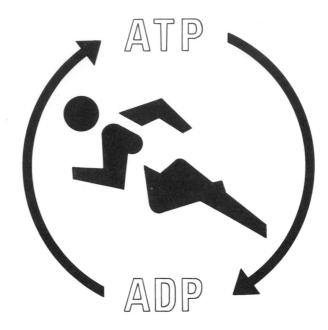

Figure 3.10. Logo of the International Committee of the Biochemistry of
Exercise

Drawing parallels between our use of currency and the body's use of
ATP helps to explain the biochemistry (Figure 3.12). Before currency
was devised, trading had to be done by barter; services or goods were
exchanged directly. This is not a flexible system, for the 'seller' might
not require the goods or services offered by the 'buyer'. Money overcomes this difficulty. The seller exchanges his goods or services for
money which can then be used to buy *any* goods or services required.
Similarly, ATP can be produced in a variety of reactions and used to
drive *any* energy-requiring process in the cell. It links energy production to energy utilization, just as a currency links working to purch-
ases (Figure 3.13). ATP can best be likened to 'cash in the pocket'—
relatively small in amount but readily replenished from storage fuels,
just as cash is drawn from the bank.

There are of course differences between financial transactions and
the way that the cellular energy budget is managed. The body is 'old
fashioned' and does not permit credit. If an athlete does not eat and so
does not obtain the fuels for generating ATP, performance will suffer.
A second difference between ATP and currency is that money can be

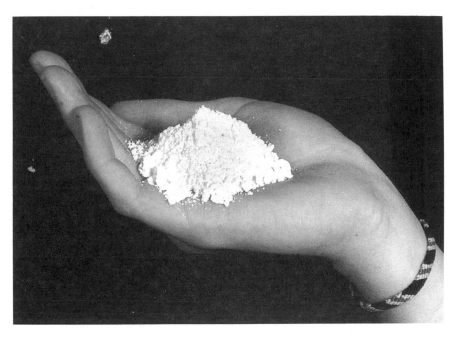

Figure 3.11. This amount (10 g) of ATP is turned over (i.e. made and broken down) each *second* by an athlete running the marathon. Imagine the size of a person who actually *stored* energy as ATP. The total amount of ATP in the muscles of an average person is around 60 g

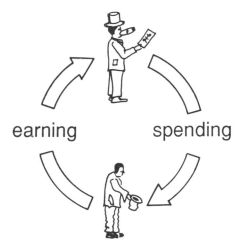

earning spending

Figure 3.12. A human 'currency' analogy of the ATP/ADP energy cycle

transported whereas ATP must be used in the cell in which it is produced. All cells, therefore, must be able to generate ATP from fuels.

One final point emerges from this analogy. In recent years business executives or their financial advisers have begun to appreciate the need for a good understanding of economics; unfortunately, most athletes and their advisers chase gold medals without understanding energy economics.

Although ATP is the central intermediate in biological energy conversions, the major *source* of the energy for movement is the stored

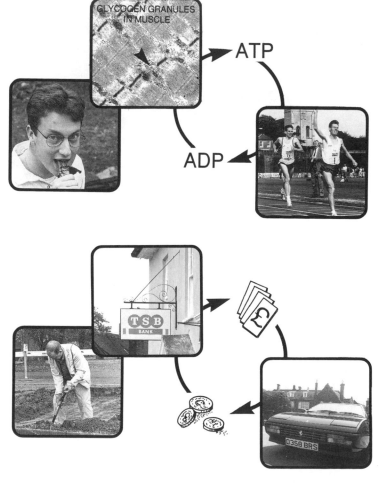

Figure 3.13. An extended human currency analogy

fuels—fat and carbohydrate—which are derived from food, and it is to them that we turn in Chapter 4. The amounts of fuel stored and the rates at which it is mobilized impose limitations on most, if not all, athletic endeavours. By implication, therefore, any effect that training has on these procedures will influence performance.

Chapter 4

Filling the Fuel Tanks

It takes less than one hour for a jumbo jet to take on enough fuel for a transatlantic flight. Once aboard it is simply stored until needed since the elaborate processing required to produce aviation fuel from crude oil has already been carried out at the oil refinery. Like fuel for a jet plane, food provides the athlete with the energy needed for movement but, unlike fuel for the plane, some refining must take place on board.

The 'on-board' processing of food is, like the chemistry involved in the oil refinery, a complicated process. It starts with eating itself, and the athlete aiming to produce the best 'athletic' fuel must choose his or her 'crude' fuel carefully. The connections between the nutritional quality of food and the quality of the refined products are explored in Chapter 11. Since a greater part of our food consists of the storage fuels of other organisms, the simplest strategy might seem to be to store them unchanged, but this is not possible since only small molecules can be absorbed from the intestines into the blood. Since storage fuel molecules are large, they must be broken down by digestion before they can enter the body's tissues (Figure 4.1). Fuel storage in the body involves re-assembling the small molecules to form larger molecules, with chemical modifications needed to suit them better for storage in the human body.

THE PERFECT STORAGE FUEL

The perfect storage fuel should have the following characteristics:

- A high chemical energy content, so that enough energy can be stored on board without it being too heavy.
- Chemical stability, so that it does not break down before it is needed.

- Capacity for rapid mobilization, so that it can be made available for the muscles as quickly as required.
- Ability to generate ATP without the production of toxic end-products.
- High molecular weight or insolubility to avoid osmotic complications (i.e. the movement of water in or out of a cell in response to a change in the concentration of dissolved materials in the cell).

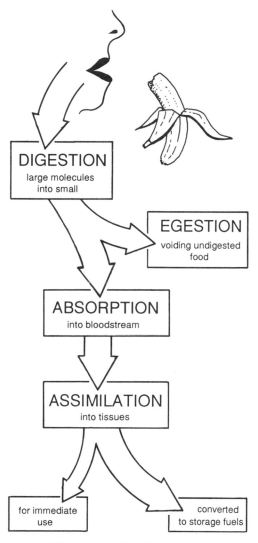

Figure 4.1. Food processing

By these criteria, the perfect storage fuel does not exist; no single substance scores highly enough on all counts. The solution, therefore, is to store more than one kind of fuel and to switch from one to another as circumstances dictate. Each of the three important storage fuels— *glycogen* (carbohydrate), *triglyceride* (fat) and *phosphocreatine* (phosphagen)—has its own special part to play in the athlete's energy budget. If meaningful science-based advice is to be given to the athlete, knowledge of the special roles that these storage fuels play in different athletic events is essential.

GLYCOGEN: PACKAGED GLUCOSE

Glycogen is a carbohydrate composed of many thousands of glucose units polymerized into a gigantic tree-like molecule (Figure 4.2). The significance of this tree-like structure is that large amounts of glucose can be rapidly released from the ends of its branches—just as the leaves of the tree can be shed rapidly when the temperature drops in autumn. Most of the glucose that is used for the synthesis of glycogen comes from starch—the major carbohydrate in the human diet and abundant, for example, in bread, potatoes, pasta, rice and cereals. This starch is digested in the intestines to release glucose, which is absorbed into the bloodstream. From the blood, the glucose is taken up by tissues, such as muscle and liver, where it is built up into glycogen.

Glucose itself is not an ideal storage fuel. Although it is present in the blood, where it provides a fuel for many tissues, the actual amount is quite limited; there is barely sufficient to keep an élite marathon runner going for just one minute. One of the reasons why glucose is not stored is that it is chemically reactive and, even at levels normally found in the blood, it can react with certain proteins to change their structure and impair their function. In the glycogen molecule, the reactive groups of glucose are masked so they cannot react with proteins. Another disadvantage of glucose is that, if a storage fuel were to consist of small molecules, the number of molecules would change rapidly when the fuel was used, causing severe osmotic problems. The 'tree-like' glycogen molecule is a very successful solution to both problems.

Although glycogen is a successful solution to these problems, it is not the perfect fuel. In the first place its energy content, 16 kJ/g, is only modest—less than half of that found in fat. Secondly, this value is for pure, dry glycogen, but this does not occur in cells where it

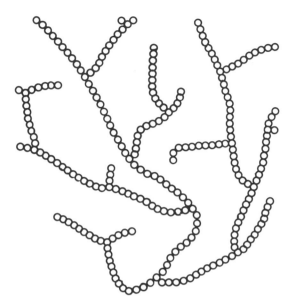

Figure 4.2. Part of a glycogen molecule. Each circle represents a glucose unit, of which up to a million may be present in a single molecule of glycogen. Within muscle fibres, glycogen molecules associate with the enzymes involved in their synthesis and breakdown form glycogen particles which are visible under the electron microscope

associates with proteins and water to form glycogen granules. The amount of additional water is large enough to makes its mark on the bathroom scales since a full 'load' of 500 g of glycogen is accompanied by an additional 1500 g (3 lb) of water. The biological significance of this is apparent from the fact that, if an average man stored all his fuel reserves as glycogen instead of fat he would weigh twice as much! Consequently, most of the fuel reserves in the body consist of fat rather than glycogen.

In fact, 600 g of glycogen, at most, is stored in the muscles of a typical male athlete, some 500 g of which is in muscles used in running. Although glycogen is likely to be the major fuel in middle- and long-distance track events, this amount is insufficient to provide enough energy for a whole marathon. A calculation based on the rate of oxygen consumption during a simulated marathon run in the laboratory indicates that élite marathon runners consume about 5 g glycogen per minute, so that they have on board barely enough to last 100 min. Although rest, plus a carbohydrate-rich diet prior to the event, may boost glycogen stores, other fuels must be used to complete the race.

A further 100 g glycogen is stored in the liver, where its main function is to maintain an adequate concentration of glucose in the blood between meals. This glucose is not primarily used by muscles and, although some of it undoubtedly is used during marathon and ultra-marathon events, the bulk must be conserved for use by tissues that are unable to use other fuels. Paramount amongst these is the brain, which uses about 5 g glucose each hour. During the overnight fast a significant proportion of liver glycogen is mobilized as glucose for use by the brain; an early-morning carbohydrate-rich breakfast helps to restore it.

TRIGLYCERIDE: CONCENTRATED ENERGY

Chemists refer to fats (and oils) as triglycerides because each molecule consists of a glycerol unit and three fatty acid units (Figure 4.3). It is these fatty acids which contain most of the chemical energy; indeed their structure is very similar to that of the hydrocarbons in fuels such as petrol (gasoline). Typically they contain between 16 and 22 carbon atoms and if all of these (except those at the ends) are attached to two hydrogen atoms, the fatty acid is said to be saturated (i.e. with hydrogen). If a pair of adjacent carbon atoms are linked by a double bond (with the elimination of two hydrogen atoms) the fatty acid is unsaturated. The chemistry is explained in Figure 11.3 (p. 230) but this is more than a chemical detail, for triglycerides composed of unsaturated fatty acids tend to be liquid at room temperatures, i.e. they are *oils* rather than *fats*. Of greater significance is the fact that certain polyunsaturated fatty acids—those with more than one double bond—despite being needed for the formation of cell membranes and other cellular constituents, cannot be made by humans from saturated fatty acids. Consequently, they must be present in the diet and are known as *essential fatty acids* (see p. 231–232).

The triglycerides stored in the body contain a mixture of saturated and unsaturated fatty acids and have an energy content of approximately 35 kJ/g—more than twice that of glycogen. Furthermore, triglycerides are stored 'dry', so that they are by far the most efficient way to store fuel. This is of particular benefit to the ultra-marathon runner, who cannot store anywhere near enough glycogen to fuel these events. It is, however, the very high energy content of fat that makes reduction of body weight during periods of 'dieting' very difficult; even

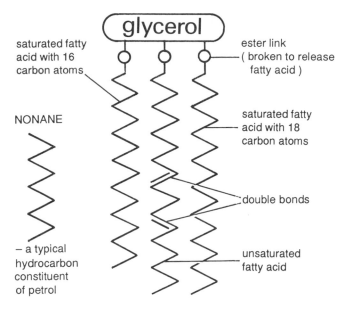

Figure 4.3. Anatomy of a triglyceride molecule

a severe restriction of energy intake produces only a small loss of body fat. The best that can be achieved safely is about 2 lb per week.

Fat is stored mainly in special cells called adipocytes, each of which contains a droplet of triglyceride that occupies almost the whole cell (Figure 4.4) An adult male may contain 100 000 000 000 such cells, which cluster together to form adipose tissue, the primary function of which is to store chemical energy. Adipose tissue does not form a discrete organ, like the kidney, liver or lung, but is widely distributed through the body. It is found beneath the skin, around major organs such as the heart and kidneys, in the abdominal cavity and between muscles. Some fat is stored in certain muscles but in comparison with adipose tissue the amount is very small.

When compared with glycogen, the quantities of fat stored are large and can be embarrassingly so. Typically an average 70 kg male will store 8 kg of fat, and an average woman of 60 kg nearly twice as much. This additional fat in the female is stored in the upper thighs, buttocks and hips, breasts and back of the upper arms. The large capacity for fat storage, coupled with its greater energy content, means that an average man stores enough fat to survive 6 or more weeks of starvation or run non-stop for 3 days and nights *at an élite marathon runner's*

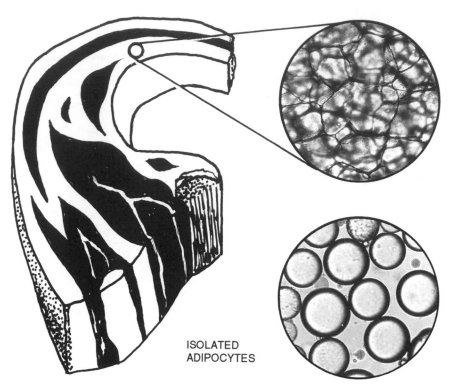

ISOLATED
ADIPOCYTES

Figure 4.4. The best place to see adipose tissue is a butcher's shop. Photograph of cells from adipose tissue kindly provided by Dr Caroline Pond, the Open University, Milton Keynes

Box 4.1   Apples or pears?

No exercise physiologist, or even biochemist, would claim that all muscles are similar. Each appears to have evolved exquisitely for its particular role in the whole animal. So why should adipose tissue be different? We now know that it is not.

Adipose tissue occurs not just anywhere but in a limited number of specific locations, including the breast, the upper regions of limbs, on the calf, at the back of the neck, on each side of the base of the spine (buttocks) and at a number of well-defined sites in the abdomen. These

_ continued _|

— *continued* —

locations appear common to all mammals but the proportion of fat in each varies between species, with humans, especially males, having by far the largest paunches. Indeed the conspicuous difference in adipose tissue distribution between the sexes is almost uniquely human, although its significance is not clear. In addition to these anatomical sites, between about 4% and 15% of dissectible fat in humans is found within muscles.

There is increasing evidence that each of these fat stores has a somewhat different function. The adipose tissue within muscle, for example, is the most metabolically active and readily removes triglyceride from the blood for storage. It is also particularly sensitive to the action of the 'exercise' hormones adrenaline, noradrenaline and insulin, so it is these deposits which supply most of the fatty acids to the muscles of hard-training athletes.

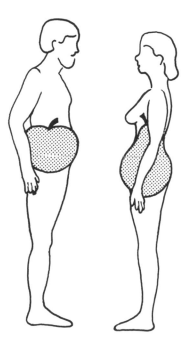

Figure 4.5. A common difference in the distribution of adipose tissue in men and women. Men usually expand their adipose tissue around the waist to give an 'apple' appearance, whereas women usually expand in the region of the hips to give a 'pear'-shaped appearance (a difference readily observable on any beach)

— *continued* —

— *continued* —

By contrast, adipose tissue in the lower abdomen is less metaboli-cally active but it does have considerable potential for growth, as many middle-aged men discover to their dismay. An intriguing corre-lation has been found between their characteristic 'apple' shape (Figure 4.5) and susceptibility to coronary heart disease and diabetes. The connection appears to be that abdominal fat is readily mobilized under stress and that the fatty acids released increase fat deposition in the arteries.

Women are different. A much larger proportion of their adipose tissue is in the groin and hip region, making them typically more 'pear' shaped. These stores are less likely to be mobilized in times of stress but are much more susceptible to female sex hormones releasing fatty acids when pregnancy and lactation make their demands. Pear-shaped people, men as well as women, appear less susceptible to the harmful consequences of moderate obesity.

pace (Figure 4.6). But, hang on, no one can do that! Even the 24 h ultra-marathon (approximately 120 km) has to be run at a pace roughly 60% of the best marathon pace. The problem is that the fat fuels cannot be used by the muscle at a rate fast enough to sustain the high power output required to support the pace of the normal marathon (80–85% of $\dot{V}O_{2\,max}$). The reason for the slow use of fat is that fat fuels are not soluble in water, so in order to be carried in the blood they must be combined with proteins—an association which probably slows their uptake by muscle.

So the athlete has two fuel tanks: a small one in the muscles which contains glycogen and which can generate ATP rapidly, and a much larger fuel tank containing fat which can be drawn upon steadily but which provides ATP at only about half the maximum rate of that from carbohydrate (Figure 4.7).

Fuel storage is possible whenever the chemical energy content of ingested food exceeds the current demand for energy. Although both fuel 'tanks' can be filled from carbohydrate food, the carbohydrate 'tank' cannot be filled from fat in the food, since the human body has no means of converting fats to carbohydrates. Consequently, it is important that runners, especially middle- and long-distance runners, eat *appropriate foods* at *appropriate times* to keep their glycogen 'tanks' as fully charged as possible.

During the period immediately after exercise, ATP requirements are, of course, much lower than during the exercise but still above the

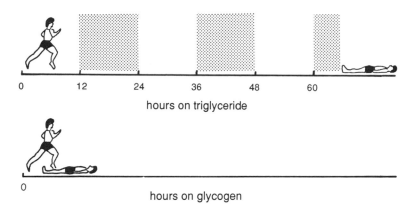

0   12   24   36   48   60

hours on triglyceride

0

hours on glycogen

Figure 4.6. Triglyceride stores are vastly greater than glycogen stores

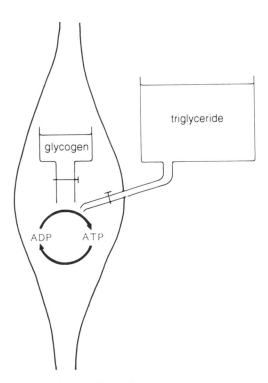

Figure 4.7. Alternative fuels. Note that in some muscle small amounts of triglyceride are stored as droplets within muscle fibres as well as in adipose tissue

resting level, probably because of the energy needed to repair damage caused by exercise, to convert glucose to glycogen in the muscle and to reset the body's metabolism to the resting level. Such moderate rates of ATP generation are easily satisfied by fat oxidation, so that any available glucose, especially that derived from carbohydrate in the food, can be converted to glycogen to refill the glycogen tanks. But this high rate of fat oxidation only occurs for a short time (2–3 h) after exercise is finished so this is the time, therefore, to take on board as much carbohydrate as can be converted to glycogen during this period. Suggestions for snacks and meals rich in carbohydrate suitable for consumption after a race or a training session will be found in Part II(D).

MAKING THE FUELS AVAILABLE

Fuel in the tanks of a plane or car has only to be pumped into the engines for oxidation to provide the energy, but in humans things are more complicated; the fuels must be mobilized. This involves breaking down the large storage compounds into smaller ones that can be oxidized to generate ATP. Glycogen is broken down to sugars (or sugar phosphates) and fat is broken down to fatty acids. Since most of the fat (triglyceride) is stored in cells remote from muscle it must be transported in the blood before it can be used.

Box 4.2   One of our enzymes is missing

It is well known that we do not appreciate what we have until it is missing. We take our metabolism, orchestrated by several thousand different enzymes, each speeding up a different chemical reaction, very much for granted. But patients seen by Dr B. McArdle around 40 years ago were having problems. After a few minutes of quite steady exercise they developed severe pains and cramps in their muscles and had to stop. However, if they began exercising very steadily, after a few minutes they could increase their power output to levels well above those which had caused discomfort previously and maintain this pace for a considerable period of time.

It turned out that these patients lacked the enzyme glycogen phosphorylase in their muscles—the first enzyme involved in the break-

continued

┌─ *continued* ─────────────────────────────────┐

down of muscle glycogen—so were unable to use muscle glycogen as a fuel. After a couple of minutes, the small stores of glucose and phosphocreatine (p.90–91) in the muscle would become exhausted and ATP levels would fall. Unable to generate more ATP anaerobically the patient would suffer severe discomfort. However, if they accepted the discomfort and continued to exercise at a low intensity, this stimulated the supply of blood to their needy muscles and delivered oxygen and alternative fuels, such as glucose and fatty acids. Once glucose, fatty acids and oxygen were available from outside the muscle, exercise could continue aerobically for a prolonged period, albeit at a steady pace.

Chemists are very skilled at manipulating chemical reactions to make the product they desire, but the task of organizing thousands of reactions, simultaneously in a small test-tube, at constant temperature, would be quite beyond even the most able. Yet that is precisely what each of us is doing right now in our muscles, breaking down large molecules, building up others and generating ATP from stored fuels. And we are able to do so because we possess enzymes.

Reactions can only take place if the products have less energy than the reactants, but if this were the only criterion all possible reactions would occur simultaneously and we would, quite literally, go up in smoke. In fact, for each reaction, there is an energy barrier over which reactants have to be 'kicked' before the reaction can occur. Chemists overcome the barrier by supplying energy, usually in the form of heat, or by using their ingenuity to devise reactants for which sufficient activation energy is available at room temperature. Organisms use enzymes, nature's own catalysts, which speed up chemical reactions by lowering the activation energy needed (Figure 4.8). The activation energy barrier for a reaction is analogous to a mountain separating two valleys. Given enough energy it is possible to get from one valley to the other by climbing the mountain, but it takes time and only a few people can do it. However, once a tunnel is built through the mountain, even granny can make the journey. In a similar way, an enzyme provides a 'tunnel' between substrates and products.

Enzymes have two biologically important properties: they are specific, catalysing just one reaction or a small group of related reactions, and they are fragile. Both properties arise from the fact that enzymes are proteins. Their fragility means that they will only work under certain conditions and are inactivated by high temperatures, extremes of acidity or alkalinity and many chemicals. Some of these chemicals

└───────────────────────────── *continued* ─┘

continued

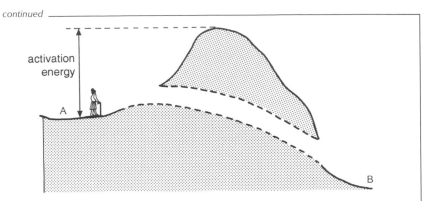

Figure 4.8. An enzyme provides a reaction pathway with reduced activation energy, but for the reaction to occur at all the product at B must have a lower free energy level than the reactant at A

are bad news, for their effect is irreversible and they can poison an organism by knocking out critical enzymes; cyanide, for example, blocks the enzyme that reacts with oxygen in Figure 4.11. Other substances which reversibly decrease enzyme activity serve as regulators of body chemistry. Through the action of such regulators, the activity of one enzyme, and hence a whole metabolic pathway, can be adjusted according to the rate of other processes occurring in the cell (Figure 4.9).

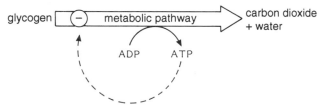

Figure 4.9. Negative feedback. The broad arrow represents a sequence of enzyme-catalysed reactions. At rest, little ATP is used so its concentration begins to rise. This reversibly inhibits an enzyme near the beginning of the pathway and slows down the rate of ATP production. When exercise begins, the ATP level begins to fall, reducing the inhibition and allowing an increased rate of ATP synthesis. In this way, the concentration of ATP is maintained between narrow limits

Changing the level of key enzymes in the fibres of the muscle and other cells of the body is one of the ways in which the body adapts to increased demand for energy. Such changes, stimulated by training, allow the specific fuel necessary for the type of running undertaken to be brought into play quickly and effectively.

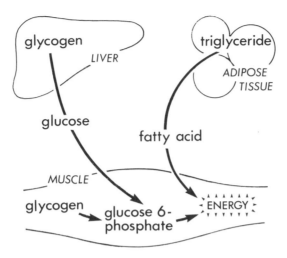

Figure 4.10. Mobilization of fuels

Mobilization of glycogen involves the splitting off of glucose units in the form of glucose phosphate, as a result of a chemical reaction with phosphate in a reaction catalysed by the enzyme phosphorylase. In muscle, this glucose phosphate enters directly into the ATP-generating sequence of reactions known as glycolysis, which provides ATP directly to the myofibrils (Figure 4.10). The fact that glycogen is actually inside the muscle cells means that it is immediately available to provide ATP whenever contraction occurs—one of the factors that makes muscle glycogen the most important fuel for the track athlete.

Fat, too, is hydrolysed. Each triglyceride molecule can react with three molecules of water in a reaction catalysed by the enzyme lipase to produce glycerol and three fatty acid molecules. Although the latter can pass out of the adipocyte into the blood they are, unlike glucose, insoluble in water and so cannot be simply carried in the blood plasma—the watery liquid between blood cells. The problem is overcome by the presence in blood plasma of the protein albumin, which adsorbs fatty acid molecules onto its surface. Albumin transports fatty acids in much the same way that haemoglobin transports oxygen (see pp.145–146), picking them up in adipose tissue where their concentration is high and releasing them in muscle where it is low. The fatty acids then enter muscle fibres, where they are oxidized and the energy released is harnessed to form ATP. The mobilization of fat to provide fatty acids for use by muscle is especially important in prolonged endurance events such as the ultra-marathon.

The important question for the athlete is, how far do these stores of fuel limit performance and can any limitation be extended by diet or by training? The encouraging answer is yes but, to understand how, we need some more information on how the all-important ATP is generated from these storage fuels.

GENERATING ATP

If you doubt whether glucose contains chemical energy try putting a match to a small pile. You may find it easier to carry out your experiment on table sugar (sucrose), which is chemically very similar to glucose. The ensuing reaction between the glucose (or sucrose) and oxygen gives out enough heat energy to maintain the flame and in a short time all the sugar has been converted to water and carbon dioxide, both given off as gases. Precisely the same overall reaction occurs when glucose is burned in exercising muscle; the same products are formed and the same amount of energy is released. But there are, of course, differences. In the body there is nothing equivalent to the match to raise the temperature of the glucose to start the reaction, so the body relies on special catalysts—enzymes—which speed up reactions in living cells so much so that they can take place at body temperature. These reactions are known collectively as metabolism.

Enzymes can be re-used over and over again for the same reaction but each kind can only catalyse one particular reaction, so a very large number of different enzymes are present in each cell. The product of one enzyme-catalysed reaction becomes the starting material for the next, and so on, forming a chain of reactions known as a *metabolic pathway*. These metabolic pathways, operating in sequence, serve to break glucose down to carbon dioxide and water. The salient features of each pathway are listed below and Figure 4.11 shows how they fit together:

Glycolysis
- Glucose molecules are split into two pyruvate molecules.
- A small amount of ATP is formed.

Krebs cycle (tricarboxylic acid cycle)
- Pyruvate is oxidized to carbon dioxide.
- Many hydrogen atoms (represented by H in Figure 4.11) are split off.

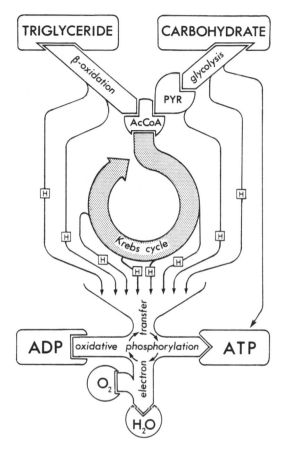

Figure 4.11. Metabolic pathways. Each of the broad arrows represents a sequence of enzyme-catalysed reactions. Abbreviations: PYR, pyruvate; AcCoA, acetyl coenzyme A

Electron transfer and oxidative phosphorylation
- The hydrogen atoms, in combination with carrier molecules, are oxidized by oxygen to produce water.
- Energy released is used to synthesize large numbers of ATP molecules.

Overall, this can be represented by two equations:

$$\text{glucose} + \text{oxygen} \rightarrow \text{carbon dioxide} + \text{water}$$
$$\text{phosphate} + \text{ADP} \rightarrow \text{ATP} + \text{water}$$

For each glucose unit of glycogen that is oxidized in this way, 37 molecules of ATP are formed.

An additional pathway, beta-oxidation, breaks down fatty acids (from triglycerides) and feeds the products into the Krebs cycle so that their oxidation too can generate ATP. Each of these pathways consists of many enzymes, and one of the benefits of training is to increase the amounts of these enzymes in muscle fibres.

Although this detailed biochemistry might seem out of place for an athlete or coach, subsequent chapters will show how it can help to explain fatigue, account for the limitation in the amount of training that can be done at any one time and demonstrate the key role of diet in athletic performance.

A MATTER OF CONTROL

There is enough ATP in the leg muscle of a man to support just one second of full-speed sprinting, and a housefly could remain airborne for a mere one-tenth of a second on its complement of ATP. Since a fall of more than 50–60% in the ATP content of a cell is probably sufficient to cause its death, it follows that ATP synthesis must keep pace with its consumption. This means that in the leg muscles of an élite sprinter, the rate of ATP synthesis must increase several thousand-fold in just two or three seconds. One factor controlling this change is the ATP concentration itself; the slight fall in ATP concentration occurring at the onset of exercise sets in motion a sequence of events that results in an increase in the rate of the metabolic pathways that produce the ATP. Conversely, when exercise ceases, the level of ATP rises and this results in a decrease in its rate of production (Figure 4.9). Such a negative feedback system maintains cellular ATP concentrations fairly constant, in much the same way as a thermostat keeps the temperature of a room constant. An improvement in the effectiveness of the mechanisms that regulate such processes is another area in which training will help (see pp. 96).

MANAGING WITHOUT OXYGEN

Although details of the chemical changes occurring in metabolic pathways might seem of little significance to the runner, hidden in the overall view of metabolism (Figure 4.11) is a feature of considerable consequence to all athletes and of supreme importance to sprinters.

Oxygen is only used in the final stages of the process. It pulls electrons from the hydrogen carriers symbolized as [H] and in so doing makes enough energy available to add a phosphate to ADP and so produce ATP. Without this essential role of oxygen almost none of the energy released in the stepwise breakdown of fats or carbohydrates could be used to generate ATP. *Almost* none? Look carefully at the right-hand side of the diagram. A lone arrow sneaks down from glycolysis to ATP, showing that some ATP can be made without oxygen, i.e. anaerobically. Although the flow of blood to the muscles during exercise is increased dramatically, it is logistically impossible to get enough oxygen to the muscles for oxidation of fuels to provide enough ATP to satisfy the maximum power output. Additional energy can then be obtained by increasing the rate of this so-called anaerobic process. The significance is enormous when it is realized that oxygen supply can be a major factor limiting the performance of middle- and long-distance athletes.

Table 4.1. Calculated maximal rates of ATP formation in human muscle based on maximal activities of key indicator enzymes under aerobic and anaerobic conditions

		Calculated maximum rate of ATP formation from glucose or glycogen (μmol/ min per gram fresh weight)	
Group	Sex	Anaerobic glycolysis	Oxidation via Krebs cycle
Untrained	Male	208	26
	Female	174	32
Medium-trained	Male	182	42
	Female	178	38
Well-trained	Male	144	52
	Female	122	58

Maximum rates of ATP formation are calculated as follows: for anaerobic glycolysis 6-phosphofructokinase activity is multiplied by 3; for oxidation by the Krebs cycle, oxoglutarate dehydrogenase activity is multiplied by 18. It is well established that the capacity for anaerobic glycolysis is decreased by endurance training, but the significance and value of this are unknown.
From Blomstrand, E., Ekblom, B. and Newsholme, E. A. (1986). Maximum activities of key glycolytic and oxidative enzymes in human muscle from differently trained individuals. *J. Physiol. (Lond.)*, **381**, 111–118.

The 100 m sprinter obtains almost all the energy required for this event from anaerobic metabolism and, surprisingly, even trained endurance runners have a greater capacity to generate ATP anaerobically than they do aerobically (Table 4.1). If enough glycogen is left in the muscle at the end of the race, a marathoner can still sprint to the tape! But there is a price to pay, in fact several, for this anaerobic ATP generation. Indeed it is the trade-offs between aerobic and anaerobic metabolism that make middle-distance running such a skilled activity.

Look yet again at Figure 4.11. The first problem is that only glycogen can give rise to ATP anaerobically and that glycogen stores are small. Fat, although abundant, can only be broken down if oxygen is present. The second problem is that anaerobic metabolism releases only a small fraction of the energy available—enough to form just three ATP molecules per glucose unit of glycogen compared with 37 from complete oxidation. So, too heavy a reliance on anaerobic metabolism will deplete glycogen stores very rapidly. Although the anaerobic conversion of glycogen to lactate provides only 3% of the ATP turned over in a 10 000 m race, it consumes almost one-third of the glycogen stores (Table 4.2). If the contribution of the anaerobic process rose just slightly, to 4%, there would probably be insufficient glycogen to complete the race, the pace would fall and the runner would have to withdraw. High rates of anaerobic metabolism are, therefore, only possible in sprint events.

The third problem with anaerobic metabolism, in fact a major drawback and the one that actually prevents sprinters from sprinting for longer, is the accumulation of end-products. Aerobic metabolism produces only water and carbon dioxide, which cause no problem. The carbon dioxide passes from the muscles into the blood and is then vented from the body through the lungs. Water can also be lost from the lungs but may be retained to help avoid dehydration. In contrast, the immediate products of anaerobic metabolism are pyruvate and reduced hydrogen carriers which, in the absence of oxygen, cannot be oxidized to generate ATP. Under anaerobic conditions, and in the presence of appropriate enzymes, they react together to form lactic acid and to regenerate the reduced hydrogen carriers needed for the continuation of glycolysis (Figure 4.12). The accumulation of lactic acid in a muscle rapidly decreases its pH (a measure of acidity; the lower the number, the more acid) to a point where all its enzymes would stop working and the cells would die. Such a build-up is prevented by the developing fatigue—a safety mechanism which slows the pace, decreases the demand for ATP and therefore decreases the rate of the

Table 4.2. Estimates of the contribution of aerobic and anaerobic metabolism of glycogen to energy provision for different track events

Distance of event (m)	Percentage contribution to ATP formation from aerobic metabolism	Amount of glycogen used (g/kg muscle)	Percentage glycogen used by:	
			aerobic metabolism	anaerobic metabolism
800	50	7.7	7	93
1 500	65	8.3	20	80
5 000	87	17.6	36	64
10 000	97	19.3	72	28
Marathon	100	20	100	0

The total amount of glycogen present in human muscle is about 20 g/kg muscle. The method for calculation is given in Table 4 of Newsholme, E. A., Blomstrand, E. and Ekblom, B. (1992). Physical and mental fatigue: metabolic mechanisms and importance of plasma amino acids. *Br. Med. Bull.*, **48**, 477–495.

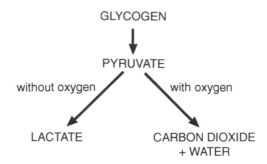

Figure 4.12. Metabolic processes for energy formation

anaerobic process which generates the acidity. This is further discussed in Chapter 6.

PHOSPHOCREATINE: SHORT-TERM BOOST

There are times when power output just has to be maximal: the sprinter's explosion from the blocks; the middle-distance runner's sprint for the tape; the cheetah's acceleration to 45 mph in 2 s; the chase for the ball to score the winning goal; the party-goer's dash for the last train. But glycolysis alone cannot take place rapidly enough to supply sufficient ATP to support such burst activities. That they can take place at all is due to the existence of a reservoir of high-energy

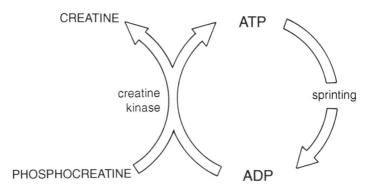

Figure 4.13. Regeneration of ATP using phosphocreatine

Box 4.3   The sprinting lobster

Next time you visit an aquarium, watch the lobsters. They move backwards amazingly fast by a 'flick' of their abdomen. This flick is caused by the contraction of the abdominal muscles and, for the lobster, it represents an escape mechanism. The fuel used to provide the ATP is phosphoarginine, serving in the lobster the same purpose as phosphocreatine in humans. The abdominal muscles of the lobster, so good to eat, have a very low capacity for anaerobic glycolysis but an *enormous* activity of the enzyme arginine kinase and at least four times more phosphoarginine than there is phosphocreatine in the muscle of man. Indeed, the lobster is totally dependent upon this fuel

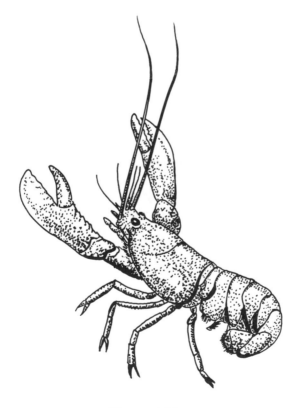

Figure 4.14.

continued

— *continued* —

for its escape reaction. Phosphoarginine (and phosphocreatine) stores can generate ATP faster than glycolysis but the amount that can be stored is strictly limited. It would be interesting to know if athletes who are very fast 'off the mark' have a particularly high activity of creatine kinase for this supercharging boost. Is 'speed off the mark' due to 'lobster-like' energy generation?

phosphate called phosphocreatine which is present in the muscles involved. This can be called upon to rephosphorylate ADP very quickly and so maintain adequate levels of ATP despite exceptional demands. In short sprints, the simultaneous use of both phosphocreatine and glycogen enables peak power output to exceed 3000 watts.

To generate ATP from phosphocreatine and ADP requires only one reaction, catalysed by the enzyme creatine kinase (Figure 4.13). Like other enzymes, creatine kinase is not fussy about the direction in which it works, so that during recovery from the sprint it catalyses the reformation of phosphocreatine from ATP and creatine. In invertebrates, phosphoarginine does the same job as phosphocreatine and both are known as *phosphagens*.

The significance of phosphocreatine to the athlete is that, unlike ATP, it *can* be stored in the muscle, ready and available to rephosphorylate ADP in an instant! The quantities are small (enough in leg muscles for perhaps 5 s of sprinting) but it can be used very rapidly in sprinting races, in sprinting to the tape in longer races and in climbing hills in marathons and ultra-marathons. If ATP is likened to cash in hand, and storage fuels to a deposit account, then phosphocreatine is the piggy-bank on the mantelpiece—it is filled slowly, a few pence at a time, but can be blown on a single night out (Figure 4.15). The single 'night out', however, at the end of the 5000 or 10 000 m race, may be the difference between a gold medal and finishing well down the field!

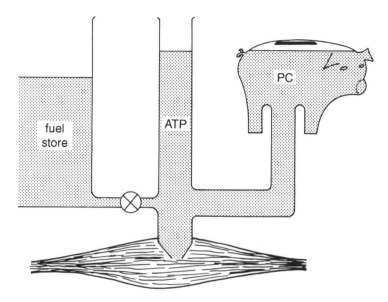

Figure 4.15. The phosphocreatine investment—a small reserve which can rapidly regenerate ATP

Box 4.4   Legal dope

Athletes dream of being able to boost their performance with a food supplement—something which is normally in the diet so cannot easily be banned. Of course there is still the risk that taking large quantities will cause undesirable side-effects but many are willing to take that risk. Most food supplements were researched in the 1970s but one—creatine—has hit the headlines more recently and may be quite widely used.

Phosphocreatine—the phosphorylated form of creatine—provides the means of regenerating small quantities of ATP extremely rapidly, so boosting short-duration activities (see p. 96). The discovery by Dr Eric Hultman in Stockholm that depletion of phosphocreatine caused fatigue in sprinters led to the possibility that raising the level of creatine in muscle would raise the level of phosphocreatine and lead to an increase in sprinting performance. Creatine is both made in the body (from the amino acids arginine, glycine and methionine) and gained from the diet; non-vegetarians get around 2 g per day from the meat

_____ continued _|

— continued —

they eat. The question is, would eating more creatine increase the amount in muscle? The total creatine content (creatine plus phosphocreatine) of muscles typically varies between 25 and 40 μmol/g, with the higher levels correlating with the consumption of a very meat-rich diet containing 12–15 g creatine per day. But ingesting such large amounts of meat would create other dietary problems for the athlete, so attempts were made to provide creatine in pure form. Doses of 5 g creatine hydrate taken five or six times a day for 2 or more days elevated total creatine levels to the upper part of the normal range. An even larger increase was seen if exercise was carried out immediately after taking the creatine, and the elevation was better sustained if smaller doses were taken over a longer period.

Preliminary studies indicated that the observed rises in muscle creatine content increased power output by about 5–7%, presumably due to enhanced phosphocreatine levels. Whether this would benefit longer events such as the 800 m and the 1500 m, in which phosphocreatine plays a small but important role, has yet to be established.

Chapter 5

Fuel Management

If the New Jersey race were a Marathon Trials of the mind, Gompers could lay fair claim to an uncontested spot on the team. But is it possible to overintellectualize the simple act of running? After all, the centipede stumbled when forced to concentrate on its biomechanics. And Yogi Berra, exhorted to think at the bat, stood paralysed while three strikes whizzed across the plate. Hadn't the Africans and other Third Worlders proved that athletes can excel without knowing the blood pH?

'Yes, of course,' says Dr Newsholme, pausing to exhale in a slow, deliberate manner. 'Yet I would argue that the Africans would be even greater if they had a scientific background. More to the point, I would argue that all runners gain a greater enjoyment and appreciation of their sport when they understand it more fully.'

Andy Barfoot, interviewing one of the authors about the career of Paul Gompers, a contender for the American marathon team for the 1988 Olympic Games, in *Runners World*, April 1988, pp. 73–77.

You drive into the filling station and have to choose from which pump to fill your car: high octane, low octane, leaded, unleaded or even diesel. Different vehicles run best on different fuels. In contrast, the human body is an all-purpose vehicle, capable of many different activities each of which, as hinted at in the previous chapter, needs a different fuel or combination of fuels. Although it is not necessary for the athlete to fill up with very specific fuels, the type of food eaten does have a large effect on correct fuel store repletion for training and competition (see Chapter 11). Food choice is important but variation is possible since we possess 'on-board' fuel-processing capabilities. We can break down the appropriate food to its essential components and then build up the required food stores.

Provided that the fuel tanks are appropriately refilled, training can help the athlete to use the fuels in the correct combinations for the particular activity being carried out and at the rate which offers the best performance. If improved manipulation of fuel stores gives even a 1% advantage, it will provide the competitive edge over rivals.

In this chapter we examine in detail how each fuel contributes to energy generation in different events, and start by summarizing the options for ATP generation:

- From phosphocreatine.
- From glycogen anaerobically.
- From glycogen aerobically.
- From blood glucose.
- From fatty acids.

Each of these 'fuel options' has advantages and disadvantages in terms of the rate of ATP production, the duration of the physical activity that they can support and the accumulation of waste products. It is impossible to find a single running event in which just one fuel is used; a combination is invariably needed. This lays particular emphasis on the control mechanisms which permit smooth switches from one fuel to another or which permit the use of several fuels in combination. It is probable that it is just as important to train these control mechanisms as it is to train the aerobic capacity; we simply know less about how to go about it.

100 METRES

Of the standard track events the 100 m sprint is unique in that it is run almost entirely without oxygen (Table 5.1). There is enough phosphocreatine in leg muscles to account for about half the ATP needed and it has been assumed for many years that this phospho-creatine would be used first in all the sprints. However, recent research has shown that maximal sprinting performance can occur only when both phosphocreatine and glycogen are used simulta-neously, each contributing about half of the energy required (Figure 5.1). It is likely that, in all events, phosphocreatine contributes most to the formation of ATP in the first second or two that it takes to increase the rate of glycogen breakdown and glycolysis but thereafter, in the sprints, both fuels are used. It should be noted that in the sprints the rate of glycolysis must increase by a factor of at least 1000—an increase which will take at least a second or two to establish.

Why should 100 m sprints be run almost entirely anaerobically—a mode of metabolism which yields less than 10% of the ATP available from complete oxidation? The essence of sprinting is speed. The ability to sprint evolved not to win gold medals but to save life; the faster he

Table 5.1. Proportion of ATP derived from aerobic metabolism in various events

Event (m)	Percentage of ATP derived from aerobic metabolism
100	<5
200	10
400	25
800	50
1 500	65
5 000	87
10 000	97
Marathon	100

It should be noted that these values are estimates based on available biochemical information and they will undoubtedly vary from athlete to athlete. Adapted from (i) Bangsbo, J., Gollnick, P. D., Graham, T. E. *et al.* (1990). Anaerobic energy production and O_2 deficit–debt relationship during exhaustive exercise in humans. *J. Physiol. (Lond.)*, **422**, 539–559; (ii) Newsholme, E.A., Blomstrand, E. and Ekblom, B. (1992). Physical and mental fatigue: metabolic mechanisms and importance of plasma amino acids. *Brit. Med. Bull.*, **48**, 477–485.

or she ran, the greater the chance of escape from predatory animals! Speed depends primarily on muscle power which, in turn, depends on the number of fibres that can be crammed into the muscle. If these fibres were to operate aerobically they would need a blood supply which delivered oxygen to each fibre, and this would mean not only increasing the diameter of arteries and veins but also increasing the number of capillaries (possibly by a factor of two). All this would

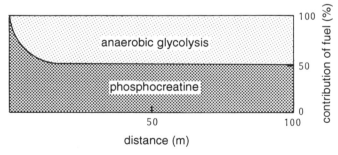

Figure 5.1. Fuels used in the 100 m*

*This diagram and the other fuel utilization charts in this chapter are based on biochemical expectations rather than experimental evidence

diminish the space available for the contractile machinery on which
power output depends. Anaerobic glycolysis and the enzyme creatine
kinase do not depend on blood supply and so require much less space.
They provide plenty of ATP for the sprinter although only for a short
period of time. Despite the poor long-term energy 'economics' of the
anaerobic process, it does provide the optimum power solution for
escape—and hence for winning sprint races.

Although little oxygen is breathed in during the 10 s or so that it
takes to run 100 m, the sprinter remains out of breath for some time
after the race. Most of this increased breathing serves to 'blow off'
carbon dioxide in order to reduce blood acidity (see Chapter 6). This
increased ventilation rate is stimulated not only by the increased acid
load in the blood but also by the actual movement of the limbs. Even
very light exercise, provided that the limbs are moved fully, results in
a considerably enhanced post-exercise ventilation rate. It would

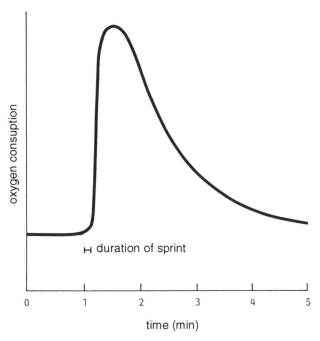

Figure 5.2. Raised oxygen uptake persists for a time after sprint activity.
However after prolonged vigorous exercise increased oxygen uptake may
persist for a very long time—perhaps for as much as 12 hours. From Maehlum,
S., Grandmontagne, M., Newsholme, E. A. *et al.* (1986). Magnitude and
duration of excess postexercise oxygen consumption in healthy young subjects.
Metabolism, **35**, 425–429

appear that signals from receptors within the muscles stimulate the respiratory centre within the brain.

Not only does the ventilation rate increase after exercise but oxygen consumption itself rises (Figure 5.2). Why should more oxygen be consumed after the 100 m event than during it? This increased oxygen uptake has been described as repaying the oxygen debt, implying that oxygen has somehow been used from a store during the race and must subsequently be replaced. This, however, is only a minor part of the answer. A better description of this oxygen is *recovery oxygen*, for most of it is used to decrease the lactic acid content of the blood raised as a consequence of the anaerobic activity. A high proportion of this lactic acid is turned back into glucose in the liver, in an ATP-requiring process known as gluconeogenesis. Much of this ATP is provided by additional aerobic metabolism in the liver (Figure 5.3), which accounts for some of the recovery oxygen. The recycled glucose is returned by the blood to the muscles, where its conversion back into glycogen also requires ATP and accounts for more of the recovery oxygen. This extra oxygen uptake occurs after all events but it is most obvious immediately after short intense bursts of activity as in the sprints. After

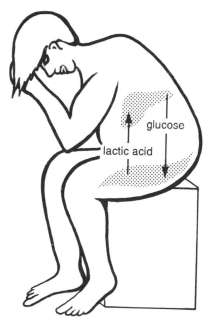

Figure 5.3. Immediately after vigorous exercise, lactic acid from the blood is carried to the liver, where it is converted into glucose. Much of this glucose returns to the muscles, where it is converted to glycogen for storage

longer events, recovery oxygen uptake is less intense but continues for many hours to allow metabolism to return slowly and gradually to normal and to ensure repletion of the glycogen stores in the muscle.

200 METRES

As with the 100 m sprint, both phosphocreatine and glycogen (anaerobically) are used simultaneously (Figure 5.4). If, however, after about 150 m the phosphocreatine store has been exhausted, the pace must decrease by about 10%. Aerobic metabolism will make some contribution to ATP formation in this event but it is likely to be small (10–20%). The recent knowledge that phosphocreatine is so important in sprinting has raised the question of the possible means for increasing the levels of phosphocreatine in muscles. Research in Sweden has provided evidence that eating large amounts of creatine can indeed increase the levels of phosphocreatine in muscles of athletes (Box 4.4).

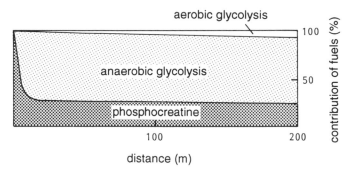

Figure 5.4. Fuels used in the 200 m

400 METRES

The 400 m is a specialized event; few élite 400 m athletes excel at any other distance (Table 5.2). The reason may be biochemical, since it is likely that *three* modes of ATP generation make significant contributions to the energy required for this event (Figure 5.5).

A little over 10% of the energy comes from phosphocreatine and ideally, after its use in the first second or two, the remainder should

Table 5.2. Names of athletes who won gold medals in two sprints at the same Olympic Games

Year of Olympic Games	Winner of two events for			
	100+200 m	100+400 m	200+400 m	400+800 m
1896	–	Burke	–	–
1904	Hahn	–	–	–
1906*	–	–	–	Pilgrim
1908	Craig	–	–	–
1912	–	–	–	–
1928	Williams	–	–	–
1932	Tolan	–	–	–
1936	Owens	–	–	–
1956	Morrow	–	–	–
1976	–	–	–	Juantorena
1984	Lewis	–	–	–

*The 1906 Games are known as the intercollated Olympic Games.

be eked out to supplement the other sources of ATP as the race progresses. Inability to store sufficient phosphocreatine to make a greater contribution to energy provision is one factor which contributes to fatigue in this event, but a more important limitation is lactic acid accumulation, discussed more fully in the next chapter. To reduce this latter problem, it is estimated some 25% of the ATP needed in the 400 m is generated aerobically from the oxidation of muscle glycogen. What emerges from this analysis is that training regimes for the 400 m must be designed to improve the relevant control mechanisms for integrating these three processes, as well as training each process maximally.

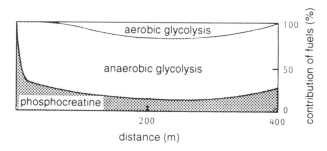

Figure 5.5. Fuels used in the 400 m

MIDDLE DISTANCES: 800 METRES AND 1500 METRES

For both the 800 m and 1500 m events, phosphocreatine and anaerobic glycogen metabolism make contributions to ATP generation (Figures 5.6, 5.7) but aerobic metabolism now becomes increasingly important, providing about 50% of the energy required in the 800 m and about 65% in the 1500 m (Table 5.1).

The main advantage of aerobic metabolism is that much less glycogen is used for the same amount of ATP produced. Indeed, if muscle glycogen were used totally anaerobically it would last (at the sprinter's pace) no more than about 1000 m! Since aerobic metabolism requires oxygen, the muscles of middle-distance athletes are provided with a good blood supply. This has the additional advantage that the lactic acid formed from anaerobic metabolism can now escape from the muscle into the blood, where its acidity can be taken care of by buffers that are much more effective than those in the muscle. This means that some anaerobic conversion of glycogen to lactic acid can occur

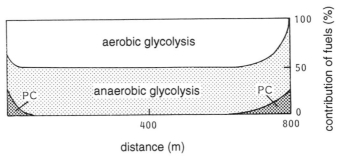

Figure 5.6. Fuels used in the 800 m

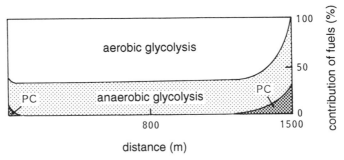

Figure 5.7. Fuels used in the 1500 m

without risking the onset of fatigue due to acidity. Middle-distance runners have less muscle than sprinters but they possess a higher proportion of slow twitch fibres in their muscles (see p. 43) to support this increased reliance on aerobic metabolism. However, they pay a price in terms of speed; these fibres contract less rapidly than fast oxidative fibres.

With increased reliance on aerobic metabolism in these events an additional metabolic possibility opens up—the use of fatty acids as a fuel. Although fatty acids cannot be utilized rapidly enough to satisfy the entire aerobic capacity of a muscle, there does not, at first sight, seem any reason why they should not be used as well as glycogen. Further consideration, however, makes this possibility less attractive. An important limiting factor in middle-distance runners is the oxygen supply to the muscles, but oxidation of fatty acids requires almost 10% more oxygen to produce the same amount of ATP when compared to the oxidation of glycogen (Figure 5.8). Therefore, if fatty acids are used to provide some of the ATP, oxygen consumption would have to increase. If this is already maximal, i.e. the oxygen consumption is limiting performance, less glycogen would be oxidized, the rate of ATP production would fall and the pace would drop. Fatty acids should, therefore, not be used by middle-distance runners. Since it is a biochemical fact that whenever fatty acids are available in the blood they will be oxidized in preference to glycogen, it is important that middle-distance runners do nothing to increase fatty acid mobilization either during or before a race. This can be prevented by sensible eating prior

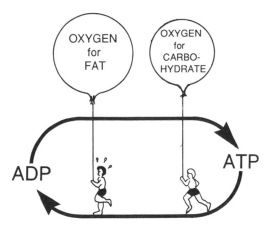

Figure 5.8. The release of energy from fat requires more oxygen than the release of the same amount of energy from carbohydrate

Table 5.3. An estimate of percentage contribution of different fuels to ATP generation in different events

Event (m)	Percentage contribution to ATP generation				
		Glycogen		Blood glucose (liver glycogen)	Triglyceride (fatty acids)
	Phosphocreatine	Anaerobic	Aerobic		
100	50	50	–	–	–
200	25	65	10	–	–
400	12.5	62.5	25	–	–
800	6	50	44	–	–
1 500	a	25	75	–	–
5 000	a	12.5	87.5	–	–
10 000	a	3	97	–	–
Marathon	–	–	75	5	20
Ultra-marathon (80 km)	–	–	35	5	60
24 h race	–	–	10	2	88
Soccer game	10	70	20	–	–

aIn these events phosphocreatine will be used for the first few seconds and, if it has been resynthesized during the race, in the sprint to the tape.

From Newsholme, E.A., Blomstrand, E. and Ekblom, B. (1992). Physical and mental fatigue: metabolic mechanisms and importance of plasma amino acids. *Brit. Med. Bull.*, **48**, 477–495.

to the event. For example, a small carbohydrate-rich snack eaten some 90–120 min before the event will decrease fatty acid mobilization because the glucose in the snack will cause the release of insulin, which prevents the mobilization of fatty acids from adipose tissue. However, the timing of this carbohydrate-rich snack has to be precise since insulin not only suppresses fatty acid mobilization but can also decrease glycogen breakdown in the muscle and lower the blood glucose level (rebound hypoglycaemia). Since glycogen is the major source of energy for the athlete in this event and severe hypoglycaemia can cause fatigue, the snack must not be taken too close to the event. The best advice we can give to the athlete is to experiment. Do you perform better if the snack was eaten 60, 90, or 120 min previously? More detailed advice on the kind and amount of food to be eaten before or after training and competition is given in Part II(D).

Note that, despite the fact that blood contains almost 1 g glucose per litre, little of this is actually used by muscles; the main fuel is glycogen. It follows, therefore, that despite advice given in some magazines, taking glucose just before or during a middle-distance track race will be of no value since there will be insufficient time for it to be assimilated into glycogen. It must be taken much earlier and preferably as a carbohydrate-rich snack.

LONG-DISTANCE TRACK EVENTS: 3–10 KILOMETRES

Glycogen is the only fuel of significance in these events (Figure 5.9) and most of the energy is obtained from its aerobic metabolism; we estimate 87.5% for 5 km and 97% for 10 km. Nonetheless the contribution from anaerobic metabolism is still important and can make the difference between winning or losing. The loss of pace that must follow

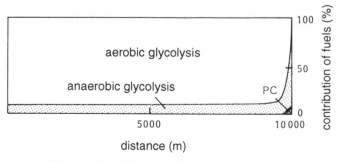

Figure 5.9. Fuels used in the 10 000 m

from the adaptation of the muscles to aerobic metabolism is remarkable. If an athlete could run aerobically without sacrificing muscle fibres for blood vessels and if slow twitch fibres could be persuaded to contract as fast and with as much power output as fast twitch-oxidative fibres, the 10 km race could be won in about 17 min. No training schedule, drugs or genetic engineering will ever realize this biochemist's dream!

It would be naive to assume that a muscle capable of making energy available both aerobically and anaerobically would achieve its full aerobic capacity before *any* anaerobic metabolism occurred—the control mechanisms are just not that good. In fact, anaerobic metabolism becomes increasingly important as aerobic capacity is approached. Figure 5.10 shows this response, but it also shows that the rise in lactate is slow until a certain intensity of work (i.e. running speed) is reached. Above this intensity, which has been called the *'anaerobic threshold'* or *'lactic acid turnpoint'*, lactate levels in both the muscle and blood rise dramatically. Below this pace, anaerobic metabolism still occurs but not at a sufficiently high rate that processes for removing the lactic acid from the muscle cannot cope. Some of the lactic acid produced at this lower rate will be taken up by other muscle fibres that are not fully active, and that which escapes into the bloodstream will be removed by other organs, including the liver.

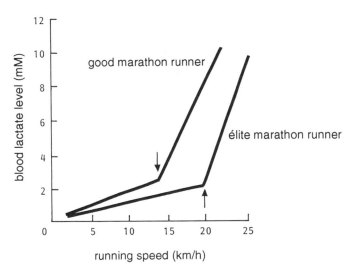

Figure 5.10. Arrows indicate the anaerobic threshold or lactic acid turnpoint. Data from Noakes, T. (1992). *Lore of Running*. Oxford University Press, Cape Town

Running at a pace just below this threshold prevents a large accumulation of lactic acid in the active muscles so that performance is not impaired—a consideration to be taken into account not only in competition but also in training.

In some studies, the rather arbitrary level of 4 mM lactate in the blood has been used to define the onset of significant anaerobic metabolism. This is sometimes known as OBLA (onset of blood lactate accumulation) but may not be such a good predictor of endurance performance as the lactic acid turnpoint. The lactic acid turnpoint is expressed as the percentage of the maximum aerobic capacity that can be achieved before the blood lactic acid level rises sharply. This may be quite low for the untrained athlete but it is increased by training, particularly peak training, and may attain values between 75% and 90% of the $\dot{V}O_{2\,max}$.

Most of the phosphocreatine initially present in muscle will have been used in the first few seconds of the race, but in long events such as these a very small proportion of the ATP formed during the event may not be used directly to power contraction but to resynthesize phosphocreatine. In this way, energy is put back into the 'piggy-bank' to be withdrawn for spending on the 'sprint to the tape'. Training may well increase both the store of phosphocreatine and ability to refill this store during a race.

MARATHON AND ULTRA-MARATHON

For reasons already made clear, these events must be run entirely aerobically. A full marathon needs about 700 g carbohydrate, more than is stored, even after carbohydrate loading (see p. 226–227), in all

---

Box 5.1   Birth of the marathon

Pheidippides was one of the hemerodromoi—intercity messengers of Ancient Greece. Humans can travel faster than horses over rough ground, so runners were an important part of the communication system in Ancient Greece. In 490 BC, when invasion of Athens by the Persians was imminent, Pheidippides was dispatched from Marathon to Sparta with a message requesting help (Figure 5.11). It is recorded that he arrived in Sparta (about 140 miles away) the day after setting out. His mission was in vain but the Athenians managed to defeat the

continued

continued

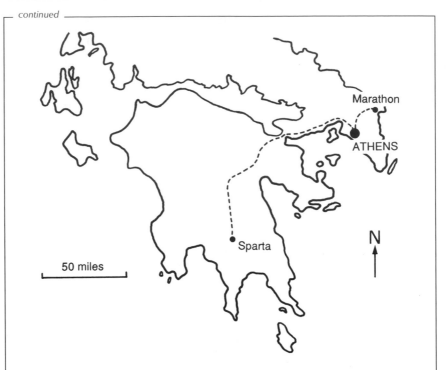

Figure 5.11. Map of Greece showing Pheidippides' runs

Persians at Marathon without help from the Spartans. Pheidippides was once more called upon to carry a message, this time to Athens, some 26 miles distant, in order to prevent the Athenians surrendering to the Persian fleet. It was to commemorate this latter feat that Baron de Coubertin included a race from Marathon to the Olympic stadium in Athens in the first modern Olympic Games in 1896. The thousands of athletes competing in today's popular marathon races all over the world should be grateful that their event is based on Pheidippides' second running feat and not his first! It is, however, possible to commemorate Pheidippides' run from Athens to Sparta in the annual 246 km Spartathlon, which has to be completed within 36 h.

A disquieting aspect of the report of Pheidippides' achievement is that, after giving his message to the Athenians, he dropped dead from his exertions. Hardly the fate of an experienced professional runner! In fact, the historical account of the events given by Herodotus makes no mention of Pheidippides' death. Herodotus was writing only a generation after the run and it seems unlikely that he would have failed

continued

— *continued* —

to record such a dramatic incident. It was left to Lucian, writing well over *six centuries* later, to invoke artistic licence and embellish the story with Pheidippides' death. The British poet Robert Browning, understandably, incorporated this dramatic conclusion in his poetic tribute to Pheidippides and so became responsible for the general acceptance of this version of Pheidippides' death. Browning's poem ends:

> So is Pheidippides happy for ever,—the noble strong
>   man
> Who could race like a God, bear the face of a God, whom
>   a God loved so well;
> He saw the land saved he had helped to save,
>   and was suffered to tell
> Such tidings, yet never decline, but, gloriously as he
>   began,
> So to end gloriously—once to shout, thereafter be
>   mute:
> 'Athens is saved!'—Pheidippides dies in the shout for
>   his meed.

The first marathon race was won by a Greek postal messenger, Spiridon Louis, who ran from Marathon to the Olympic stadium in Athens, almost 25 miles, in a time of 2 h 58 min 50 s, equivalent to about 3 h 10 min for the current distance. Of the 25 (male) starters, only nine finished, eight of whom were Greek, but its place in the modern Olympics was ensured. Races took place in the USA soon after the first Olympic Games; in New York, on 20th September 1896 and in Boston on 19th April 1897, with the latter becoming an annual event from that time. Surprisingly, the distance was not precisely set and varied around 25 miles. In the London Olympics of 1908, the distance from the start at Windsor Castle to the Royal Box in White City Stadium was 26 miles but, at the request of Queen Alexandra, the start was moved back to the edge of the rough lawn so that the Royal Family could get a better view. The total distance was then 26 miles 365 yards. This was fixed as the internationally accepted marathon distance as late as 1924. The first marathon for women at the Olympic Games was run in September 1984 in Los Angeles (see Chapter 8).

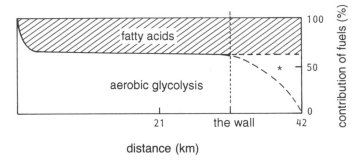

Figure 5.12. Fuels used in the marathon. *Indicates that contribution from fatty acids increases when glycogen stores exhausted

the muscles of the body. Furthermore, some of this glycogen store is in muscles that are not called upon to work maximally during the marathon. Although there is an additional store of about 100 g glycogen in the liver, some of this will be needed by the brain. So marathon runners appear to have a fuel problem. The solution is to draft in fatty

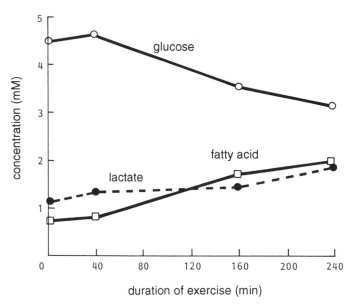

Figure 5.13. Changes in the concentration of glucose, fatty acids and lactate in blood during sustained exercise. Note that concentrations depend on the balance between the rates of mobilization and utilization. Most of the energy will be provided by glycogen stored within the muscle. See Newsholme, E. A. and Leech, A. R. (1983). *Biochemistry for the Medical Sciences*, p. 373. Wiley, Chichester

acids to supplement the carbohydrate (Figures 5.12, 5.13). Between 10% and 50% of the energy required to run the marathon is probably obtained from fatty acid oxidation, with the proportion varying markedly in different athletes. The lowest contribution will occur in the muscles of an élite runner who has raised muscle glycogen levels to the highest possible by reducing the intensity of training for at least a week, by completely resting for 3–4 days before the race and by eating an appropriate diet.

There is no shortage of fat in the average human; 12–15% of body mass in the average man and twice this in the average woman is fat. Élite long-distance runners may not be average, with men having as little as 5% of their body mass as adipose tissue and women about 10%, but even this is plenty, for the marathon could be run on as little as 300 g fat even if it were the only fuel. Although fat has a high energy content, it is not the ideal fuel because of the relatively low rate at which fatty acids can be taken up and oxidized within muscles. Some idea of this limitation can be gained from examining ultra-marathon performances; fat is virtually the only fuel available for the later

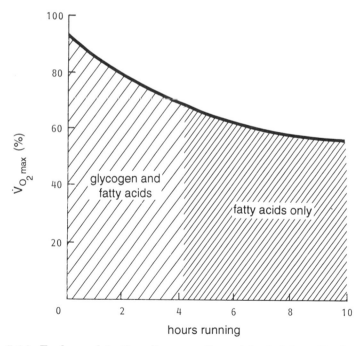

Figure 5.14. Fuels used in the ultra-marathon. Adapted from Davies, C. T. M. and Thompson, M. W. (1979) Aerobic performance of female marathon and male ultramarathon athletes. *Eur. J. Appl. Physiol.*, **41**, 233–245

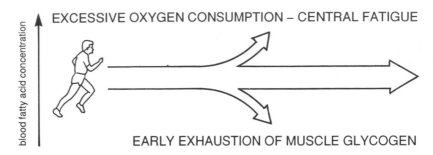

Figure 5.15. Running the metabolic tightrope. Problems arise if too much or too little fatty acid is mobilized

periods of such long-duration runs when the pace falls to around 50% of the athlete's aerobic capacity (Figure 5.14). As the élite marathon runner races at a pace equivalent to about 85% of $VO_{2\,max}$ much of this oxygen will be consumed by the oxidation of glucose in glycogen, but fatty acid oxidation plays a significant role. Since both glycogen and fat must be used, getting the balance correct is of vital importance to each runner (Figure 5.15). Too high a level of fatty acid in the bloodstream will increase the rate of fatty acid oxidation and consume too much oxygen, which could result in a decrease in pace. But this is not the only problem with elevated blood fatty acid levels—they may also bring on central fatigue, as described in Chapter 6.

It is likely that very long training runs of 20 miles or more help to establish the correct rate of fatty acid mobilization for each individual marathon runner and help to avoid early fatigue (see p. 189).

Chapter 6

When the Running Has to Stop

In 1954, Roger Bannister became the first man to run the mile in less than 4 min. Yet, although one of the favourites for the 1500 m race in the 1952 Olympic Games, Bannister did not get a medal. Shortly before the Games it was announced that there would be semi-final heats in the 1500 m race. Bannister had not prepared for three hard races in 3 days. Bannister describes his fatigue in the final few hundred metres:

> My legs were aching and I had no strength left to force them faster. I had a sickening feeling of exhaustion and powerlessness as Barthel came past me, chased by McMillen . . .

The Comrades marathon is run from Pietermaritzburg to Durban (or vice versa), in South Africa, a distance of 90 km (54 miles). Tim Noakes describes his experience in the event:

> My legs, detecting the first signs of an ailing will, begin their own mutiny, their tactics carefully prepared. They inform me that this is far enough. Geographically, they argue, the race is two-thirds over. Why, they ask, must they continue to run, knowing that from here each step will become ever more painful, ever harder? After all there is always next year. Through the blanket of developing fatigue, I begin to appreciate the logic behind these questions; begin to feel the attraction of that haven of rest at the side of the road, the bliss of not having to take even one more step towards Durban. Around me, I know that each runner is engaged in this same battle. In common suffering, we are alone to find our individual solutions.

Thus, for the athlete, fatigue is the overwhelming necessity to reduce pace. Physiologists define it more objectively as the inability to maintain power output; i.e. the amount of energy expended per second has to decrease.

Although fatigue may sound like the scourge of athletics, it is, literally, a life-saver, for fatigue is the safety device which switches off the power when our conscious mind has rejected gentle or even severe hints of impending doom. In so doing, fatigue prevents our own metabolic activities from causing irreversible damage to our bodies. Experienced athletes judge the race so that they finish *just* within limits set by their own susceptibility to fatigue. Training extends these limits by modifying muscle, by manipulating metabolism and by changing mental approaches, but it can never abolish them. How near athletes come to causing damage by pushing too hard is not known but there are examples of athletes who after winning one major event or breaking a world record never repeat this performance. Could this be due to the extent of the damage caused by refusing to accept the tell-tale signs and signals of fatigue?

The idea that fatigue is simply due to 'running out of energy' is too naive to be of value. Indeed it would be surprising if fatigue in events as diverse as the 200 m and the marathon had a common cause. Frequently, however, the explanation does involve fuel mobilization and utilization and at least five biochemical causes have been identified, although even this list is unlikely to be complete:

- The depletion of phosphocreatine in muscle.
- The accumulation of protons (acid) in muscle.
- The depletion of glycogen in muscle.
- Hypoglycaemia (a marked lowering of blood glucose level).
- Changes in the concentration of key amino acids in the blood.

There are, of course, many other reasons for being unable to run— a damaged muscle, a sprained ankle, a blistered foot, hyperthermia, a viral infection—but these are pathological, not physiological. Psychological limitations in performance are discussed in Chapter 10, but it is likely that such limitations may exert part of their effect via one or more of the biochemical causes listed above. Although the first three causes of fatigue relate directly to the muscle, the last two involve the brain. The brain appears to be able to detect changes in the levels of normal constituents of the blood and responds by increasing the sensitivity of the runner to fatigue, so that the runner gives up more easily than otherwise.

FATIGUE AND PHOSPHOCREATINE

At least one form of fatigue strikes very early in sprints. It reduces power output almost from the starting blocks but unlike some other

Table 6.1. World record times for sprints. The 'flying start' 100 m was timed in a 100 m relay event

Event	Time (s)
100 m (Carl Lewis)	9.86
100 m ('flying start' (Carl Lewis)	8.91
200 m (Pietro Minnea)	19.72
Best possible 200 m	18.77

forms causes no perceived discomfort. Examination of world record times for the sprints highlights the problem (Table 6.1). It is obvious that you cannot 'predict' a best time for the 200 m race simply by doubling that for the 100 m race, since the 100 m includes an acceleration phase that does not occur in the second 100 m of the 200 m race. What we need is a time for the best 'flying 100 m', to add to the 100 m record. Carl Lewis's achievement in the 1984 Los Angeles Olympics provides the necessary data since he clocked 8.91 s on his leg of the 100 m relay, having already accelerated for the changeover. Adding this to the world record for the 100 m gives a 'best possible predicted' time of 18.77 s for 200 m—nearly a whole second faster than the current world record. Does this mean that 200 m runners are not doing their stuff? Of course not, it just shows that fatigue occurs even during a race as short as 200 m, although some of this difference is caused by the bend in the track in the 200 m. And this is true fatigue, as defined above—an inability to maintain the 100 m pace for 200 m. It indicates an approximate 5% decrease in power output, which may not seem dramatic but would cause a potential victor to finish last in the 200 m race.

So we are looking for the factor that operates in the first few seconds of a sprint, and the obvious candidate is phosphocreatine depletion. Laboratory experiments with human quadriceps femoris muscles, stimulated electrically so that fatigue originating in the brain can have no effect, confirm that the concentration of phosphocreatine falls very rapidly when the blood flow is restricted (Figure 6.1). Such biochemical knowledge allows us to suggest the following 'manipulation' to achieve maximum performance in sprinting:

- Maintain and, if possible, increase the phosphocreatine store in muscle, most effectively done by strength-training and by ingesting creatine prior to the competition (Box 4.4).

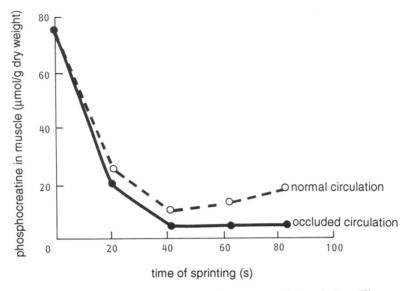

Figure 6.1. Muscle phosphocreatine levels in 'scientific' sprinting. The muscle was stimulated 70% of the maximal during intermittent tetanic contractions at 1.6-second intervals. The large fall in phosphocreatine level at the first time point suggests that this could be responsible for the observed decreased power output. From Hultman, E. and Spriet, L. L. (1986). Skeletal muscle metabolism, contraction force and glycogen utilization during prolonged electrical stimulation in humans. *J. Physiol. (Lond.)*, **374**, 493–501

- Completely rest the leg muscles for some minutes prior to the race to encourage repletion of phosphocreatine stores, since some may have been used in the warm-up.
- The faster the glycolysis rate can be increased in the first seconds of the sprint, the less the phosphocreatine reserves will be depleted and the longer they will remain available to maintain their 'supercharge' effect. Controlled nervous tension before the race will help to stimulate glycolysis and raise its rate towards its maximum capacity as soon as possible after the race begins.

Maintenance, or restoration, of phosphocreatine levels is probably also important in providing fuel for the finishing sprint in longer races, from 800 m upwards.

AVOIDING AN ACID BATH

Lactic acid is so named because it is formed by the action of bacteria on lactose, or milk sugar, and is responsible for the sour taste of soured

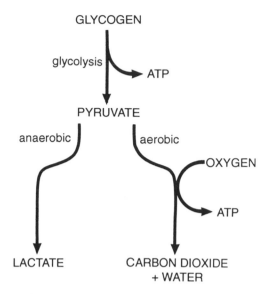

Figure 6.2. The anaerobic alternative

milk. Bacteria produce their lactic acid in exactly the same way as we do and for the same reason; to generate ATP in the absence of oxygen (Figure 6.2).

Lactic acid causes problems precisely because it is an acid, defined by chemists as a compound which releases a hydrogen ion (also known as a proton) in water. This dissociation can be represented by the equation:

$$\text{acid} \rightarrow H^+ + \text{base}^-$$

where H^+ is the hydrogen ion (or proton) with the $^+$ signifying the loss of an electron, now gained by the base. In the case of lactic acid this dissociation produces lactate ions:

$$\text{lactic acid} \rightarrow H^+ + \text{lactate}^-$$

When the athletics commentator describes the sprint to the tape by saying that the athlete finished in 'a sea of lactic acid', this is not strictly so, for the lactic acid dissociates and it is the protons which cause fatigue. In fact, the protons and the lactate ions are produced at different stages in glycolysis but it would be unduly pedantic to insist that the sprinter finished in 'a sea of lactate ions plus protons' and, for much of this book, we too will refer to lactic acid.

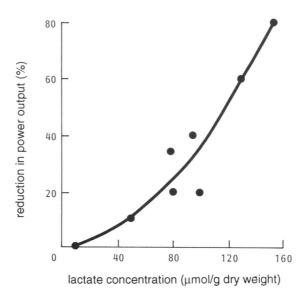

Figure 6.3. As lactic acid accumulates in muscle, so power output falls. From Hultman, E. and Spriet, L. L. (1986). Skeletal muscle metabolism, contraction force and glycogen utilization during prolonged electrical stimulation in humans. *J. Physiol. (Lond.)*, **374**, 493–501

The problem with protons is that they can associate with other bases to produce acids, and changing a base into an acid can have some serious consequences, especially when the base is a protein (Figure 6.4). Proteins bear numerous basic (as well as acidic) groups on their surface and the distribution of these plays an important part in determining the functions of the protein, be it an enzyme catalysing a critical reaction in energy generation in muscle or a component of a myofibril involved in cross-bridge formation (Figure 6.5). If the number of protons binding to a protein is changed, it will probably work less well (Figure 6.5). We don't know precisely which proteins are most sensitive to this interference or how their malfunction is perceived as fatigue, but the important thing for the runner is knowing how to overcome the increasing acidity of the muscle, or, more realistically, how to delay it.

One answer to the proton problem lies in buffers. These are bases which 'mop-up' protons by combining with them:

$$\text{buffer}^- + \text{H}^+ \rightarrow \text{Buffer–H}$$

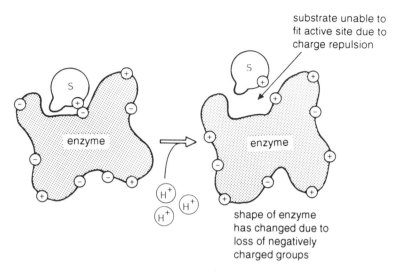

Figure 6.4. Addition of protons (i.e. a fall in pH) will remove some negatively charged groups and make additional positively charged groups on the protein. Raising the pH will reverse these changes

After the sprint is over, the buffer will release the proton in a reverse of this reaction and other processes will then remove the protons, so that the buffer is recycled ready to accept more protons when necessary. The problem for the athlete is that there is not much buffering capacity within the muscle; enough to absorb protons for only about 10–15 s of maximal glycolysis from glycogen even in top-class sprinters. Sprint training should increase the buffering capacity within the

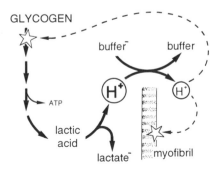

Figure 6.5. Fatigue-producing effects of protons arising from glycolysis

muscle but only by a small amount, and it may be that a further
important biochemical characteristic of the 400 m runner is an
unusually high buffering capacity within the muscles.

If capillary density in muscle is high, as it will be in middle-distance
athletes, the protons will leave the muscle and enter the bloodstream,
where they encounter a much larger buffering system based on bicarbonate (hydrogencarbonate) ions. This buffer absorbs protons according to the equation:

$$HCO_3^- + H^+ \rightarrow H_2CO_3$$

hydrogen-   carbonic
carbonate   acid

Much the same happens when you take Alka-Seltzer or 'bicarb'
(sodium hydrogencarbonate, formerly known as sodium bicarbonate)
to reduce acidity in the stomach after over-indulgence. The beauty of
the hydrogencarbonate buffer is that the carbonic acid produced
readily decomposes into water and carbon dioxide:

$$H_2CO_3 \quad \rightarrow \quad H_2O + CO_2$$

carbonic   carbon
acid   dioxide

This carbon dioxide is lost from the body through the lungs (or from
the stomach by burping if antacids have been taken by mouth). This
allows more carbonic acid to form and so extends the buffering capacity. But the system is much more subtle than this because an increase
in the blood acidity or carbon dioxide level actually stimulates breathing, so that more carbon dioxide is lost from the body via the lungs.
The main sources of the hydrogencarbonate ions in the blood are the
liver and kidney, so that these organs and the lungs operate between
them a push–pull system to rid the body of excess protons (Figure 6.6).

The effect of protons (or carbon dioxide) on the rate of breathing can
be used by the endurance athlete to detect when acid begins to
accumulate, i.e. when the anaerobic threshold has been reached. This
is known as the ventilatory turnpoint and can be seen as the position
where the curve suddenly changes when a graph of breathing rate
against pace is drawn (Figure 6.7).

What any sprinter wants to know is whether buffering capacity can
be increased. The answer is a qualified yes! Strength training
increases buffering capacity. And bicarbonate can be taken by mouth

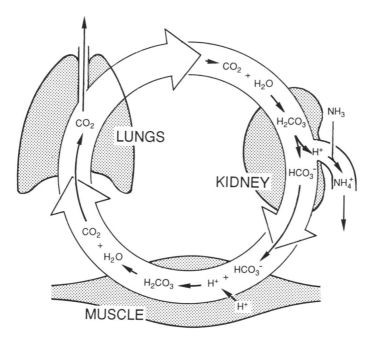

Figure 6.6. Most of the hydrogencarbonate ion (HCO_3^-) is made in the kidney and combines with protons from muscle to form carbon dioxide, which is excreted from the lungs. An enzyme ensures that the reactions involving carbon dioxide, water and hydrogencarbonate ions occur rapidly. In the kidney, released protons combine with ammonia to form ammonium ions (NH_4^+), which are excreted into the urine. The ammonia arises in the liver and reaches the kidney via the blood (chemically combined into a non-toxic form)

prior to the race, although in some experiments in which this has been attempted improvements in performance have been accompanied by vomiting—an unfortunate side-effect.

For the middle-distance runner the answer to the problem of acid build-up is to improve blood supply to the muscles, for it is the blood which flushes lactic acid out of the muscles to be neutralized by buffers in the bloodstream. Improved vascularization, i.e. an increase in the number of blood vessels, in muscle, is one of the benefits of aerobic training.

For the 400 m runner the benefits are less clear cut. On the one hand, anything that decreases proton build-up in muscle should delay fatigue, but if myofibrils and muscle bulk are lost because of the increased space occupied by mitochondria and blood vessels, speed

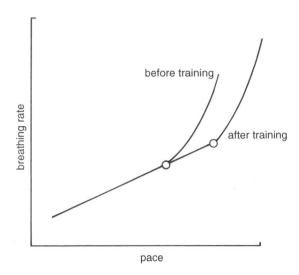

Figure 6.7. The ventilatory turnpoint. The breathing rate increases linearly with pace until the turnpoint is reached, when breathing rate increases much more rapidly. This is due to the increased rate of release of lactic acid from muscle. This is equivalent to the anaerobic threshold, although it may occur at a slightly higher pace than if blood lactate is measured (see pp. 106–107)

will be sacrificed. This serves to re-emphasize the point that, even biochemically speaking, the 400 m race is a very difficult event.

THE MIDDLE-DISTANCE BALANCING ACT

In middle-distance events, anaerobic metabolism generates ATP in addition to that produced from aerobic metabolism, so the optimum strategy for the middle-distance runner would appear to be to run close to the anaerobic threshold (pp. 107). Most of the ATP should be produced aerobically, with the contribution of anaerobic metabolism kept below the rate at which lactic acid can be flushed from the muscles. Acid accumulation is tolerated in the shorter races only because in them less acid will be formed than in the longer events.

As distances increase, however, another factor must be taken into account; the amount of glycogen stored in muscles. Once again a simple calculation makes the point. The glycogen stored in muscles would take the runner, on average and at marathon pace, some 30 000 m before it ran out, assuming totally aerobic metabolism. The same amount of glycogen would only last for about 2000 m if used totally anaerobically at the marathon runner's pace, and less if the pace were increased, underlining the inefficiency of anaerobic glycolysis in terms of ATP production. What this means in practice is that, in the 10 000 m race, glycogen depletion can be a limiting factor if more than *about* 3% of the ATP is generated anaerobically (see Table 5.1).

Tapering of training, sensible rest for a few days before the event plus appropriate nutrition (pp. 219–221) will ensure that glycogen stores are fully loaded prior to competition. This is just as important for middle-distance and long-distance track athletes as it is for marathon runners!

THE MARATHON

> After 18 miles, the sensations of exhaustion were unlike anything I had ever experienced. I could not run, walk or stand, and even found sitting a bit strenuous.

So wrote David Costill* after his first marathon.

Inexperienced marathon runners frequently suffer severe fatigue some time after 18 miles. So strong is the urge to stop running that this phenomenon has been dubbed 'hitting the wall'. Its explanation is relatively simple; at this point muscle glycogen reserves are totally depleted. The only other fuel available is fatty acids in the blood, but these can only be used at a rate which provides about half of the energy per minute in comparison with the rate provided by glycogen. The result is that pace must also slow to about 50% of what it had been which, for many non-élite marathon runners (e.g. '8-minute milers'), is about 1 mile in 16 minutes—no more than walking pace!

This emphasizes the importance of mechanisms to increase the content of muscle glycogen prior to the event. These include a sensible diet in the days before the marathon, a reduction in training time and intensity (tapering), a satisfactory warm-up to avoid anaerobic metabolism at the start of a race, maintaining if possible a steady pace throughout the event and taking carbohydrate-containing drinks during the event.

---

*David Costill is a physiologist who has done much work in the field of sports science, published several books (see Further Reading and Bibliography) and is an élite veteran swimmer.

Box 6.1   It all depends on glycogen

Imagine sitting on a cycle ergometer—a device which ensures that your hard work gets you precisely nowhere, and pedalling like mad until, after 1½ h, you are totally exhausted. In the cause of science that is precisely what a group of Stockholm volunteers were persuaded to do. To make matters worse for the subjects, blood samples and muscle biopsy samples (see Chapter 2) had to be taken at intervals. They had, however, the satisfaction of knowing that their bodies had provided, for the first time, a clear picture of what fuels were being used during sustained exercise and good scientific evidence for one cause of fatigue. The muscle biopsy samples showed that not only did

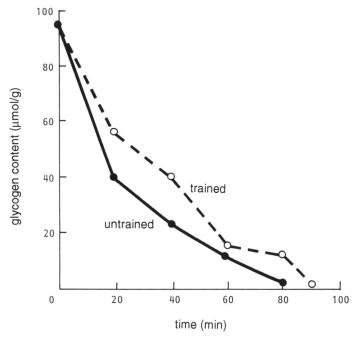

Figure 6.8. Volunteer Stockholm firemen pedalled until they were exhausted, at which time their muscle glycogen had fallen to zero. Trained subjects appeared to be able to use glycogen more economically, probably because they convert less glycogen to lactic acid. From Hermansen, L., Hultman, E. and Saltin, B. (1967). Muscle glycogen during prolonged severe exercise. *Acta Physiol. Scand.*, **71**, 129–139

continued

continued

the glycogen content of their quadriceps muscle fall steadily during the exercise but that exhaustion occurred when almost all of it had been used up (Figure 6.8).

This was the first scientific evidence that showed conclusively that glycogen levels in muscle are important in fatigue, and from this has grown our appreciation of its role as a fundamentally important fuel for the longer track events and endurance races.

FATIGUE AND BLOOD GLUCOSE

Ultra-marathon runners pose an interesting question in relation to fatigue. These runners are able to run continuously for many hours, during which time their oxygen consumption gradually falls to about 50% of their maximal capacity, corresponding to a very large, if not complete, dependence on fatty acids as a fuel, once their glycogen reserves are exhausted. At this stage, it becomes important that blood glucose is strictly conserved for the brain, which can use no other fuel under these circumstances. An important characteristic of ultra-distance runners, and presumably one that is enhanced by training, is their ability to restrict the rate of glucose utilization by muscle to the rate at which it can be produced within the body, for if they did not their muscles would rapidly reduce their blood glucose concentration to zero! Nevertheless, hypoglycaemia—a very low blood glucose concentration—remains a major hazard, and to avoid this it is advantageous for the ultra-marathon runner to take glucose or other carbohydrate-containing drinks during the race.

Recent studies have shown that glucose supplementation is beneficial for prolonged periods of cycling, and can support a high rate of cycling despite low levels of muscle glycogen. It may be that maintenance of a normal blood glucose level is able to ward off fatigue for a period of time after glycogen depletion. These studies suggest that glucose-containing drinks would also be of advantage in the marathon, at least for non-élite marathon runners, and for the ultra-marathon.

One of the consequences of hypoglycaemia is fatigue, but in this case it is a response of the brain rather than the muscles and for this reason is known as *central* fatigue. It appears to arise as the brain interprets the decrease in the blood glucose level as a danger signal and takes steps to decrease power output; the effort to maintain power output becomes progressively greater, so that only the mentally tough can

Box 6.2   The executive's lunch

What do fast-living business executives and élite marathon or ultra-marathon runners have in common? Not a lot (fortunately) but both can run (literally in the case of the athlete) into the problem of hypoglycaemia—too little glucose in the blood. Glucose is virtually the only fuel used by the brain and, if its concentration in the blood falls much below half of its normal value, the brain is affected. Signs and symptoms include sweating, weakness, visual disturbance, clouding of the consciousness and coma. These are, at best, unpleasant and at worst, very dangerous.

Two mechanisms prevent hypoglycaemia from intruding into everyday life for most of us. First, the glycogen in the liver acts as a reservoir to maintain blood glucose levels within normal limits. When the blood glucose level falls, more glycogen is broken down to produce glucose in the liver, and this glucose is released into the blood (the liver glycogen reserves are re-formed after a meal). Hormones, particularly insulin, play the major role in regulating these processes, and diabetics who accidentally inject more insulin than they need also run the risk of hypoglycaemic coma. The second source of glucose, also from the liver, arises from gluconeogenesis—a process in which glucose is manufactured from non-carbohydrates such as lactate and some amino acids which are present in the bloodstream.

The problem of the marathon runner, and particularly that of the ultra-marathon runner, is that the prolonged demand for glucose exhausts liver glycogen reserves and tends to divert all of the glucose produced by the liver to muscles rather than the brain. Fortunately, in most situations control mechanisms intervene to prevent this occurring. Somewhat surprisingly in marathon races there have been very few cases of severe hypoglycaemia. However, in the 1982 Boston marathon Alberto Salazar and Dick Beardsley battled out the last 10 miles and Salazar won in a record time of 2h 8 min 5 s, only 5 s ahead of Beardsley. After completion of the marathon, Salazar became hypoglycaemic but, after receiving an intravenous infusion of a glucose solution, rapidly recovered. And in the first women's Olympic marathon race in the Los Angeles Games, Gabriella Anderson-Scheiss completed the last few hundred metres in the stadium in a state of clouded consciousness, due not to hyperthermia but to hypoglycaemia. She too responded quickly to intravenous glucose.

So why should the business executive suffer? To begin with, in his

_____ continued _|

― *continued* ―

or her haste to get to the office on time, breakfast was missed. Despite the sedentary lifestyle, this long fast may have depleted glycogen stores by lunchtime. But this should be no problem, since the liver will now produce glucose from other non-carbohydrate compounds in the blood and this 'new' glucose should sustain the executive even if lunch is missed. Unfortunately, the last insult to the body is to down a couple of gin and tonics instead of, or prior to, lunch without realizing that alcohol is a potent inhibitor of gluconeogenesis—the process in the liver that produces glucose. So with no liver glycogen left, with no glucose being produced in the liver and no lunch, but a continuous demand for glucose by the brain, muscle and other organs, the blood glucose level falls. The business executive becomes weak, uncoordinated, makes wrong decisions and even collapses into a coma. Fortunately, as with marathon runners, the blood glucose level can quickly be restored with an intravenous drip, provided medical help is at hand. However, if the unconscious state occurs in an isolated office, or while crossing a busy road, it can be life-threatening. Perhaps because of the stress of air travel, there have been several reports of such hypoglycaemic incidents on long-haul flights. Knowledge of biochemistry is important therefore, not only for the athlete, coach and sports physician but for everyone!

keep going. In the final stages of the race, hypoglycaemia will impair pace and orientation and may even cause loss of consciousness.

FATIGUE AND AMINO ACIDS

Of all the chemical compounds comprising our bodies, proteins are the most versatile by far. They enable us to move, catalyse processes within cells, defend us against disease, serve as internal messengers and literally hold us together. For these diverse functions, thousands of different proteins must be made, each a polymer of amino acids linked in a different but precise order (Figure 11.5). These amino acids are the product of the digestion of the proteins in the food we eat, and an adequate supply is particularly important during growth, as the parental admonition 'meat before the sweet' implies. Even after maturity, amino acids continue to be required to replace those lost by metabolic conversion in the continuous cycle of degradation and resynthesis of proteins which keeps body components in pristine condition.

It is a fact that adults in the developed countries consume more protein than they need. This excess protein cannot be stored as such but the amino acids produced from these proteins can be used by the liver for generating ATP. Another circumstance in which amino acids are used as fuels is in prolonged starvation, when they arise from the breakdown of structural proteins in the body—hopefully not a condition that will affect the athlete. Most amino acids destined for use as fuels are first converted, in the liver, to glucose, which can either be used immediately or stored as glycogen. Very-long-distance runners may even get some extra glucose for their muscles during their long runs in this way, but the main purpose of this glucose-producing process (gluconeogenesis) is to maintain the blood glucose level so that those tissues which can use no other fuel, especially the brain, will survive.

Out of a total of 20 different types of amino acid that make up proteins, three—valine, leucine and isoleucine—have a more direct fuel-providing role in muscle. These are the branched-chain amino acids (BCAAs), which are oxidized in muscle rather than in the liver (Figure 6.9). Although oxidation of these amino acids does provide some ATP, the amount is rather insignificant on a runner's scale of values. The impact of BCAAs on the runner is more subtle and involves several apparently unrelated factors: another amino acid, the brain and a piece of biochemistry that seems at first far-removed from the power-house of the runner's muscles.

The amino acid is tryptophan, which is used by the brain not as an energy source, nor merely as a building block for protein synthesis, but as the starting point for the synthesis of 5-hydroxytryptamine, or 5-HT as it is more conveniently known. This is one of a growing list of neurotransmitters, now numbering 40 or 50 substances, the function of which is to carry messages within the brain by 'ferrying' information across the junctions between nerve cells (see Chapter 12). Variations in the level of a neurotransmitter in brain neurones can cause problems: too little message and the connection fails; too much message and the connection persists for too long. Such disturbances in the transfer of information in the brain can cause changes, sometimes dramatic ones, in behaviour. An increase in the level of 5-HT in the brain is known to cause tiredness, improve the quality of sleep and improve mood, as well as causing a decrease in aggression.

So how do the BCAAs enter this story? The connection is that both tryptophan and the BCAAs enter the brain through the same carrier

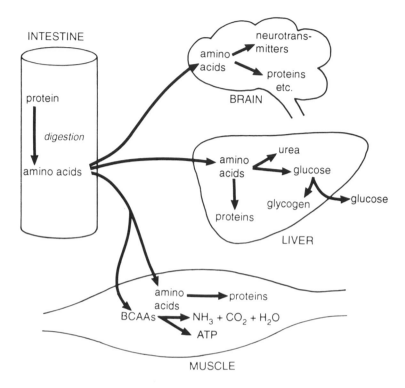

Figure 6.9. Summary of amino acid metabolism (BCAAs=branched-chain amino acids)

system and so compete with one another (Figure 6.10). If the concentration of BCAAs in the blood increases, less tryptophan will enter the brain, so the level of 5-HT will fall, resulting in less tiredness and an increase in aggression. In prolonged exercise, however, the level of BCAAs in the blood falls since they are taken up by muscle as a fuel. Consequently, more tryptophan can enter the brain and, so the argument goes, more 5-HT will be made. This could well account for the fact that exercise makes you feel tired and improves the quality of sleep. However, this mental 'relaxation' could also increase the mental effort necessary to maintain pace in athletic activity. Such central fatigue can affect anyone who participates in cycling, soccer, football, rugby, baseball, tennis, squash, boxing—in fact anyone who undertakes prolonged exercise. It may even play a part in explaining the

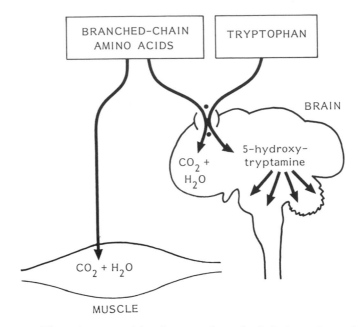

Figure 6.10. There is competition between branched-chain amino acids and tryptophan for entry into the brain. As more branched-chain amino acids are used by muscle, so more trytophan enters the brain

phenomenon of excessive arousal in athletes prior to competition which decreases performance (pp. 202).

If it does, a solution is at hand—dietary manipulation. Consumption of drinks rich in BCAAs should restore vigour to athletes whose performance is being depressed by an excess of brain 5-HT. Research has indeed provided evidence that BCAAs benefit performance, and a new sports drink which contains these amino acids is now available (see Box 11.4). What could be a better justification for understanding as much as possible about the metabolism of the athlete?

Chapter 7

Maintaining the Supply Lines

Winston Churchill, in Volume XI of his book The Second World War, *wrote of the advance of the Allied troops in the struggle for Europe in 1944, 'the number of divisions that could be sustained, and the speed and range of their advance, depended however entirely on harbours, transport and supplies . . . but food, and above all petrol, governed every movement'.*

As an army depends on the strength of its supply lines, so muscles depend on their supply of fuels and oxygen. These are delivered by blood—the body's general-purpose transport medium, which also carries waste products, such as carbon dioxide and lactic acid, away from muscles.

The physiology of the lungs and the circulatory system, and the way they function, has formed the focus of most books on sports science for reasons which are not difficult to see. Historically, the working of the heart and lung was understood, at least in broad terms, long before the chemistry of energy provision was elucidated. There is also no doubt that physiological aspects are much easier to explain to the non-scientist—an athlete can sense increases in heart rate or the depth of breathing but has no 'feel' for glycogen breakdown or a change in the rate of ATP turnover. However, in athletic performance, physiological and biochemical events are both important, neither one more than the other. Both involve many processes which could limit the rate at which energy is made available to muscles and, having described some of the biochemical limitations in previous chapters, it is to the physiological aspects that we now turn.

THE HEART OF THE SYSTEM

To move any fluid through a circuit of tubes a pump is needed; the human body has two, neatly packaged together in the heart. Each pump consists of two muscular chambers: a thin-walled atrium and a

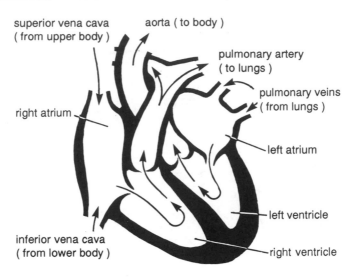

Figure 7.1. Diagrammatic section through heart showing route taken by blood

much thicker-walled ventricle (Figure 7.1). While the heart muscle relaxes between beats, blood flows simultaneously from the venae cavae into the right atrium and from the pulmonary veins into the left atrium. As these fill, some of the blood passes on into the adjacent ventricles. Suddenly the two atria contract, forcing the blood they contain into the ventricles. Almost immediately the thick muscular walls of the ventricles also start to contract. The sharp rise in pressure of the blood within the ventricles causes the valves between atria and ventricles to slam closed and blood is forced into the arteries. As the pressure in the ventricles falls, the heart relaxes, so that blood again flows into the atria to begin the cycle once more. While the heart is relaxed, blood is prevented from flowing back into the ventricles by the semi-lunar valves.

Each time the heart contracts, blood from the right side is expelled along the pulmonary artery to the lungs, where it is re-oxygenated— this is the action of one pump. On its return, through the pulmonary vein, this blood is directed to the left side of the heart, ready in the next contraction to be expelled through the aorta for distribution through the branching system of arteries to all parts of the body—this is the second pump. The heart muscle itself gets its share of oxygenated blood through the coronary artery, which branches from the aorta near its origin. Any restriction of blood flow through the coronary

Box 7.1   The fatal clot

The heart is as aerobic an organ as any in the body. If the supply of blood to any part of it fails, the muscle affected can no longer produce enough ATP to keep working, so that the normal rhythm falters and the pumping mechanism may fail or the heart may stop beating. The immediate cause of such a heart attack is usually the lodging of a blood clot in a narrowed coronary artery, but it is anticipated by changes which take place over a whole lifetime (Figure 7.2).

The narrowing occurs because of fatty deposits occurring in the artery walls; atherosclerosis. The primary event is probably damage to the thin layer of endothelial cells lining the artery. Factors thought to cause this include high blood pressure, tobacco smoking, viruses or a high concentration of cholesterol in the blood. This damage attracts white blood cells to this area, and in the confined space within the arterial wall they take up cholesterol-containing particles and die. The death of these cells releases factors that attract more white cells and causes smooth muscle fibres in the wall of the artery to multiply.

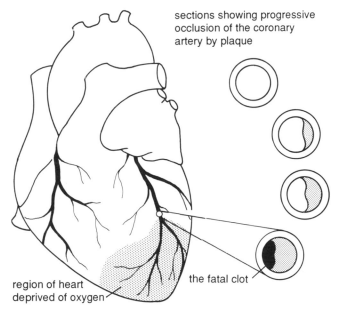

sections showing progressive occlusion of the coronary artery by plaque

region of heart deprived of oxygen

the fatal clot

Figure 7.2. Heart attack caused by blocking of a coronary artery

continued

— *continued* —

As a result of this damage, the muscle layer becomes thicker and more fibrous, often reducing the diameter of the vessel to a small fraction of its original dimension. The scene is now set for the fatal clot. Clotting of blood is normally initiated by platelets—small bodies in the blood derived from cells but very much smaller than red blood cells. When platelets come into contact with damaged tissues they burst, releasing chemicals which set blood clotting in motion. There are mechanisms in the blood to disperse such clots but, if they should occlude an artery before this happens, it could be too late.

Fortunately there are a number of things you can do to prevent this fatal sequence occurring in your heart. First, do not smoke, for not only do components of tobacco smoke cause arterial damage, but the nicotine inhaled and absorbed stimulates the heart, causing it to 'idle' at a slightly higher speed. Furthermore, the carbon monoxide produced enters the blood, where it combines with haemoglobin to prevent it binding oxygen. Around 8% of a 30-a-day smoker's haemoglobin is 'permanently' out of action for this reason. The second precaution is to reduce the amount of animal fat you eat. This is associated with increased blood levels of cholesterol, particularly the bad form of cholesterol, known as low-density lipoprotein (LDL) cholesterol, which is associated with an increased risk of atherosclerosis and coronary artery disease. Thirdly, if your blood pressure is chronically high, take steps to reduce it. This may be achieved through changes in diet and lifestyle or by taking appropriate hypotensive drugs. The final advice is to take reasonably vigorous exercise such as running, jogging, fast walking, cycling, rowing or swimming, all of which if performed for 20–40 min will be aerobic and therefore will benefit the heart.

artery has serious consequences and, if a branch should become blocked by a blood clot, muscle beyond the blockage will stop contracting. If a major branch of the coronary artery is occluded the whole heart may stop beating and, if it fails to restart, the heart attack will have been fatal (Box 7.1).

In order to pick up or release materials such as oxygen, blood must pass through capillaries. A glance at Figure 7.3 shows that, for most organs, blood passes through only one series of capillaries on each journey from heart back to heart. (An exception is the hepatic portal vein, which takes blood from the intestines directly to the liver.) The

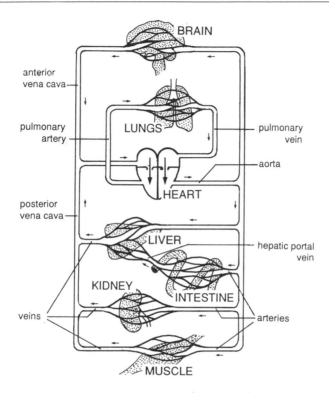

anterior
vena cava

pulmonary
artery

pulmonary
vein

aorta

posterior
vena cava

hepatic portal
vein

veins

arteries

BRAIN

LUNGS

HEART

LIVER

KIDNEY

INTESTINE

MUSCLE

Figure 7.3. General plan of the circulation

significance of this arrangement is two-fold. First, each tissue gets its
share of freshly oxygenated blood and, secondly, the pressure, which
falls considerably as blood overcomes the high resistance of a capillary
bed in one tissue, can be raised again by the heart before it suffers a
further drop in another capillary bed.

CAPILLARY ACTION

In one sense, the most important elements of the cardiovascular
system are its smallest: the capillaries. A single capillary is a very fine
tube, no more than one-hundredth of a millimetre in diameter and only
just wide enough for a red blood cell to squeeze through. But capillaries
do not come singly. They come in branching and converging networks
or capillary beds, each fed by a branch of an artery known as an
arteriole and drained by a venule (Figure 7.4). Since the total cross-

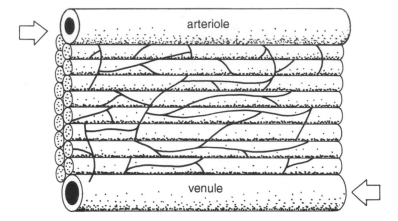

Figure 7.4. Diagrammatic representation of a capillary bed in muscle

sectional area of a capillary bed is large, the blood slows down as it passes through. The second and a half that blood spends in the average capillary provides ample opportunity for the effective exchange of materials between blood and the muscle fibre. The exceptionally thin cells which form the capillary walls also hasten this process.

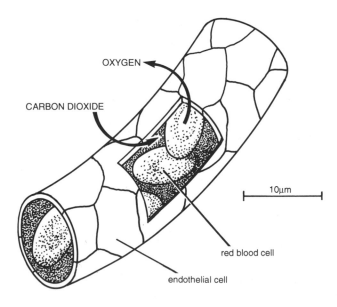

Figure 7.5. Gas exchange in a capillary

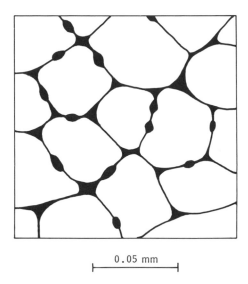

0.05 mm

Figure 7.6. Diagram based on a transverse section of human gastrocnemius muscle showing distribution of capillaries between fibres

Just as water always flows downhill, so molecules diffuse from where they are at a higher concentration to where their concentration is lower. This means that, for example, in muscles, oxygen molecules move out of the capillaries into the fibres, while carbon dioxide molecules move in the opposite direction (Figure 7.5). Diffusion is a slow process and is therefore only effective over short distances, but every muscle fibre is supplied with at least one capillary, and slow-twitch fibres may have several (Figure 7.6). One of the benefits of training (other than sprint training) is that it increases the number of capillaries for each muscle fibre, i.e. the capillary density, and so reduces the distance an oxygen molecule must diffuse. This increases the rate of delivery of oxygen to the muscle and hence increases the rate of ATP generation from the aerobic system.

DISTRIBUTING THE BLOOD

Arteries have thicker, more elastic and more muscular walls than do veins. Their thickness gives them the strength to withstand high blood pressure as they convey blood from the heart to the organs, and their elasticity is important in smoothing out blood flow from a pulsating heart. The expulsion of blood from the heart causes a pressure wave which travels along the major arteries at least 10 times faster than the flow of blood within them. This is the pulse which can be felt wherever a major artery passes close to the body's surface, notably at the wrist, temple and neck. The pulse rate equals that of the heart beat but is often easier to measure.

With exercise comes the demand from the muscles for more oxygen and that means more blood. The arterioles, which supply each capillary bed in the muscle, contain in their inner wall circular muscle fibres. When these smooth muscles relax, the pressure of the blood dilates them and allows faster blood flow to the muscles so that, during exercise, not only does cardiac output rise (see below) but the muscles receive a larger share of the blood. Indeed, even the flow through individual capillaries is regulated by pre-capillary sphincters so that the distribution of blood can be precisely controlled even in a single muscle. Because flow rate is inversely proportional to cross-sectional area, quite small changes in diameter lead to large changes in flow. In resting muscle only about one capillary in 30 or 40 is open, so the potential for increasing blood flow is enormous. However, blood cannot be in two places at once and if more is flowing through muscles, less will be available for other tissues. The same consideration applies when you are running a bath and someone else in the house turns on another tap. Your bath fills more slowly. In your body, the brain is the organ least tolerant of a reduced blood supply, and to protect its blood supply compensatory vasoconstriction must take place. This is the reduction in blood flow to organs such as the intestines, kidneys and liver, brought about by constriction of sphincters in their arterioles and capillaries (Figure 7.7). Vital as these organs are, their metabolic activity can be temporarily reduced without serious ill effect, although this may be responsible for the indigestion and nausea which some people experience during and after vigorous and prolonged exercise. One benefit of training might be that the body 'learns' just how far it can cut down the blood supply to these organs without serious consequences.

Exercise is not the only situation which leads to blood redistribution. On a very cold day, despite warming-up exercises, your hands and face may be white and cold to the touch. The whiteness indicates a lack of blood, brought about by constriction of the arterioles supplying capillary beds in your skin while, at the same time, arteriovenous shunts open to bypass the capillaries. Since blood transports heat from deep within your body to the surface, this mechanism drastically reduces heat loss. Now run the race. All, or almost all, of the chemical energy

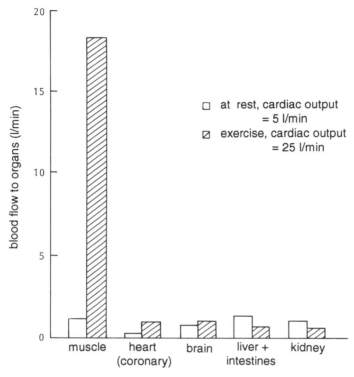

Figure 7.7. Changes in blood flow to organs during vigorous exercise

Box 7.2   Are humans diving mammals?

An extreme example of vasoconstriction occurs in seals and other marine mammals when they dive. Some species can remain submerged for nearly half an hour, although they normally surface much more frequently. On submergence the animal empties its lungs to reduce buoyancy and reduces the flow of blood to all its organs except the brain. The muscles of diving mammals contain larger amounts of myoglobin (an oxygen-binding protein) than the muscles of human beings. Although this oxymyoglobin provides a 'store' of oxygen, there is, nevertheless, extensive reliance on anaerobic metabolism during the dive. With circulation restricted mainly to the heart and brain, the heart rate drops dramatically (Figure 7.8)—a condition known as bradycardia.

_____ continued __|

continued

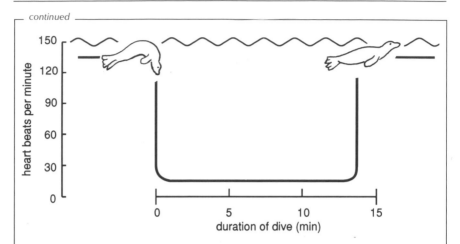

Figure 7.8. Bradycardia in diving seal. Data from Blix (1976)

A corresponding, but less dramatic, bradycardia can be demonstrated in human beings by splashing cold—and it must be cold—water on the face and chest. Could this have any adaptive significance? It is tempting to relate it to a number of incidents where humans have unexpectedly survived long periods of submersion. Take for example the case of a young boy who was trapped in a car which ran into a Norwegian fjord. In this well-documented case, the car was under water for 27 min under circumstances where it is extremely unlikely that the boy had any access to air. It is generally accepted that irreversible brain damage occurs within 3 min of the brain being deprived of oxygen but, despite being unconscious when rescued, 6 months later the only sign of his experience was impaired peripheral vision. Had compensatory vasoconstriction helped him by directing his minimal oxygen supplies to his brain? It is a strong possibility, for the episode is by no means unique and all cases of survival after prolonged immersion have involved cold water and a young person.

used to fight your way around the track is converted to heat and the body must get rid of it in order to prevent a catastrophic rise in body temperature. Blood will flow through your skin as much as a hundred times faster, giving you a rosy, or even flushed, complexion as the heat is lost to the atmosphere.

Veins, too, are rather more than simple tubes which return blood to the heart. Smooth muscle bands surround some veins, and contraction

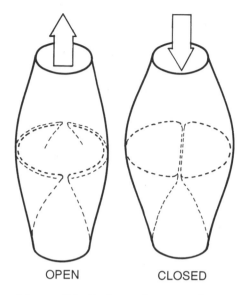

OPEN   CLOSED

Figure 7.9. Pocket valve operation

of these muscles helps venous return to the heart. In addition, the larger veins possess valves—pairs of simple pocket-like flaps which allow blood to flow towards the heart but impedes its flow back (Figure 7.9). During exercise, the thin-walled veins are continually being squeezed by the muscles through which they pass, and with the valves preventing back-flow each squeeze adds to the force propelling blood towards the heart and so assists venous return. One of the benefits of 'warming down' after exercise may be to promote this venous return and accelerate lactic acid removal from the blood and muscles. The importance of this auxiliary pump is most clearly appreciated when it fails—and the soldier on parade faints. While he has stood perfectly still, no venous pumping has taken place, less blood has returned to the heart so less blood can be pumped out and blood pressure falls, or, in medical terms, postural hypotension occurs. In response to an inadequate oxygen supply the soldier's brain ceases to maintain tone in his postural muscles and the soldier assumes a horizontal position. Although embarrassing, the faint solves the problem by reducing the hydrostatic pressure against which the heart has to pump blood to the brain, so the brain now receives its necessary supply of blood.

A similar tendency to faint can arise soon after a long run or an intensive training session, especially if you stand for any length of time, waiting for the prize-giving ceremony or talking to someone at a party after the event. Unlike the soldier, however, you can easily sit down, increasing the rate of venous return to your heart and relieving the problem. In this case, the low blood pressure may be caused by muscular vasodilation persisting well after the exercise has finished. A similar effect can sometimes be experienced after a hot bath, when skin vasodilation has reduced the volume of blood returning to the heart. Fainting is a safety device, an inelegant last resort when other mechanisms to maintain blood flow to the brain have failed. If this is the cause of fainting or feeling faint after exercise, it is quite natural and does not indicate any underlying pathology in the athlete. Nonetheless, if fainting occurs without a satisfactory explanation and if it occurs more than once, it would be wise to seek medical advice.

CONTROLLING THE SYSTEM

Your cardiac output at rest is likely to be around 5 l/min whether you are a trained athlete or not. In a good club athlete this might rise to 25 l/min to provide the extra oxygen needed during vigorous exercise, but endurance-trained élite athletes can achieve cardiac outputs of between 35 and 40 l/min—the discharge from a typical fully open bathroom tap. Part of this is the result of an increase in heart rate, up to a maximum of about 200 beats/min (70 beats/min is a 'normal' resting frequency for untrained subjects) and part is the result of a large increase in stroke volume, i.e. the amount of blood expelled by the heart per beat. The resting stroke volume of trained endurance athletes may approach 200 ml—more than twice that of their untrained counterparts—partly due to their larger heart volume (cardiac hypertrophy) and partly due to more complete emptying. In consequence, many athletes have resting heart beat frequencies below, and even well below, 55 beats/min.

The importance of variation in stroke volume rather than heart beat frequency alone is dramatically demonstrated by patients who use implanted pacemakers to stimulate their hearts, which would otherwise beat irregularly or unreliably. Since most pacemakers deliver their stimuli at a constant frequency, the heart rate does not change even during exercise. These patients can, nevertheless, undertake moderate exercise without difficulty due to the increase in stroke volume.

Keeping just the right amount of blood circulating through different parts of the body under varying conditions is a complicated business. Blood pressure, for example, must be confined within narrow limits:

too high and blood vessels are damaged; too low and the brain is starved of oxygen. Yet as the middle-distance athlete bursts from the start, oxygen consumption can rise more than 40-fold in a few seconds. The cardiovascular centre which coordinates the responses to these demands is part of the hindbrain—a region which is responsible for the automatic control of all vital processes. The centre is made aware of the state of the system it controls through input from receptors, primarily those monitoring blood pressure and carbon dioxide concentration. To change these parameters, signals initiated in the cardiovascular centre pass via motor nerves to the effectors; both cardiac muscle itself and the smooth muscle fibres in the arterioles (Figure 7.10). Superimposed on all this is the ability of the heart to change its output in direct response to the change in blood pH (a decrease in pH increases the heart rate) and hormones such as adrenaline (which increase heart rate).

Negative feedback is the principle behind the control of virtually all physiological processes (and, indeed, most non-biological ones). A rise in some value sets in motion events which decrease that value while, conversely, a fall results in its increase, with the consequence that the quantity remains virtually constant. Perhaps the most familiar example of negative feedback is that controlling room temperature in a modern house. If the temperature rises above a pre-determined level,

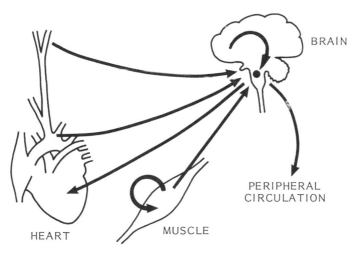

Figure 7.10. The cardiovascular centre receives input from arterial receptors, higher centres of the brain and from exercising muscle itself. It coordinates changes in cardiac output and in the flow of blood through peripheral tissues, including muscle

the thermostat cuts off the supply of heat and hence the temperature falls. Conversely, when the temperature falls below this pre-determined level, the heating is turned on and this raises the temperature.

The most important blood pressure receptors are those found in the carotid sinus, situated in the neck where the carotid artery divides to supply different parts of the brain. Being close to the brain these receptors relay particularly important information back to the cardiovascular centre. In response to information that pressure has fallen, the frequency of impulses passing along the vagus nerve increases in order to stimulate the pacemaker region of the heart. Conversely, a rise in blood pressure results in signals being sent to the heart via the sympathetic nerve to effect a reduction in pacemaker stimulation and to bring about a consequent fall in cardiac output.

So what happens if vigorous exercise is undertaken? Through the action of the 'muscle pump', working muscles speed the return of blood to the heart. This results in greater filling and extension of the ventricles, which respond—and this seems to be a fundamental property of cardiac muscle—by contracting more powerfully. The result is an increase in stroke volume. At the same time, the increase in muscle activity will raise the carbon dioxide concentrations in the blood, which will have a two-fold effect. It will be detected by the cardiovascular centre and lead to an increase in heart rate, and it will also have a local vasodilating effect in the muscles themselves. The increased blood flow which results will tend to reduce blood pressure and this, too, stimulates the cardiovascular centre. Add to all of this the fact that nervous stimulation of the heart alters the relationship between ventricle expansion and force of emptying and it can be seen that there is an exceedingly complex interplay of factors. The result is not chaotic, however, but a very smooth and appropriate response of cardiac output to the changing demands.

It is even possible for demand on the heart to be anticipated to produce an even smoother response as noradrenaline is released from the endings of the sympathetic nerves which innervate cardiac muscle. In fact, this neurotransmitter plays a much larger part in stimulating the heart before a big race than does the chemically related but better-known adrenaline. This hormone, which affects the heart in the same way as noradrenaline and which is a favourite of athletic commentators, is released from the adrenal glands in times of stress and is carried round the body in the blood.

PUMPING IRON

Muscles can generate energy without oxygen, but short sprints are the only events run almost entirely anaerobically (see Table 5.1). In all other events, oxygen is crucial and is supplied to working muscles by the blood. But blood is mostly water and a litre of water will dissolve only about 3 ml oxygen at body temperature. With a blood volume of around 5 litres this would carry barely enough oxygen to support the body for 5 s at rest! Clearly the athlete has a lot to thank haemoglobin for, since this iron-containing protein binds so much oxygen that a litre of blood can contain more oxygen (200 ml) than a litre of air! This oxygen is held by the haemoglobin in loose chemical combination, so that when oxygen concentration is high, as it is in the lungs, the haemoglobin takes on a full load of oxygen. In working muscles, by contrast, the oxygen concentration is low, so that most of the oxygen separates from the haemoglobin and becomes available for the muscle.

Box 7.3   Getting a grip on oxygen

An iron atom in the right circumstances can form chemical bonds with six other atoms. In haemoglobin four of these bonds are provided by the chemical framework which holds the iron atom in its centre. This complex, known as haem, is bound through the fifth bond formed by the iron atom to the protein globin which enfolds it. The sixth and final bond is the one that gives haemoglobin its special role, for it has the vital task of binding an oxygen molecule. So effectively does it do this that 1 g haemoglobin can hold 1.34 ml oxygen. But binding with oxygen is only part of the story; an equally important part is letting the oxygen go, and it is the protein part of haemoglobin that determines just how strongly the oxygen binds.

The amount of oxygen bound depends on the concentration of oxygen around the haemoglobin (Figure 7.11). As the oxygen concentration rises so more is bound until in the lungs, where oxygen concentration is at its highest, virtually 100% of the haemoglobin is carrying oxygen. It has turned into oxyhaemoglobin. As the blood passes from the lungs and into tissues, such as muscles, which use oxygen, the oxygen concentration falls and so the haemoglobin unloads its oxygen.

Can we pump without iron? Although blood transfusions are an essential part of modern medicine it has long been a goal to produce

continued

— *continued* —

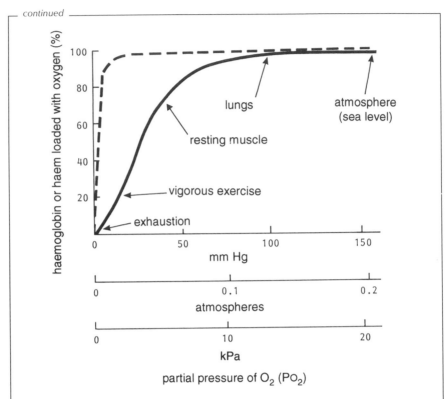

Figure 7.11. Dissociation curves for oxyhaemoglobin and oxygenated haem (broken line) showing relationship between oxygen concentration and the amount of oxygen carried

an artificial blood substitute with infinite shelf life, total sterility and lacking compatibility problems. Synthesizing haem presents no fundamental problem but without globin to control its properties it would be quite useless. Even if globin could be produced in useful amounts, its presence in the blood outside red cells would produce problems. The most promising solution is a most unnatural molecule called perfluorodecalin—a relatively simple hydrocarbon in which all the hydrogen atoms have been replaced by atoms of fluorine, an element which very rarely occurs in living organisms. It is an excellent solvent for oxygen and it is biochemically inert, but it is not water soluble and must be emulsified prior to injection into humans. Unfortunately the emulsifying agent is not so chemically inert and is removed slowly by the liver, which may eventually be damaged.

Haemoglobin is not found free in the blood but packaged into the red blood cells, of which there are more than three hundred million in each drop of blood. Each day a total of 100 000 000 000 blood cells die in a healthy human due to 'wear and tear'. This may sound horrendous but it is less than 1% of the total, and such losses are easily sustained provided that the red cell manufacturing plant (operating, somewhat unexpectedly, in the marrow of limb bones) is working properly. If it is not, anaemia results and the oxygen-carrying capacity of the blood falls. This causes an increased dependence on anaerobic metabolism, leading to a general feeling of lethargy and an inability to cope with even relatively low-intensity exercise—a particularly disastrous situation for the athlete. For most of us this is unlikely to happen unless our diet contains insufficient iron to make enough haem—the iron-containing complex which lies at the heart of each haemoglobin molecule. Most of the iron released from dead red blood cells is retained by the body and efficiently recycled, but loss of blood can result in iron deficiency. Women with heavy menstrual blood loss and particularly those on a vegetarian diet, which contains relatively little iron and may lack the vitamin B_{12} which is needed for the uptake of iron into the body, are particularly at risk. In such cases, iron supplementation may be needed (see Chapter 11).

If oxygen supply to muscles can limit performance in all events except sprints, you might expect endurance training to increase the haemoglobin content of blood. An easy way of detecting such a change is by measuring the haematocrit, i.e. the percentage of total blood occupied by cells. A single drop of blood provides a sufficient sample if sucked into a capillary tube and centrifuged to sediment the cells (Figure 7.12). No increase in haematocrit is observed, however, in trained athletes; indeed some show a 1–4% lower haematocrit after intense training—a condition which has been dubbed 'sports anaemia'. In fact, such athletes will have an enhanced oxygen-carrying capacity, for another consequence of endurance training is an increase in total blood volume by as much as 15%.

It is possible that training does not increase the haematocrit because such an increase could carry with it some disadvantage. Whatever this disadvantage may be, it does not appear to operate in the short term since athletes experimenting with 'blood doping' or 'blood boosting' have shown improvement in performance. The success of this proce- dure depends on the fact that when blood is removed from the body more red cells are produced to replace the loss. If the removed blood is stored and later re-infused, the haemoglobin content can be raised by as much as 10%. Further details of this illegal manipulation, which

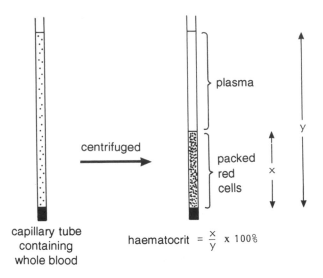

$$\text{haematocrit} = \frac{x}{y} \times 100\%$$

Figure 7.12. Determination of haematocrit. Normal values are 40–52% for males and 36–48% for females

can enhance performance for several weeks, are presented in Chapter 13. High haematocrits do occur for prolonged periods in those who live at very high altitudes, but there is anecdotal evidence that such high haematocrits may be harmful.

Box 7.4   Too much of a good thing?

Imagine you are on the beach. You breathe right out then fill your lungs. Just how much air you take in will depend on your vital capacity—say yours is 4 litres. At sea-level, these 4 litres contain around 1.1 g oxygen (depending on the actual temperature). Now travel, in your imagination, to the top of Mount Everest (8848 m above the beach). The same deep breath will contain barely 0.5 g oxygen. The composition of the air will be the same but the pressure has fallen and with it, in proportion, the amount of oxygen. Blood leaving the lungs is no longer fully oxygenated, so tissues may not be able to get all the oxygen they need. Everest *has* been climbed without the use of additional oxygen (for the first time on 8th May 1978, by Peter Habeler and Reinhold Messner) but most expeditions have used oxygen in spite of the immense logistic problems of carrying it to where it is needed.

continued

┌─ *continued* ──────────────────────────────────

If you actually live at a high altitude rather than just visit in your imagination, real changes will take place in your blood to compensate for the lower amount of oxygen. In particular the amount of haemoglobin will increase and become apparent as an increased red blood cell count or haematocrit. A variety of mechanisms bring this about, ranging from a short-term release of additional cells from storage in the liver and spleen to genetic adjustments occurring over generations. Residents of Aucanquilcha in the Andes, which at 5500 m above sea-level is the highest permanent human settlement, have a haemoglobin content of up to 23 g/100 ml, compared with an average of 15 g/100 ml for sea-level residents. Without this adaptation they could not work at such altitudes. However, most suffer chronic mountain sickness characterized by failure of the left side of the heart. This is the side that pumps blood around the body and it is likely that the damage is caused by the increased resistance to flow provided by their 'thicker' blood. Habitual blood dopers and athletes taking the hormone erythropoietin (EPO) (pp. 294) beware!

OVERHEATING

During training or racing an athlete expends a considerable amount of chemical energy, almost all of which appears as heat. For example, during a marathon the rate of heat production can be more than 1 kW or at least 13 times greater than that at rest. This would be sufficient to raise core body temperature, normally close to 37 °C (98.4 °F) by 1 °C every 8 minutes. In normally active, healthy adults, core temperature rarely rises above 38 °C. Higher temperatures indicate hyperthermia but moderate hyperthermia is by no means life threatening; vigorous exercise can raise core temperature to 40 °C, and rectal temperatures as high as 41 °C have been reported for runners completing a 3-mile race without apparent ill effect. Indeed some body warming is probably beneficial when such demands are placed on muscle chemistry, and chemical reactions usually proceed faster as the temperature increases. The real danger is that hyperthermia will lead to heat-stroke when the mechanisms which normally operate to limit a rise in body temperature themselves fail. A core temperature of 42.5 °C is generally considered fatal unless treated within minutes.

Heat-stroke is characterized by irritability, aggressive behaviour, disorientation, unsteady gait and a glassy stare. These signs and symptoms are not specific to heat-stroke and can, for example, be caused by dehydration when it is then sometimes known as heat exhaustion. Indeed dehydration compounds the problem of insufficient heat loss since it reduces sweating. There are reports of fatalities or near-fatalities for which heat-stroke is blamed, but correct diagnosis of the condition is difficult. In the Empire Games in Canada in 1954, the British runner Jim Peters collapsed in the final 400 m of the marathon on a very hot day. When a British cyclist, Tom Simpson, died in the Tour de France in 1959, the heat-stroke may have been precipitated by amphetamines (see pp. 280) and Alberto Salazar was sufficiently near death in August 1978, after a road race, to be administered the last rites.

To prevent hyperthermia, heat produced in the muscles must be lost from the body, and this means transporting the heat from the core of the body to its surface—the skin. By increasing the flow of blood through the skin heat is lost from the body not only by convection and conduction, but also, and most importantly, as a result of evaporation of water. In fact, a litre of sweat, if evaporated fully and not just dripped off the body, can remove about 2400 kJ of heat, so that just over 3 litres would be needed to remove all the excess heat generated in a marathon. The unfortunate aspect of this is that blood needed to carry heat to the skin and water to sweat glands is not being used to carry oxygen to muscles. Regrettably performance must suffer.

Heat-stroke is most likely to occur on a hot, humid day because the air is then unable to hold much more water vapour, so little evaporation can occur. What precautions should be taken when training or racing under such conditions? Fluid should be taken before and during the race; splash the body with water before the race and in the longer events at every feeding station. Soak your headband and T-shirt, if you wear them, for evaporation from these surfaces will carry away a considerable amount of heat. During interval training, this can be done in the rest periods.

The problem of hyperthermia is compounded by dehydration; a fluid loss as little as that corresponding to 1% of body mass produces a detectable impairment of temperature regulation. Unfortunately, the sensation of thirst in man is not immediately sensitive to dehydration so that it cannot be relied upon and, once dehydration has set in, matters go from bad to worse. Therefore fluid should be consumed prior to training or competition and during the activity even though you may not feel thirsty.

To detect hyperthermia, feel the skin at the top of the chest; if it has become warm and dry the runner should slow and obtain liquid as soon as possible. Unfortunately this test is not always reliable and athletes who feel unwell for a period of time on hot, humid days should stop running and take medical advice.

ENVIRONMENTAL INTERFACE

Twenty-one per cent of the air around us is oxygen, but getting it into the body presents some difficulties. Many simple organisms, such as the earthworm, absorb oxygen through their skin but we cannot use this method, for several reasons. Our oxygen demand is very much greater than that of a worm, not only because we, and especially the athletes among us, are more active but also because we maintain our body temperature well above that of the environment. That means a high energy demand even at rest, and most of it is generated through processes that use oxygen. To obtain oxygen fast enough by diffusion we would need a very large and a very thin (and therefore delicate)

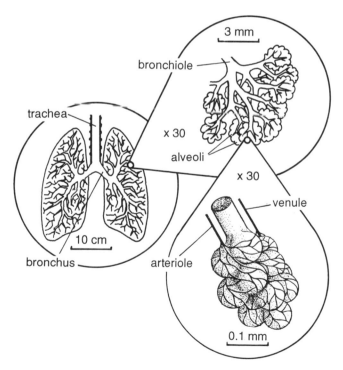

Figure 7.13. Fine structure of the lungs

surface. Our skin is barely 2 m² in area and far from delicate. By contrast, our lungs consist of over 50 m² of the most delicate membranes, neatly protected in a firm rib-cage. Furthermore, this internal surface can be kept moist, thus aiding gas diffusion, without excessive water loss by evaporation. The lung is a remarkable organ; its surface consists of millions of tiny sacs, each of which receives a branch from the main airway and is intimately surrounded by a capillary bed (Figure 7.13). Changes in chest volume, achieved through contraction and relaxation of the diaphragm and intercostal muscles, flush air in and out of the lungs. During its brief stay in the lungs, the oxygen content of the air falls from 21% to about 14.5% as haemoglobin 'pulls' the oxygen into the blood. Conversely the carbon dioxide content rises from almost zero to 5–6%.

VITAL AND OTHER CAPACITIES

The maximum usable volume of the lungs is defined as the vital capacity (Figure 7.14). It is measured by taking the deepest possible breath and exhaling completely into a device for measuring gas volume. Vital capacity depends on age, size, sex and general pulmonary health. It is generally within the range 3–6 litres, and endurance runners are likely to have vital capacities at the upper end of this range, partly as a result of training.

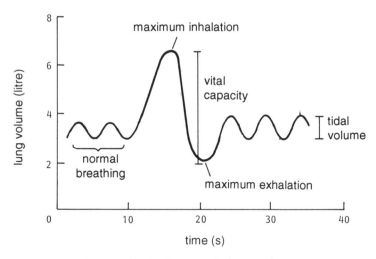

Figure 7.14. Changes in lung volume

At rest, only about half a litre is drawn in and expelled in a single breath. This is known as the *tidal volume* and is typically taken about 15 times per minute. This rhythmic pattern of breathing appears to be generated within the respiratory centre of the brain and is modified according to demand for oxygen as a result of information received from receptors in the aorta and carotid arteries. Somewhat surprisingly, these receptors are stimulated not by a fall in oxygen concentration but by an increase in carbon dioxide concentration, and it is the latter which causes a rise in the rate of breathing. Changes in the oxygen concentration itself have much less of an effect on breathing but, since a fall in blood oxygen concentration is normally associated with a rise in carbon dioxide concentration, the mechanism works well. It can, however, be fooled. Rebreathing air from a closed bag through soda-lime to remove carbon dioxide fails to stimulate the respiratory centre even when the oxygen content of the blood falls to dangerously low levels.

When exercise demands it, oxygen supply is increased both by increasing the frequency of breathing and the depth of breathing. The product of tidal volume and number of breaths per minute gives the minute volume. Training increases the maximum minute volume that can be achieved, so that volumes greater than 120 l/min can be achieved by endurance runners during their races. Training also improves the efficiency of gas exchange between air and blood across the membranes of the lung.

Box 7.5   Putting a figure on fitness

No single measure of fitness is possible, because fitness means different things to different people. To the sportsperson it means being in optimum condition for the chosen activity; to the executive it means feeling good or extending active life. Tests of fitness all involve imposing a defined stress and measuring the response. The questions of what stress and what response are not easy to answer but in practice generally depend on the equipment available and the reliability required.

Anaerobic 'fitness' can be assessed by timing how long it takes to sprint up a measured flight of steps and calculating the rate of energy expenditure as described in Figure 3.2 (p. 52). If a cycle ergometer is available the Wingate test can be carried out, in which the subject

continued

continued

performs 30 s of all-out supra-maximal exercise against a frictional load depending on body mass (75 g for each kilogram mass). From the data recorded not only can peak power output be measured but the time to reach peak, the average power output over the 30 s and the rate of fatiguing can also be determined.

The assessment of aerobic fitness is of wider interest, for this is the fitness associated with health benefit. Indeed fitness assessment (and improvement) is now big business at health clubs all over the country (Figure 7.15). The most useful criterion of aerobic fitness is undoubtedly $\dot{V}O_{2\ max}$—the maximum rate at which oxygen can be used. Since expired air has to be directed into a spirometer which measures flow rate and oxygen content it is essential to have the

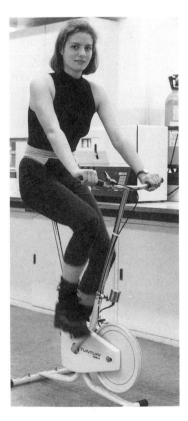

Figure 7.15.

continued

— continued —

subject stationary. As exercise intensity is increased following a standard protocol so oxygen consumption, displayed on a digital read-out, increases. The aim is to increase the intensity until no further increase in rate of oxygen consumption is seen—not easy with the untrained subject for whom the discomfort of severe exercise often forces premature withdrawal from the test before $\dot{V}O_{2\ max}$ is achieved.

For many purposes it is adequate to use a more accessible form of exercise and to predict $VO_{2\ max}$ from readily measurable parameters. A widely used predictive test is the step test in its various forms, in which the rise in heart rate is measured as the subject steps on and off a bench. In the Queen's College version of this test, subjects step on and off a 16¼-inch high bench 24 times per minute (22 for women) and measure their pulse rate for a 15 s period between 5 and 20 s into recovery. The stepping is done regularly in synchrony with a metronome set to 88 or 96 beats/min. After multiplying the rate by four it is compared with values on a reference table (Table 7.1) drawn up from studies in which step-test performance has been compared with more vigorous means of assessing $\dot{V}O_{2\ max}$.

Minute volumes are not difficult to measure, but as predictors of endurance potential they are limited because they measure how much oxygen is taken into the lungs, rather than how much is *used* by the tissues. Most (about 65%) of the oxygen entering the lungs also leaves in the exhaled air.

Of more direct significance to the athlete is the aerobic capacity $\dot{V}O_{2max}$—the maximum rate at which oxygen is used by the body (Figure 7.16). Aerobic capacity is usually expressed in relation to body mass, and an élite endurance male athlete may well have an aerobic capacity of about 80 ml/kg per minute, whereas an average value for a 20-year-old man would be about 45 ml/kg per minute. An élite endurance female athlete would have a $\dot{V}O_{2\ max}$ of 65–70 ml/kg per minute. Exceptionally high values for the $\dot{V}O_{2\ max}$, in excess of 90 ml/kg per minute, have been recorded for a few cross-country skiers and road cyclists. $VO_{2\ max}$ can be increased by training, typically by around 25%.

Athletes and their coaches have long searched for a simple-to-measure factor to provide an index of athletic performance that could be used to select potential élite athletes or monitor training progress. The best endurance athlete is not necessarily the one with the highest

Table 7.1. Relationship between step-test performance and $VO_{2\,max}$

| Heart rate | $VO_{2\,max}$ (ml/kg per minute) | |
	Men	Women
120	60.9	–
124	59.3	–
128	57.6	42.4
132	55.9	41.4
136	54.2	40.7
140	52.5	40.0
144	50.9	39.2
148	49.2	38.5
150	48.3	38.1
152	47.5	37.7
154	46.7	37.4
156	45.8	37.0
158	45.0	36.6
160	44.1	36.3
162	43.3	35.9
164	42.5	35.5
166	41.6	35.1
168	40.8	34.8
170	39.9	34.4
172	39.1	34.0
176	37.4	33.3
180	35.7	32.6
184	34.1	31.8
188	–	31.1
192	–	30.3
196	–	29.6

Based on work by W. D. McArdle. Statistically there is a 95% probability that the predicted $VO_{2\,max}$ will be within 16% of the true value.
From McArdle, W. D., Katch, F. I. and Katch, V. L. (1991). *Exercise Physiology: Energy, Nutrition and Human Performance.* Lea and Febiger, Philadelphia/London.

$VO_{2\,max}$, although it helps. A somewhat better indicator is provided by combining it with measurement of anaerobic threshold—the percentage of $VO_{2\,max}$ at which blood lactate concentration dramatically increases (pp. 106). Again training will raise this value, and a high value of the anaerobic threshold (e.g. 90%) is excellent news for the endurance athlete. Combine these with a measurement of Achilles tendon elasticity (see p. 61), which is less easily made, an assessment

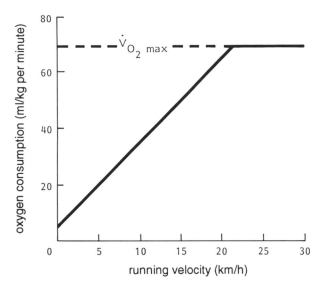

Figure 7.16. Aerobic capacity

of psychological make-up (Chapter 10) and an ability to select and eat a sensible diet (Chapter 11), and you might have an index of potential athletic performance!

Chapter 8

The Female Runner

Women's sports are all against the law of Nature.
Pierre de Coubertin (founder of the modern Olympics) (1902).

Traditionally, sport has been the prerogative of the male and has served as a laboratory for the socialization of the boy into the man in society. At the same time, the behavioural and physical demands of strenuous and competitive sport have been the antithesis of what femininity supposedly represents. The real fear of society has been that the participation of the female in such activities would masculinize her behaviour. The general assumption has been that the female who found such experiences gratifying was not quite 'normal', that there must be something wrong with her glands, and that she was trading off her feminine selfhood for such participation.
Dorothy V. Harris and Susan E. Jennings (1976).

However, society still reinforces the value of physical activity for men and only tolerates sports for women. Exercise, for men is supposedly good, making them stronger, more competitive and more manly. For women the turn-of-the-century medical view that 'sport wasted vital force, strained female bodies and fostered traits unbecoming to "true womanhood"' still persists.

Jerilyne C. Prior (1990).

The view that female participation in sport in general, and track athletics in particular, is abnormal persists, despite the fact that women are no longer satisfied to contemplate with awe the achievements of the male but have become able, competent and enthusiastic competitors in their own right. Of the 23 000 runners who completed the 1991 London Marathon, 3000 were women. Although this is still a fair step from equality in numbers, it does represent a considerable achievement in the mere 21 years since women have officially been allowed to run marathons. Nina Kuscsik's review of the fight for acceptance of females in athletic competitions provides some of the background to this achievement.

GETTING IN ON THE ACT

The modern Olympics were devised by men for men; in 1896 anything else would have been quite shocking. Nevertheless a woman did, it is claimed, run unofficially with the 25 male competitors in that first marathon. Melpomene finished the 40 km course (the standard distance, 42.195 km, was not fixed until 1924) in about 4½ h. Although women were able to compete in Olympic events such as tennis and swimming, it was not until the Amsterdam Olympics of 1928 that three track events—the 100 m, 800 m and 4 × 100 m relay—were opened to women, together with the discus and high jump. As it turned out, this first women's Olympic 800 m event was to set back the course of women's athletics by many years since some of the participants in that race collapsed. Although the failures probably resulted from inadequate preparation (as they would have done for male athletes) they inevitably received more publicity than the winner, Lina Radke, from Germany, who completed the race in 2 min 16.8 s, and they provided support for the view that women should not be allowed to participate in such events. Indeed the 800 m event for women was not reinstated until the 1960 Olympic Games.

The 1960s brought an increased questioning of the role of women in society in general and the realization that running long distances was no more harmful to women than to men. Since this realization did not extend to the governing bodies of athletics, the decade was one of 'unofficial' female participation, particularly in the marathon.

In December 1963, two women from California, Lyn Carman and Merry Lepper, hid at the start of the Western Hemisphere Marathon in Culver City, California, and 'jumped into' the race when it started. Irate officials failed to prevent them completing the race and Lepper finished in 3 h 37 min 7 s. In 1964, a Scottish woman, Dale Greig, set an unofficial world best of 3 h 27 min 45 s, and was the first woman to break the 3 h 30 min barrier. During the race, an ambulance followed her all the way! Roberta Gibb Bingay 'jumped in' at the start of the 1966 Boston Marathon and completed the race in 3 h 21 min, ahead of two-thirds of the otherwise all-male field, and this became news across the USA. Male prejudice was apparent in the race director's comment: 'Roberta Gibb Bingay did not run in the Boston Marathon, she merely covered the same route as the official race while it was in progress.' In 1967 Kathrine Switzer applied to run in the Boston Marathon without indicating her sex. She was assumed to be male and turned up for the race wearing a hood. When the hood was removed to reveal her sex at the beginning of the race, the race director ran after her but was unable to catch her!

The number of unofficial female participants in marathons now began to increase dramatically. Finally, in October 1970, the Road Runners Club of America (RRCA) arranged the first marathon for women in the USA, the RRCA National Women's Marathon Championship. Six women started and, of the four finishing, Sara Berman was fastest. Two women completed the New York City Marathon in September 1971 in less than 3 h, Beth Bonner in 2 h 55 min 22 s and Nina Kuscsik in 2 h 56 min 4 s. In December 1971, in Culver City, Cheryl Bridges lowered the world's best time to 2 h 49 min 40 s.

In April 1972 women were allowed to participate in the Boston Marathon. In October 1973, West Germany held their first national women's marathon and they also hosted the first international marathon for women, in Waldniel, on 22nd September 1974. In 1979, Grete Waitz broke the 2 h 30 min barrier and Joan Benoit from the USA won the first Olympic marathon race for women in Los Angeles in 1984 in 2 h 24 min 52 s. The current (1994) world's best time is held by Norway's Ingrid Kristiansen: 2 h 21 min 6 s in the London Marathon in 1985.

RUNNING FOR ALL

While the last 20 years have seen women's times for all events improve dramatically, bringing them closer to the men's best times for the various distances (Table 8.1), they have also seen a great increase in the number of women participating in running at all levels. For most, personal best times are far more important than world records. In the many hundreds of marathon events held annually in the USA, Britain and other parts of the world, there will be joggers as well as élite women runners. In Britain, waves of female club runners, often highly motivated and trained, are helping to increase the standard of women's running across the country and, from these, élite runners of the future will emerge.

If speed, or lack of it, is no longer a barrier to participation then neither is age. It is now not uncommon for there to be several women in the 50-plus age group taking part in any particular race and maybe one or two from the 60 or even 70-plus age groups. And as the cohort of middle-aged women runners moves up to the higher age brackets there will be even more 'elderly' women participating in races.

This change, from running being an élitist sport to a sport for

Table 8.1. World records (h:min.s) for men and women for track events and the marathon in 1960 and 1990

Event	1960 Men	1960 Women	1960 Women as % of men	1990 Men	1990 Women	1990 Women as % of men
100 m	10.0	11.3	88	9.92	10.49	95
200 m	20.5	22.9	89	19.72	21.34	92
400 m	44.9	53.0	85	43.29	47.60	91
800 m	1:45.7	2:04.3	85	1:41.73	1:53.28	90
1 500 m	3:35.6	4:25.0	81	3:29.46	3:52.47	90
3 000 m[a]	7:35.2	8:46.6	86	7:29.45	8:22.62	89
5 000 m[a]	13:13.0	15:48.5	84	12:58.39	14:37.33	89
10 000 m[a]	27:30.80	34:01.4	81	27:08.23	30:13.74	90
Marathon	2:15:16	3:40.22	61	2:06.50	2:21.06	88

[a]Later than 1960 for women.

everyone, happened less quickly in Britain and Europe than in the USA, where in many places almost equal numbers of male and female athletes participate.

Competition is not everything and many women have taken up running and other endurance sports (e.g. fell-running, cycling, swimming, triathlons, biathlons, orienteering) for the personal challenges involved and the benefits of running, which include:

- Improvement in mood.
- A sense of well-being.
- An improved ability to control body weight.

WOMEN: A RACE APART?

There is variation between all individuals, so it could be said that a truly 'fair' race is never run. Some competitors start off with better innate ability, some with better training, some with better fuel stores, some with better shoes and clothing. To separate all these variables would be impossible, but to achieve a degree of fairness, competitors are separated into different classes, according to age for example, so juniors race against juniors and veterans against fellow veterans. Similarly women run against women and men against men.

Because of anatomical and physiological differences, women cannot achieve the same power output as men (assuming that factors such as 'natural ability', training and diet are equal). If women do ever achieve the same or better times than men, they will have done this by training harder and working harder than the male. The main differences between males and females that affect athletic performance are physiological (see Chapter 7) and include the following:

- Cardiac output is about 10% less in a woman than in a man of the same body size, owing to a slightly smaller heart volume.
- The volume of blood is about 20% lower in the female for the same body weight.
- For the same volume of blood, women have about 10% less haemoglobin.
- The wider pelvis of a woman decreases mechanical efficiency by increasing the angle of the thigh bone to bring the knees closer together.
- For the same body weight, the average female possesses about 10% more fat than the average male, which increases the load to be carried.
- The vital capacity (pp. 152) of a woman is about 10% lower than that of a man.
- The Achilles tendon, which is important in the elastic recoil of running, is shorter in women.
- The menstrual cycle imposes physiological and psychological stresses on a woman's body and mind which may decrease athletic performance in some athletes.

The suggestion that women have a greater ability to oxidize fatty acids so as to give them an advantage in prolonged endurance events has not been refuted. The research indicated no difference between the capacity of trained female athletes and trained male athletes to oxidize fatty acids but the capacity could be higher in untrained female muscle in comparison to the untrained male.

So, how are the women doing? None of the current women's world record holders would qualify them to compete in the men's races in the 1992 Olympic Games; however, women are currently improving at a faster rate than men, so that the gap between them is narrowing (Table 8.1). Were this rate of improvement to be maintained there will come a time when the best women would beat the best men (Figure 8.1). The steady nature of the improvements in both women's and men's records has encouraged the prediction that this might occur around the year 2035 for most events—and much sooner in the

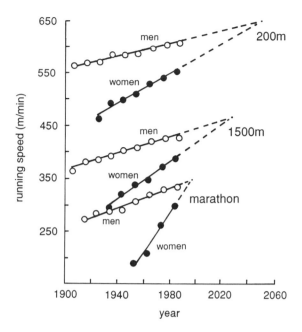

Figure 8.1. By extrapolating graphs showing changes in men's and women's record times it should be possible to predict when women will run as fast as men. This approach assumes that record times change linearly over historical time; remarkably this appears to have been the case. From Whipp, B. J. and Ward, S. A. (1992). Will women soon outrun men? *Nature*, **355**, 25

marathon. But will the faster rate of improvement for women be maintained? Because of the differences given above, this appears unlikely. The faster improvement may be explained by the fact that women entered the world of competitive athletics relatively late, so the benefits of interval training, peak training, psychological preparation and sensible nutrition have been crammed into a shorter period.

Box 8.1   Is she a woman?

If a top-class male athlete were to enter a women's event he would probably win it—and that would not be fair. Most of the time there is no doubt about the sex of a competitor but there is always the possibility of deliberate deception or an athlete having an ambiguous sexual development. In the 1932 Olympic Games in Los Angeles,

continued

continued

Stella Walsh (née Walasiewicz) of Poland won the gold medal in a women's 100 m event. Some years later she was killed in cross-fire in a gangland shoot-out in the USA and the autopsy revealed that she was in fact a man. In the 1936 Olympics in Berlin, Dora Ratjen of Germany was fourth in the high jump but was later found to be male. Sex-testing was therefore introduced and all female athletes who participate in major International Games have to present a certificate confirming their gender. Perhaps by the year 2010 (Figure 8.1), male marathon runners will be obliged to present a certificate confirming *their* gender!

The problem of the gender of athletes was considered by the International Olympic Committee (IOC) in 1964 in Tokyo and a medical commission was set up. Since the most obvious differences between men and women are anatomical, nude inspections of women participants took place. In the European Championships in Budapest in 1966 the genitalia of the female competitors were inspected by a panel of doctors; in the Commonwealth Games in Kingston Jamaica in 1966, female participants had to undergo a physical examination by a physician. Not surprisingly, there was considerable opposition to such tests, which were considered to be crude, degrading and even frightening by the female competitors. The fact that these tests were carried out during major events added further stress to the female participants. The need for such tests at that time was, however, confirmed by the fact that several female competitors from Eastern bloc countries withdrew from the European Championships in Budapest at the last minute!

In 1968, a genetic test known as the *buccal smear sex test* was introduced by the IOC Medical Commission. Of the 46 chromosomes which carry the inherited information in each human cell, just two are involved in determining sex. In females these two chromosomes are identical and are known as X chromosomes; in the male, there is a single X chromosome plus a smaller Y chromosome. Only one X chromosome is actually used in a cell, so that females can be considered to have a 'spare' X chromosome which becomes reduced to a small blob of genetic material just inside the nucleus, where it is known as a *Barr body* (Figure 8.2). If the microscopic examination of cells scraped from the inside of a competitor's cheek reveals that they have a Barr body, they are from a woman; if not, they are from a man.

Between 1972 and 1984 approximately one female competitor in 400 was excluded from an international event following a buccal

continued

— *continued* —

smear test; in the 1984 Los Angeles Olympic Games alone six such failures occurred. It is unlikely that all of these athletes had entered competitions fraudulently. Most, if not all, were suffering from some condition in which normal sexual development was impaired, such as *testicular feminizing syndrome*. Individuals with this condition are genetically male (and hence fail the sex test) but lack the protein, coded for on the Y chromosome, which prevents the development of female organs. It is now possible for tests to detect the presence of the gene on the Y chromosome which codes for this protein, thus providing an alternative 'high-tech' means of gender verification.

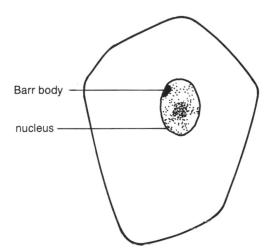

Barr body

nucleus

Figure 8.2. Epithelial cell from inside the cheek of a woman

Some experts believe that even these tests are unfair and could give false negatives. The enormous psychological problems experienced by athletes who 'fail' these tests are such that most quickly seek anonymity and disappear quickly from the athletic scene. Gender verification is such a nightmare that in 1992 the International Amateur Athletics Federation Council decided to scrap all forms of sex testing for athletes. Whether the IOC will follow this example is still under discussion.

UNDERSTANDING THE CYCLE

The menstrual cycle is a central feature of womanhood; its appearance at menarche distinguishes the woman from the girl. The fact that intense exercise can delay menarche, affect the heaviness of a period or even abolish the cycle altogether, has led, all too readily, to the conclusion that such exercise is bad for the female and should be avoided. A more modern view, however, is that these changes are temporary, reversible and normal adaptations to severe exercise and that they will disappear as soon as the intensity of exercise decreases.

In order to understand the changes that occur in the menstrual cycle and their relation to exercise, it is necessary to appreciate some of the biochemistry and physiology of the female reproductive system. Although such knowledge will not prevent changes in the menstrual cycle, it may help to provide confidence for the athlete to accept that some changes are perfectly normal for the very active female.

During her reproductive lifetime a woman produces a single egg approximately once every 28 days. If intercourse takes place in the next few days it is possible that fertilization will occur, but pregnancy will only follow if the fertilized egg successfully implants in her uterus (or womb) (Figure 8.3). For this, the uterine lining must be replaced each month to ensure that it is properly receptive at the appropriate time. This replacement involves a monthly loss of some blood—the menses or period—followed by an intensive repair phase. Timing is

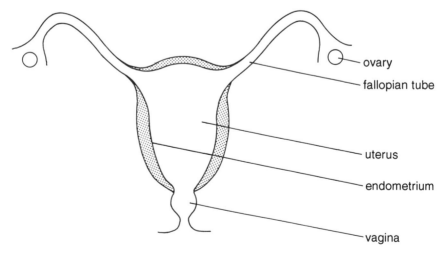

Figure 8.3. Female reproductive system

crucial, for the regenerated lining must be ready for the next egg if it becomes fertilized, and is achieved through the interplay of four hormones (Figure 8.4). Hormones are chemical messengers, released by one organ, and carried in the blood to a target organ which they affect. In this case, two of the hormones—*luteinizing hormone* (LH) and *follicle-stimulating hormone* (FSH)—are released from the pituitary, a small gland just below the brain which is strongly influenced by the nearby hypothalamus. These hormones, together known as gonadotrophins, control egg development in the ovary, release of the egg from the ovaries and the secretion of the two female sex hormones—oestrogen and progesterone—from the ovaries. This latter pair of sex hormones are steroids, chemically similar to the male sex hormone testosterone (and to the anabolic steroids abused by some athletes) but crucially different in their effects (Figure 8.5). The steroid hormones control the replacement of the uterine lining and

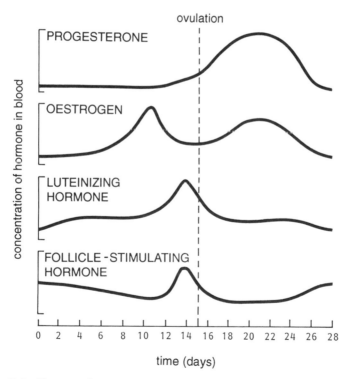

Figure 8.4. Changes in concentration of hormone in blood during the menstrual cycle

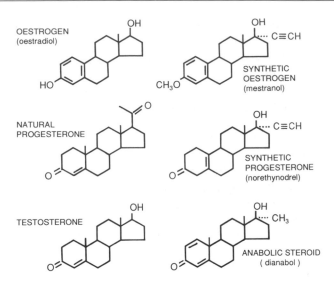

Figure 8.5. Part of the steroid family. Chemists use diagrams like these to show the arrangements of atoms within molecules. Small chemical differences alter properties in subtle ways; the synthetic sex hormones, for example, are inactivated and excreted from the body much more slowly than their natural counterparts

exert feedback effects on the pituitary to control the secretions of the gonadotrophins and thus keep the cycle going at an appropriate frequency of one per month.

At her own birth, each of a woman's two ovaries contains around a million eggs, each surrounded by a cluster of cells which form the follicle. At the beginning of each cycle, several of these follicles enlarge by developing a fluid-filled cavity which surrounds the egg (Figure 8.6) but, by the sixth day, one follicle has begun to grow more rapidly, leaving the others to wither away. This 'winning' follicle, usually produced in alternate ovaries each month, develops into a Graafian follicle. The development of this follicle is initiated by a rise in FSH during the first few days of the cycle and, as the 14th day approaches, surges in concentrations of both LH and FSH in the bloodstream result in ovulation—the ejection of the egg from the ovary. The egg is picked up by the gently moving fringes of the funnel-shaped end of the Fallopian tube and it begins its week-long journey towards the uterus, wafted by the waving of cilia lining the tube. It is during this journey that fertilization can occur, followed by the first rounds of cell division to form the blastocyst—the cluster of cells which implants in the uterine lining to continue its development into the embryo.

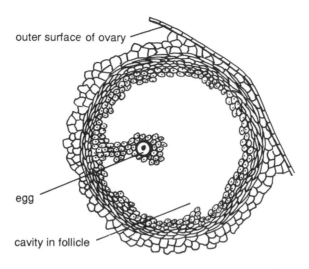

outer surface of ovary

egg

cavity in follicle

Figure 8.6. Graafian follicle before egg is released from ovary

During the development of the Graafian follicle its cells have been secreting oestrogen, and it is this steroid hormone that has played the major part in causing the surge of gonadotrophins which results in ovulation. Immediately after ovulation, the cells of the Graafian follicle multiply rapidly and it develops into a *corpus luteum* which secretes large amounts of the second steroid hormone progesterone. It is this that causes a reduction in gonadotrophin release from the pituitary (Figure 8.4). Unless fertilization has occurred, the corpus luteum begins to degenerate on about day 24 of the cycle, so that the steroid hormones are no longer produced and their rate of secretion decreases. The resultant fall in their concentration in the blood causes menstruation to occur and allows the cycle to start all over again. Should fertilization occur, however, the corpus luteum does not degenerate but continues to produce and secrete progesterone and oestrogen, maintaining high concentrations of these steroid hormones in the blood and so preventing both menstruation and the initiation of a new cycle.

The lining of the uterus—the endometrium—has a rich blood supply to provide nourishment for the implanted conceptus if fertilization has occurred. If fertilization has not, then the endometrium is replaced and it is this that results in the menstrual flow. The fall in the concentrations of oestrogen and progesterone in the blood as the corpus luteum degenerates causes alternate increases and decreases in blood flow through the endometrium. Gradually the decreases predominate and the cells of the endometrium become deprived of oxygen and die. This damage attracts white blood cells—the body's scavenger cells—which release an enzyme that breaks down the proteins holding the cells together. The tissue breaks up and is lost in the menstrual flow, together with blood released from the damaged capillaries. This blood forms about 50–75% of the menstrual flow.

During the middle part of the menstrual cycle, oestrogen stimulates epithelial cells to multiply and promotes the increased development of capillaries to bring oxygen and nutrients to the newly developing endometrium. Uterine glands also develop to secrete fluid into the uterus, ensuring optimum conditions for survival of the sperm and for implantation of the blastocyst should fertilization occur in the next cycle.

ATHLETICS AND THE CYCLE

Regular and strenuous training can affect the menstrual cycle in a number of ways, none inherently harmful and in some cases quite beneficially. As with many physiological phenomena there is considerable variation between individuals.

- *Delayed onset of menstruation.* Menarche (onset of menstruation) now occurs in the average Western girl when she is about 12 years old. In sports in which early achievement is possible and often encouraged, such as gymnastics and swimming, and in young ballet dancers, menarche is often delayed. There is no evidence that this has any harmful effect on the subsequent reproductive life of the woman.
- *Shortening of the cycle.* The menstrual cycle can be divided into four phases (Figure 8.7): the menstruation phase; the follicular phase; the ovulatory phase; and the luteal phase. Intensive exercise, including high mileage or peak training on the track, can reduce the length of the luteal phase by up to 3–4 days and so, correspondingly, the time between periods.The cause of this effect is not known but it is probably related to changes in the pattern of secretion of the hormones from the pituitary (LH and FSH).
- *Reduction of menstrual pain.* Much of the period pain and discomfort experienced by many women is caused by prostaglandins— 'internal' hormones which increase in concentration as oestrogen and progesterone concentrations fall in the luteal phase. The effect of these decreases in hormone concentrations on the levels of pros-

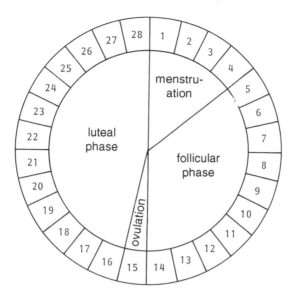

Figure 8.7. The menstrual cycle. In reality, the duration of the phases, especially the luteal phase, may be quite variable

taglandins in the uterus may be smaller after exercise but the mechanism is not known.

- *Reduction of pre-menstrual stress.* The pre-menstrual fall in these steroid hormone levels also causes, in some women, a set of responses, including irritability, depression, tenderness of the breasts, fluid retention and decrease of appetite, known as pre-menstrual stress or tension (PMT). It is tempting to speculate that the increase in concentration of the male sex hormone—testosterone—which occurs after exercise is responsible. Testosterone is secreted by the adrenal glands in the woman and some of the training effects may be due to this hormone. However, high levels may interfere in some of the actions of the female sex hormones, possibly leading to disturbance in the cycle and, in this case, less pre-menstrual stress.
- *Failure to ovulate.* If the normal cycles of changes in hormone levels are large, ovulation may not occur. In itself this is not harmful (unless the woman is trying to become pregnant) but it may be the first indication of overtraining (see Chapter 12)—a possibility that should be taken seriously.
- *Failure to menstruate.* Oligomenorrhoea (infrequent periods) and amenorrhoea (absence of periods for six consecutive months) are the

most dramatic effects of strenuous and regular exercise on the menstrual cycle. Among competitive runners, the prevalence has been reported to be as high as 50%. The precise cause of these changes is not known but it is unlikely that training itself is the sole problem; a diet with too low a carbohydrate content, emotional stress or a viral infection is often a contributory factor. While amenorrhoea is not in itself a serious condition, the associated lowering of oestrogen levels in the blood can reduce the deposition of calcium phosphate in bone. This osteoporosis weakens the bone and leads to an increased risk of bone injury—both stress and complete fractures are more prevalent in female than in male athletes. Indeed there is now serious concern that young female athletes may fail to deposit sufficient calcium phosphate in their bones at this critical stage of their development. Since calcium phosphate is lost from bone normally in the mature female and especially after the menopause, this osteoporosis can therefore become a serious problem in middle age if bone density is already low in the teens and early twenties. This problem may be exacerbated in those female runners who are also suffering from an eating disorder (anorexia or bulimia—see below). Some female athletes in North America have been reported to have bone densities in their spine as low as women in their seventies or eighties. Calcium supplementation, or even hormone replacement therapy, as prescribed by the sports physician, may be necessary. This emphasizes that the athlete, coach and physician should be aware of the problems caused by interference with the cycle—whatever the cause.

So, if athletics affects the menstrual cycle, does the cycle affect athletes? Considering the physiological changes involved, it would be surprising if this were not the case. However, the scientific studies do not produce a consistent answer; some studies indicate a better performance prior to menstruation (luteal phase), some after it and some show no difference. Indeed, of the 107 female Olympic champions in various sports who were interviewed by Ingman in 1953, only 39 athletes claimed their performance was affected during menstruation itself and two that it was improved.

Our knowledge of changes occurring in the menstrual cycle suggests that performance should be optimal either just before or just after the day of ovulation. During peak training, bone, muscles, tendons and joints are subject to intense stress. Changes in hormone levels appear to affect these tissues and there is evidence of an increased number of injuries to athletes during the menstrual period. This suggests that hard, 'quality' interval training is best avoided in the menstruation phase of the cycle and, if possible, for the couple of days preceding this period.

Another strategy is, however, available; by using the contraceptive pill, women can change their menstrual cycle rather than their training schedule. The contraceptive pill consists of a mixture of synthetic steroids that act like natural oestrogen and progesterone; when taken by mouth they mimic the normal changes in the monthly pattern of these hormones, which normally lead to ovulation (Figure 8.5). The higher and more constant levels of these steroid synthetic hormones 'trick' the woman's body into thinking that pregnancy has occurred, so that there are no further ovulations. Typically the pill is taken daily for 21 days followed by a gap of 7 days during which menstruation occurs. Athletes may be prescribed a pill which requires a break for menstruation only after 63 days. Various regimes have been devised to reduce the dose of hormones to minimize any side-effect, whilst maintaining the near 100% efficacy of this form of birth control.

The pill is often prescribed for women who suffer from disabling premenstrual tension or severe blood loss due to unusually heavy periods. Athletes may fall into these categories but, in addition, some may seek to take the pill to avoid the increased risk of injury in the premenstrual period. There is evidence that female soccer players taking the pill suffered fewer injuries during the pre-menstrual phase but, as with many pharmacological modifications of the body's normal physiology, benefits must be weighed against disadvantages and both may vary from individual to individual. This makes research very difficult to carry out.

DISORDERED EATING

For most of us, our appetite regulates our food consumption, so that normal body weight is maintained. Failure of this mechanism usually results in obesity but in some individuals, mostly women, another eating disorder may be the result.

- *Anorexia nervosa*, or self-inflicted starvation, is characterized by a morbid fear of gaining weight, which slumps to at least 15% below that expected for age and height. In extreme cases, starvation may persist until death.
- *Bulimia nervosa*, or binge eating, involves the consumption of enormous quantities of food, generally rich in carbohydrates, at a single sitting. The food is usually consumed in private and is followed by

a feeling of intense guilt and, typically, by self-induced vomiting. This can lead to dental caries, caused by frequent exposure of the teeth to the acidic content of the stomach. This condition is not infrequently preceded by a prolonged period of anorexia nervosa and may represent a different response to similar underlying causes.

Men do suffer from eating disorders but much less frequently than women. Why should this be so? Possibly because the menstrual cycle itself often disturbs eating patterns which are then exacerbated by emotional factors to which women are more prone. The typical anorexic is a bright, overachieving girl in her teens with a compulsive element to her character, although not all sufferers conform to this stereotype. Modern Western culture reveres the slim female form and, for middle- and long-distance runners, gymnasts, ballet dancers and lightweight oarswomen, a lean body with little fat is competitively advantageous. Weight-reducing diets are embarked upon and for some this leads to a total lack of control over body weight. The highest incidence of eating disorders occurs in the range 15–24-years, with studies showing the incidence of eating disorders in young ballet dancers ranging from 7% to 28%. In a study of 93 élite women runners, 37% reported anorexia, bulimia or binge eating.

In addition to the eating disorder, training can become a masochistic extension of the semi-starvation of anorexia nervosa—a punishment for the body in relation to the perceived excess of adipose tissue. The danger of this is the increased risk of injury to the soft tissue, stress fractures of the bone and of overtraining—a risk which may be further increased by the malnutrition.

In this area, above all others, the athlete's own judgement may be faulty and it is essential that some informed person—the coach, the physio or the sports physician—provides the athlete, especially the young female athlete, with appropriate health and dietary advice. It is important for such supporters to be aware of signs that might indicate an eating disorder, including:

- Severe decrease in body weight.
- Wearing loose-fitting clothes.
- Pre-occupation with food.
- Refusal to eat in company.
- Excessive concern over body weight.
- Swings in mood.
- Regular visits to the toilet after meals.
- Frequent criticism of his or her own body.

THE PREGNANT RUNNER

It used to be believed that a woman who ran during pregnancy would 'shake the foetus loose', so women were cajoled into sedentary lifestyles for 9 months for fear of damaging the baby. Then in the 1970s came the running boom in the USA, later spreading to Britain and some other parts of Europe. Many women cast aside their sedentary lifestyles in order to train for local fun races, for competitive races and for marathons. They became fitter and healthier and did not want to give up this lifestyle during pregnancy; a 9-month break from training was unthinkable! The myths and the medical profession stood their ground, however, and would not condone any real exercise during pregnancy and especially not running. A sufficient number of women, both élite athletes and 'everyday' runners, have now run during their pregnancies with no untoward effects on either themselves or their 'bouncing' babies, so that the myths surrounding this topic have been destroyed and the medical profession has been educated.

The need for care and consideration for the foetus is, of course, paramount since excessive training can lead to foetal stress. Nevertheless, for most pregnant women such fears are unfounded and it is now considered that 'sensible' exercise and training programmes involve no risk to the baby and can be beneficial to the pregnant mother, both physiologically and psychologically. For those who wish to exercise or to continue running during their pregnancy, guidelines have been put forward by the American College of Obstetricians (1989) and are summarized in Part II(B).

Since pregnant women need to exercise with care it would seem only right to ask whether they would be better advised to give up running and other exercise during pregnancy. Are there in fact any reasons why she should not stop running altogether for at least 9 months? The answer is that there are benefits to be gained from running during pregnancy, which include:

- Relief of problems normally associated with pregnancy, such as bloating, constipation, morning sickness and varicose veins.
- Reduction of the risk of excessive weight gain.
- Reduction in the length of labour by some 2½ h in the first stage and 20 min in the second stage.
- Improvement of mood.

In a 1981 Melpomene study, more than half of the 195 pregnant women subjects reported that the chief benefit of running while pre-

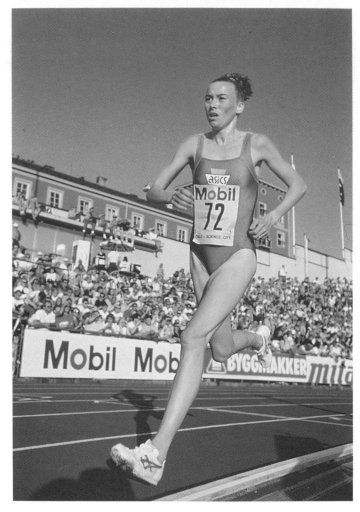

Figure 8.8. Liz McColgan winning the IAAF 5000 m Mobil Grand Prix, Oslo 1992 after giving birth to her daughter. Photograph © ALLSPORT/Mike Powell

gnant related to improved self-image. In another Melpomene study, exercising women were much less likely to suffer post-partum depression than their sedentary counterparts.

> To all of us who stay in good shape, running during pregnancy gives you something that remains in your control while everything else is changing.
> Mary Ellen Ford (a 2 h 51 min 31 s marathoner).

Chapter 9

Theory into Practice

On 6th May 1954 Roger Bannister became the first man ever to run the mile in under 4 min (3 min 59.4 s); his training consisted mainly of 400 m intervals performed each day during his lunch break. Two years earlier, Emil Zatopek won the 5000 m, the 10 000 m and the marathon races at the Helsinki Olympic Games; his daily training included ten 200 m intervals and fifty 400 m intervals in a run totalling 30 km.

These extremes of training are just two examples of the diverse approaches that athletes have used in the past to achieve excellence in their own events. Is it a case of the more training the better or is overtraining possible? To what extent should training be based on the distance over which competition will take place? How does peak training increase performance so dramatically? These are some of the questions that athletes and coaches continually ask, but does science have the answers?

We have to face the fact that it is simply not possible to start with a clean slate and devise a single perfect training scheme from first, i.e. scientific, principles. It may never be possible, or indeed necessary, since experienced runners and their coaches have been devising excellent schedules for a long time (see Part II(A)). Details differ, but they all work. What the scientific approach can do is explain what a given schedule is doing to the body, to fine-tune such schedules and to identify points where slight improvements can be made especially where they are counter-intuitive. Take, for example, the benefit of repetitive short intervals as part of the training programme for the endurance athlete; it is likely that this has a major effect on the aerobic rather than the anaerobic capacity of muscle.

In an ideal world all the benefits proposed for training regimes would have been established by experiment, but satisfactory experiments on people are difficult to do and very time consuming (see Box 13.3). Experimental studies on humans are being done and will, in time, justify (and occasionally, no doubt, contradict) established training approaches. Other scientists make use of laboratory experiments,

Box 9.1   Nature or nurture?

Much blood has been spilled in the debate over whether human attributes are inherited or acquired; can intelligence be improved by education, are homosexuals born that way and can anyone become an Olympic athlete? Most scientists hold the opinion that both nature and nurture make a contribution and would seek ways of separating their influences to establish the contribution of each.

A question frequently investigated by the sports scientist is whether a particular biochemical or physiological attribute affects performance. There are two experimental approaches to such problems: either the scientists can compare the attribute in two groups of subjects, one trained and the other untrained; or they can take one group, measure the attribute, then train the group and measure it again. In the first approach (known as a cross-sectional study) nature and nurture are not being separated; the trained group could have pre-selected themselves as athletes simply because they possessed the attribute and hence succeeded in athletics. In the second approach (known as a longitudinal study) the effect of nurture alone is being assessed, provided that the sample is large (to average out variation) and has been selected at random.

In a study of the first type, biopsy samples were taken from the quadriceps muscle of 12 sedentary and 11 trained men and examined microscopically to establish capillary density and the number of capillaries around each fibre (Figure 7.6). It was found that the trained group had a significantly greater capillary density (Table 9.1). This suggests a greater blood flow through the muscles of those who are trained compared with their sedentary counterparts, although there is other evidence that the increased capillary density leads not to an increase in flow but causes the blood to spend longer in the muscle and so release more oxygen and fuel.

In order to see whether such differences are the *result* of training, it is necessary to compare capillary density before and after training in the same individuals. One difficulty is that of persuading volunteers to part with samples of their muscle not just once but at least twice! When such a study was carried out, using different volunteers, it was found that training increased the capillary density by about 24%. Since the previous study indicated a difference of about 40%, it suggests both nature and nurture play a similar role in improving capillary density in the athletes.

often on non-human animals, which are simpler to carry out, but less easy to apply to human situations. All we can largely do for now is to use scientific understanding to elucidate the principles which underlie time-honoured training methods and try to identify limiting factors so that they might be made less limiting for the performance of our athletes.

Table 9.1. Number of capillaries in quadriceps muscle from sedentary and trained men

Condition	Number of capillaries (average)	
	around each fibre	per square mm of muscle
Sedentary	4.4	585
Trained	5.9	821

From Brodal, P., Ingjer, F. and Hermansen, L. (1977). Capillary supply of skeletal muscle fibres in untrained and endurance trained men. *Am. J. Physiol.*, **232**, H705–H712.

LIMITING FACTORS

Imagine the road which takes commuters from the city of Carchester to the dormitory town of Vanby, crossing the busy A999 and passing through the village of Busford (Figure 9.1). The maximum number of vehicles that can get from Carchester to Vanby is 2000 per hour. If any more than this start the journey only 2000 per hour reach Vanby; the remainder are delayed en route. To increase the flow of traffic engineers might widen the road. This would permit faster driving but

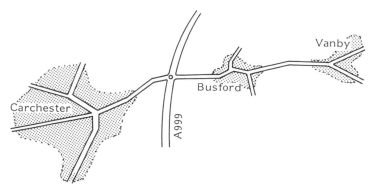

Figure 9.1. Limiting factors on a road journey (see text)

Table 9.2. Some factors which could limit athletic performance under different circumstances

---

Minute volume
Cardiac output
Oxygen transport to muscles
Anaerobic threshold
Size of fuel stores
Rate of fuel mobilization
Capacity for ATP synthesis in muscles
Muscle mass
Rate of fuel uptake by muscles
Rate of end-product removal
Control of fuel utilization
Conservation of blood glucose for brain
Maintenance of body temperature

---

would not increase flow (nor significantly shorten journey time) because congestion at the junction with the A999, and not road width, is the rate-limiting factor, i.e. the slowest step in the sequence and thus the one which determines the rate. There can only be one rate-limiting step at any one time so building a bridge over the A999 will speed traffic until another part of the road becomes rate-limiting—possibly the High Street in Busford.

The same reasoning applies to athletic performance, which depends on a long sequence of metabolic and physiological processes, each of which could be rate limiting (Table 9.2). These processes are so well coordinated that as soon as one is speeded up, another becomes rate limiting. This is why, if you are a 1500 m runner, running 1500 m over and over again is probably the least effective way of training. It will improve all the relevant factors as a set but it will not put maximum stress on each of the potentially rate-limiting processes for the event.

TRAINING FOR ANAEROBIC PERFORMANCE

The factors that affect, and thus limit, the performance of 100 m and 200 m sprinters (and to a large extent 400 m sprinters too) lie largely within the muscle fibres and in the connections, both motor and sensory, between muscle and brain. The main elements of sprint-training are short intervals (together with start-training) performed on the track, weight-training in the gymnasium and hill-training.

Training on the Track

The shortest intervals should be 30–50 m run flat out to facilitate the maximum and synchronous recruitment of fibres. One problem with massive recruitment of all fibres simultaneously is that the resulting force could damage the muscle. This is normally prevented by 'central inhibition', whereby the central nervous system overrides other considerations and prevents maximum recruitment, so limiting the power developed. Training provides 'confidence' that the muscles, tendons, joints and ligaments can handle this amount of power without damage, so that central inhibition is reduced to provide a smaller safety margin.

A second benefit of very short intervals is the training of the control systems that have to increase the rate of glycolysis at least 1000-fold in a matter of seconds. And precision in this control is essential; an understimulation of the rate of glycogen conversion to lactate by just 10% would result in the ATP concentration within the muscle falling to half in 100 m. Performance would undoubtedly suffer and the muscle would be damaged.

Longer intervals, of 100 or 150 m, will improve the use of phosphocreatine, enabling it to be used gradually over the whole distance rather than during the first few seconds. The rest periods between the intervals will allow some resynthesis of this energy reserve. Intervals of up to 300 m, with short rests, will increase the amounts of glycolytic enzymes, improve tolerance to the products of anaerobic metabolism (the protons) and 'smooth the edges' of the physiological and biochemical adaptations to this extreme form of exercise.

It is possible to argue that, for 100 and 200 m sprinters, distances greater than 200–300 m should not be run in training, since these longer distances may increase, or at least maintain, the *aerobic* rather than the *anaerobic* nature of the fibres. It is claimed that aerobic fibres are of no value to the sprinter and, since they take the place of potential anaerobic fibres, they may well be detrimental. On the other hand, it can be argued that some aerobic capacity may help the athlete to withstand prolonged training periods; research is required.

Weight-Training

Weight-training can be performed in two main ways. One is by using large weights with a small number of repetitions (known as heavy weights), while the more popular method uses smaller weights with more repetitions and often only a short rest between each series (weight circuits). The precise effects of these training methods have yet to be fully explored but we do have some indication of what they can achieve.

It is well established, for example, that heavy weight-training increases muscle bulk, on which strength depends. This occurs mainly as a result of an increase in the size of the muscle fibres due to an increase in the number of myofibrils. In addition, the number of mitochondria decreases and their volume is replaced by myofibrils, giving a further boost to strength. What is much more controversial is whether the *number* of fibres, as well as their size, increases. Some experts believe that this number is genetically determined and cannot be changed, while others consider that some increase can occur because fibres can split and then each separate split fibre grows into a new one. It is likely that weight-training will also promote fibre conversions from fast-twitch oxidative to fast-twitch glycolytic; what is much more controversial is whether conversion of slow-twitch to fast-twitch fibres can occur.

Weight-training, particularly training with heavy weights and few repetitions, appears to increase the levels of ATP, phosphocreatine and glycogen in the muscle. The increase in phosphocreatine, in particular, is enormously advantageous for the sprinter. It also increases the cross-sectional area of type IIB fibres, which not only increases the amount of contractile machinery upon which power output depends, but may also increase the buffering capacity in these fibres.

IMPROVING AEROBIC CAPACITY

Various distances are run in training for the middle-distance and endurance athletes. What these various training distances are doing for the limiting processes are summarized in Figure 9.2 and explained below.

Short Intervals (below 400 m)

One important aim of training for events of 400 m and over is to build up aerobic capacity. This involves an increase in the number and volume of mitochondria, an increase in the concentration of enzymes within the mitochondria, an increase in the capillary density and a conversion of some fast-twitch glycolytic fibres into fast-twitch oxidative. At first sight a schedule of *short* intervals, separated by short recovery times, would appear to benefit the anaerobic capacity, but

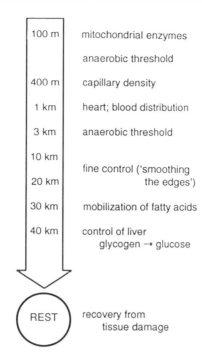

100 m	mitochondrial enzymes
	anaerobic threshold
400 m	capillary density
1 km	heart; blood distribution
3 km	anaerobic threshold
10 km	
	fine control ('smoothing
20 km	the edges')
30 km	mobilization of fatty acids
40 km	control of liver
	glycogen → glucose
REST	recovery from
	tissue damage

Figure 9.2. Training benefits from different distances

Box 9.2   Interval training: the German influence

The first really scientific approach to physical training was developed in Germany during the 1930s by Dr H. Reindell, a cardiologist who used exercise to strengthen the hearts of some of his patients. The aim was to improve the performance of the heart, and careful measurements showed that the most effective method was for the patient to run repetitive short distances with short rest periods between each—precisely what we would now call interval training. During the run, the heart rate reached 170–180 beats/min and fell below 120 beats/min during the rest periods. Reindell showed that this training increased both the size of the heart and the volume of blood expelled by the heart during each beat. He also found a marked increase in the maximum rate at which oxygen could be used by the whole body in such patients. This showed that the beneficial effects of this training

continued

┌─ *continued* ─────────────────────────────────────┐

programme were not restricted to the heart. Indeed subsequent work has shown that the greatest benefit to patients comes not from the effects on the heart itself but from the improved ability of skeletal muscle to use oxygen and fuels from the bloodstream.

In view of Reindell's work it is hardly surprising that it was the German coach Woldemar Gerschler who first systematically applied the interval-training regimes to top-class athletes. Gerschler's star pupil was Rudolf Harbig, who in 1939 took nearly 2 s off the world record for the 800 m (from the British runner Sydney Wooderson). (Harbig's record of 1 min 46.6 s was so good it lasted for 16 years; Roger Moens of Belgium broke this record only in 1955 at the Bislet stadium in Oslo—the stage for so many world records.) Soon afterwards he became the first European to hold the world record for 400 m (46.0 s) but Harbig never lived to see his records broken for, tragically, he was killed in the Second World War. Interval training, however, survived and played its part in setting new world records in the early post-war years. One of the beneficiaries was the British runner Gordon Pirie, who was advised by Gerschler and held world records for 3000 m, 5000 m and 6 miles. Other coaches adopted interval training, among them the Austrian Franz Stampfl and the Hungarian Mihaly Igloi. Stampfl advised both Roger Bannister—the world's first-ever sub-four-minute miler—and Chris Chataway, who briefly held the world record for 5000 m. During the early 1950s many of the middle- and long-distance track running records were held by Hungarians; in 1955 these included world records for 1500 m (Iharos, Rozsavolgyi and Tabori, jointly), 1000 m and 2000 m (Rozsavolgyi), 3000 m, 5000 m and 10000 m (Iharos), and in 1956 Rozsnyoi broke the world record for the 3000 m steeplechase. Although the Hungarian uprising of 1956 put an end to this run of success, Igloi had demonstrated beyond doubt the value of systematic and intensive training and of interval training in particular.

this is the very approach that benefited German middle-distance athletes in the 1930s.

The fact is that improvement of the aerobic system occurs most rapidly and most effectively when muscles are used at, or close to, their maximal aerobic capacity. At such levels of aerobic metabolism, a degree of anaerobic metabolism is inevitable, so lactic acid will build up and soon cause fatigue and restrict the training effect. This is where the intervals come in, since the rest periods allow the lactic acid to be flushed out from the muscle for buffering and removal. To encourage this flushing out of lactic acid, the 'rest' periods must be active, involving perhaps as much as 50% of the effort achieved during the interval. Once this flushing out is achieved, fatigue disappears and the next interval is possible, exerting a similar stress on the aerobic system. In this way the aerobic system is stressed over the entire period of the training session, which may last for 1–2 h.

There is a case for even shorter intervals in aerobic training, at least at the beginning of a training season. In intervals of about 100–150 m, oxygen released from myoglobin in the fibres will supplement that entering from the capillaries, so that the number of capillaries will be less likely to limit aerobic activity, allowing oxygen consumption to be very high for this short period of time. This means that great stress will be put on oxidative pathways in the fibre, with the result that the activities of enzymes in them will increase quickly. The result is aerobic training of the muscle, provided that the intervals are run almost as fast as possible. As the activity of the oxidative enzymes

---

Box 9.3 The surprising fact that short intervals benefit long-distance runners

Scientists get a special buzz from explaining counter-intuitive phenomena: events which on the surface defy common sense but which on further investigation are entirely explicable. A case in point is Per-Olof Åstrand's observation that short interval training (10-second intervals with 20-second rests) raises aerobic capacity within the muscles much more effectively than do longer intervals (1-minute with 2-minute rests). This would only be expected if the short intervals were run more aerobically than the long intervals. Can this be? Indeed it can, due to the presence in muscle of myoglobin, an oxygen-binding protein which provides a small but important store of oxygen. If we assume that only a proportion of the oxygen needed during the intervals can be delivered by the circulation, this leaves a deficit which must be 'made up' by anaerobic metabolism, and the latter will not train the aerobic system. What myoglobin is doing is providing extra oxygen to satisfy this 'deficit' so that the aerobic system can be used to its complete capacity and hence be effectively trained. Since the myoglobin store of oxygen is limited, this effect on the aerobic system will persist only for a short time (Figure 9.3). Hence during these very short

_____ continued __

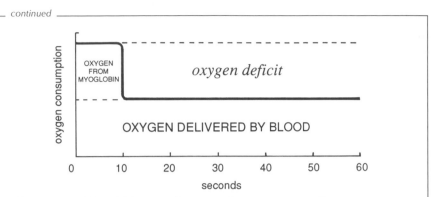

— *continued* —

Figure 9.3. Myoglobin provides a small oxygen store allowing a greater rate of oxygen usage for a short period and hence a greater training of mitochondrial enzymes. From Åstrand, P.-O. (1992). Endurance sports. In *Endurance in Sport*, Vol. II of *Encyclopaedia of Sports Medicine*, pp. 8–15 (eds Shephard, R. J. and Åstrand, P.-O.). Blackwell Scientific Publications, Oxford

intervals, almost all the ATP will be generated from use of oxygen— aerobically, so that performance will be limited by the activity of mitochondrial enzymes which therefore are more likely to be increased by this type of training. Of course, this does not mean that the longer short intervals are of no value, since for these intervals the aerobic capacity of the muscle is limited by the rate at which oxygen can be delivered, so we would expect capillary density to improve in response to this type of training.

increases, longer intervals should then be run to stress the oxygen supply system itself. Intervals of 300–400 m will increase capillary density as well as benefiting the aerobic system within the muscle fibres.

It is likely that these very short intervals will have a particularly beneficial effect on the anaerobic threshold, for the greater the capacity of the aerobic system, the better it will cope with the end-products of the first part of the metabolism of glycogen, including pyruvate. As a result, more pyruvate will enter the Krebs cycle, so less will be converted to lactate (pp. 117).

During this training, the overall aerobic capacity of the muscle should increase dramatically, as evidenced by a decrease in the time taken to run a particular interval. The more fortunate athlete may have access to lactate-measuring facilities and would find that its

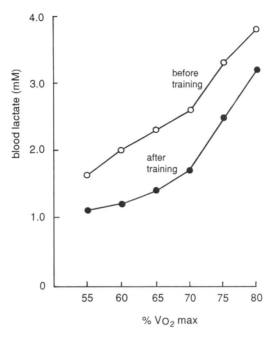

Figure 9.4. When non-athletes were trained their blood lactate levels were lower during exercise. Athletes trained for competition showed even lower levels. From Åstrand, P.-O. (1992). Endurance sports. In *Endurance in Sport*, Vol. II of *Encyclopaedia of Sports Medicine*, pp. 8–15 (eds Shephard, R. J. and Åstrand, P.-O.). Blackwell Scientific Publications, Oxford

concentration in his or her blood after a standard distance run in a fixed time fell as the level of fitness increased (Figure 9.4). The speed of recovery during the rest period is also an indication of improvement; how quickly does the pulse rate decrease to 120 beats/min timed from immediately after the interval has been completed?

Long Intervals (0.5–2 km)

Long-interval training improves three aspects of aerobic metabolism:

- Cardiac output.
- Control of blood distribution.
- Control of the rate of glycogen mobilization in muscle.

Cardiac muscle is highly aerobic and responds to the stresses of long intervals in much the same way that skeletal muscle responds to short intervals, i.e. by increasing the number of mitochondria, the amounts of enzymes within the mitochondria and the capillary density. Intervals are needed because when the heart is working very hard it relies a little more on anaerobic metabolism, and the products of this must be cleared by coronary blood during the gaps between intervals to allow the high workload to be sustained. Again, like skeletal muscle, the heart responds to exercise by enlargement of muscle fibres. This leads to an increased capacity which, together with more complete emptying, results in an increased stroke volume. For the same heart beat frequency, a trained heart can pump from two to three times the amount of blood as that of an untrained heart. Similarly to skeletal muscle, capillary density and mitochondrial volume are increased, ensuring that the aerobic capacity of the heart, which is already high, is even higher.

An increased blood flow to skeletal muscles must be accompanied by a decreased flow to 'less vital' parts of the body, including the intestines and liver. It is likely that the body will err on the side of caution, so that more blood will flow to these organs than is necessary—unless the system has been trained. Training will provide 'confidence' for the control mechanism to allow less blood to flow to these organs (vasoconstriction) and more to the muscle (vasodilation). This confidence is something that cannot be easily measured—only assessed by the performance of the athlete.

To reduce blood supply to the intestines, training (and racing) should be carried out on an empty stomach and the largest meal of the day (which should be the one that contains most protein) should be eaten some time after training has been completed.

The flow of blood to the skin will depend upon the requirement for cooling, which is governed by the rate of heat production in the body and the rate of heat loss from the body. This, in turn, will depend on the ambient temperature; on a warm day more blood must flow to the skin for cooling, so that less blood will be available for the muscles. There is little that can be done to reduce blood flow to the skin except to avoid overheating during exercise by wearing suitable clothing and pouring water over the head and body whenever it is available.

Although long-interval training may actually increase the amount of glycogen that can be stored in a muscle, its real benefit is to train the control mechanisms that regulate the rate of glycogen breakdown according to the demand for ATP. If breakdown is too fast, a valuable resource is wasted; if breakdown is too slow, performance is limited. To optimize glycogen utilization, the long intervals should be run almost as rapidly as possible but without causing total exhaustion, so that several repetitions can be completed in one training session (Part II A). Each interval will use 40 g or more of glycogen, so that at the end of a hard training session little glycogen will be left in the active muscles. Some carbohydrate should be ingested as soon as possible after the exercise has finished and a carbohydrate-rich meal (or meals) is essential before the next training session (see Chapter 11).

Longer Distances (3–20 km)

Running 3–10 km at a pace corresponding to the anaerobic threshold will tell the athlete just how fast he or she can run without the dangers of 'anaerobic fatigue' or rapid depletion of glycogen stores. Some acid production will occur, so that factors affecting its removal from blood will be trained, so improving the anaerobic threshold. Use of the stop-watch will show how well the athlete's body is responding to this training. Longer distances (15–20 km) will have to be run below the anaerobic threshold and should improve the integration of all the aerobic processes.

Very Long Distances (30 km+)

For marathon or ultra-marathon runners only, one long run of 30 km or more should be undertaken at a good pace, once a week. A run of this distance necessitates the use of some fat and so trains the ability of adipose tissue to mobilize fatty acids for oxidation by the muscles. If too much fatty acid is released, more will be oxidized by the muscle, which will then consume more oxygen, which could limit the power output. In addition, it may increase the plasma fatty acid level too much and so induce 'central fatigue' (see pp. 111–112). If too little fatty acid is released, more glycogen will be used and glycogen stores will be depleted prior to the end of the run, so fatigue will rapidly set in. It is necessary, therefore, to train the biochemical process of mobilization of fatty acid from adipose tissue so that it neither under- nor over-responds to the pace of running.

Hill-Training

Like weight-training, hill-training improves recruitment but has the advantage that it is more like normal running, so the 'right' muscles are used and therefore trained. Similar results may be achieved by running on sand. The intensity of the exercise can be varied by using hills of differing gradients, but duration is also important since some fibres will fatigue early and others will then be recruited and hence trained. Jumping up hills can also be beneficial since it increases range of movement and strengthens the body as a whole.

Altitude Training

Living at a high altitude (see Box 7.4) has an effect on the blood similar to blood-doping (Chapter 13). Both manipulations increase the haematocrit but altitude training is legal. Athletes who use this technique usually visit training centres around 1500–2000 m above sea level, where atmospheric pressure is 20% lower, so there is less oxygen in each breath. The body adapts by increasing the number of red blood cells, so that the capacity of the blood to carry oxygen increases, but this change takes some time to occur and many endurance athletes travelled early to Mexico City (2000 m above sea level) for the 1968 Olympic Games hoping they would adapt to the conditions before the events. It is not this straightforward, however, because the maximum exercise capacity is slightly decreased at these altitudes and so the intensity at which the athlete can train is reduced. Consequently, in comparison with the degree of training possible at sea level, some detraining may occur at altitude and negate the effect of the increased haematocrit. It is likely that the timing of altitude training is crucial and the precise time may be different for each athlete. The best time for altitude training would be just before the intensity of training is increased during the peak training programme.

Living and training at altitude for several months can have other effects on the muscle. The diameter of muscle fibres decreases and capillary density increases. The actual number of capillaries may also increase, so that the distance the oxygen has to diffuse from the capillary to the muscle is reduced. Perhaps, in response to this, the activities of the mitochondrial enzymes, and hence the capacity to generate ATP aerobically, increase markedly to raise the anaerobic threshold.

One disadvantageous effect of altitude is a small loss of muscle protein which may limit maximum power output. The final sprint in the 800 m, 1500 m and 5000 m events might well suffer, and timing the return to sea level in an attempt to build up muscle protein might be critical for runners in these events.

Swimming and Pool Running

Swimming has some training advantages—especially for the lower leg and ankle—kicking with flippers on helps the ankle joint. Running can also be done in the pool—either with a buoyancy aid or on the bottom of the pool. Some athletes with carry out interval training in the pool.

ROUNDING OFF

Other Muscles

Even for runners, running is not the only exercise activity of value; alternatives include circuit training, cycling, rowing and cross-country skiing. Machines for cycling, rowing or skiing are now commercially available so that, if necessary, these activities can be performed in the comfort of one's home. They can be considered as relaxation from the track or road running and have the advantage that they avoid the risk of 'impact' damage from the constant pounding. Another benefit is that they train muscles not normally fully used in running and this may be beneficial for at least two reasons:

- These muscles may fatigue more quickly than the 'main muscles' and hence limit the overall performance, particularly at a time in a race when the pace is greater than in training.
- In the very last stages of a race, when the major muscles are fatiguing, a change of gait in running may bring other small groups of muscles into play to provide power for the last few metres.

Flexibility Training

The importance of tendons as elastic stores of energy has become appreciated by athletes as a result of work by scientists such as McNeill Alexander of Leeds University. At each stride much of the energy absorbed as the front leg lands and flexes is not lost as heat but stored (mainly in the Achilles tendon and in the arch of the foot) to assist take-off on the next stride (see p. 61). It should follow from this that athletes with more elastic tendons will run more efficiency and there is some evidence that this is so. When a diverse group of 100 runners were divided into three groups according to 11 measurements of their flexibility, the most flexible group ran significantly more economically at high speeds. More recently, however, some athletes have questioned the value of very elastic tendons. A pogo stick (Figure 3.6) with a very elastic spring would be less effective because it could store less energy. There is clearly an optimum elasticity (or compliance) for tendons, and some coaches claim that too much flexibility slows runners and so do not recommend specific flexibility training.

The real problem is that 'flexibility' comprises a range of attributes, including joint mobility, which are not easily separated. Is it possible to train the elasticity of tendons? Although tendons have only a few cells it is likely that these can be influenced by exercises which place demands on the tendons so that the elastic component may be increased. Hopping and bounding exercises performed on the track or on a trampoline are considered to be most beneficial. Start with about 20 and build up to 100 bounds per session. Bounds are best done in the precompetition period. A word of caution is necessary since they can cause injury; stop if they cause any pain.

TIMING IT RIGHT

For an athlete, rest days are not just time off—they play a positive part in training schedules. Training is effectively 'controlled damage' to the muscles; when they are repaired they work better than before the 'damage'. During each week, at least one day should be devoted to complete rest without any training whatsoever, to allow full repair of this damage. This rest day should fall on the day after the heaviest training session or on the day before competition. It also makes sense to alternate heavy and light days and to vary the training activities so that one set of muscles can be recovering while another is being trained.

The practice of training once a day has become well established. It may well have evolved around a working day but today's athletes often have more time available. Should they train hard once a day, slightly less hard twice a day, or more frequently? What little scientific evidence there is suggests some benefits arise from regularly repeated training sessions during each day. For example, experiments in which muscles in the legs of rabbits were gently stimulated continuously for 24 h a day produced by far the largest increase in aerobic enzyme activities so far reported (Box 9.4). How relevant this is to the runner is less clear but it does support the view that stimulation of muscle as many times a day as possible will produce the largest effects. However, the training periods must be carefully phased to allow sensible carbohydrate-rich meals to be taken during the rest periods to replenish the all-important glycogen stores.

Training Seasons

Not only would it be physically exhausting to maintain maximum training intensity throughout the year, it would also be counter-

Box 9.4   Can rabbits help the runner?

Experiments have shown that for the best athletes the oxidative capacities of their muscles are up to three times greater than those in normal sedentary individuals. Does this represent the maximal benefit that can be obtained from all their hard training? In practice the answer may be yes but experiments on animals suggest that it could be far greater and performance might then also be greater. By stimulating particular muscles of the rabbit to contract and relax repeatedly for 24 hours a day and for several weeks, using a tiny implanted stimulator, dramatic increases in oxidative capacity are observed. A six-fold increase has been observed as measured by increases in the catalytic activities of aerobic enzymes (Figure 9.5).

Although this stimulation type of experiment is hardly feasible for training all of the muscles involved in running in humans, it suggests that the duration of training might be at least as important as the intensity. An athlete, at least an endurance athlete, might gain more from spreading the same training effort over, say, four sessions each day than by condensing it into one or two sessions.

This work on animals also underlines the importance of timing of peak training. Figure 9.5 shows that the elevated aerobic enzyme catalytic activities eventually decrease despite continued stimulation. Since it would be expected that peak performance would coincide with peak enzyme activities, the aerobic performance of such a muscle would be expected to decline after the maximum is reached. Unfortunately, the reason for these decreases in activity despite continual stimulation is not known. If the results of such an experiment are related to training of athletes it suggests that they must experiment with the length of the peak training period to obtain optimal performance.

And there is one final way in which this work could help the runner (at least in old age). As a muscle's oxidative capacity increases it becomes more like heart muscle. Stanley Salmons has obtained evidence to suggest that it might be possible to 'train' by this means some specific skeletal muscles so that they become similar to heart muscle, in particular fatigue resistant. If these muscles were close to the heart the 'treatment' could be of value to a patient suffering from heart failure. With some minimal surgery and plumbing the muscle could be persuaded to act as an auxiliary pump for the flow of blood to reduce the workload on the damaged heart.

productive. The greatest benefits come from steadily increased training effort, peaking during the competitive season, and it is on this basis that the schedules recommended in Part II(A) have been devised. Some of the principal elements for middle-distance and endurance runners are outlined below.

Conditioning

The aim of this base training is to maintain aerobic fitness without any danger of damaging muscles, so the intensity must be much less than during peak training. The athlete should avoid interval training but should run longer sessions (5–15 km) at a pace 20–25% below normal speed in the athletic season.

Pre-competition Training

Both speed and distance can now be gradually increased, so the runner is completing 10–20 km runs at 10–15% below 'peak' speed. Shorter intervals, 150–300 m, plus some longer 1–2 km intervals, can now be included but no more than once a week at first then building up to two sessions a week. Training is best done twice per day, with the long run in the morning.

Competition Training (Peak Training)

The period for peak training probably varies from one athlete to another but is usually 8–12 weeks (typically May–July in the Northern Hemisphere). The more important aspects are:

- Two or three training sessions each day.
- Intervals should be done two or three times per week and should be fast.
- These intervals should include both short and long runs, as well as hill-running and fartlek.

These intervals should be combined with 8–15 km of easy running each morning and 1.5–2.5 km intervals twice a week, and then fast 5, 8, 12 and 16 km runs (80% of the race speed). Each hard day's session should be separated by at least one easy day.

It could take between 3 and 14 weeks for an athlete to reach peak performance; individual variation is considerable. Once the athlete has attained peak performance the time at the peak will also vary, from 1 to 6 weeks. After this short period of time 'at the top', the athlete can drop from a peak performance to being almost physically incapacitated, so each coach must assess for each athlete time to peaking and the duration for peak performance. The characteristics of peaking are:

- During speed-work sessions 'the body surges forward as if by a will of its own'—there is no need to force.
- In the hour following a training session, athletes feel 'supreme vigour'.
- Everyday physical activities, such as climbing stairs, become easier.
- The athlete is increasingly sensitive to everyday situations.
- There may be heightened sexual awareness.

Why should peak performance be short lived? Training improves performance through the sequence:

$$\text{training} \rightarrow \text{stress} \rightarrow \text{damage} \rightarrow \text{repair} \rightarrow \text{improvement}$$

The type of training for peak performance may actually be doing slightly too much damage, but because of the long period of basic and

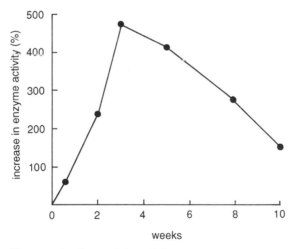

Figure 9.5. Changes in the activity of the enzyme citrate synthase in rabbit anterior tibial muscle stimulated continuously at 10 impulses per second. Similar changes were observed in other oxidative enzymes. From Henriksson, J., Chi, M. M., Hintz, C. S. *et al.* (1986). Chronic stimulation of mammalian muscle: changes in enzymes of six metabolic pathways. *Am. J. Physiol.*, **251**, C614–C632

pre-peaking training, the body can just manage to cope for a limited period. During this response, performance dramatically improves, but eventually too much damage accumulates and the body responds by invoking central fatigue to prevent irreparable damage occurring. Performance therefore declines and, if the signals are not heeded, and the athlete attempts to train harder, overtraining results (Chapter 12).

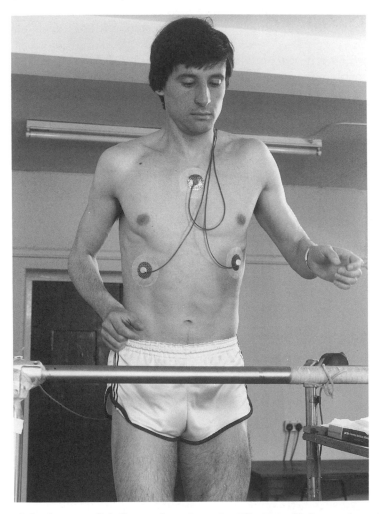

Figure 9.6. A young Seb Coe undergoing scientific tests during peak training in the Department of Sports Sciences, University of Loughborough. Photograph reproduced by kind permission of Professor Clyde Williams, University of Loughborough

Overtraining phenomena have been demonstrated in the laboratory, too. When rabbit leg muscles were stimulated continuously the activities of key enzymes of aerobic metabolism increased for several weeks but then, despite unchanged stimulation, decreased (Figure 9.5). Timing of the peak training is all important.

The athlete has, understandably, a muscle-centred view of his or her body. But muscles can only work effectively if they are supplied with fuel and oxygen, have waste products removed and are properly controlled. Training must improve the functioning of these support processes if the potential in the muscles is to be realized. This is recognized in the modern holistic approach to training in which, for example, dietary and psychological aspects play their part (see Chapters 10 and 11). In some ways, science has made a greater contribution in these areas than it has, so far, to the physical training of the muscles.

Chapter 10

The Mind and Performance

Though physiology may indicate respiratory and circulatory limits to muscular effort, psychological and other factors beyond the ken of physiology set the razor's edge of defeat or victory and determine how close an athlete approaches the absolute limits of performance.

Roger Bannister (1956).

Although it has rarely been expressed so eloquently as by Bannister, few can doubt the importance of correct mental attitude in any human endeavour taken to its limits. Yet only recently (at least, in the West) has the role of psychology in athletics been taken seriously. The situation has not been so different in medicine where, although illnesses of the mind have long been recognized, the part played by the mind in maintaining and restoring physical health is only now being appreciated. This holistic approach to medicine has its parallels in athletic training.

> Multiple regression analysis indicated that a measure of global mood and trait anxiety accounted for 45% of the variance in performance and these results support the concept that performance is associated with positive mental health.
>
> William P. Morgan *et al.* (1988).

When it comes to analysing the mind, and then modifying it, a quite different approach is needed than that appropriate to physiology or biochemistry, because behaviour is much more difficult to dissect into precise processes that can be measured quantitatively. Nonetheless, psychologists are struggling to develop means of describing and assessing human behaviour in an increasingly precise and quantitative way. In this chapter we see how these techniques have been applied to athletics and we try to define what Dr Morgan means by 'positive mental health'.

OUR BEHAVIOUR

At its simplest, behaviour can be analysed in terms of stimuli—changes in our external or internal environment that result in responses or actions. Only in the case of a true reflex does a given stimulus invariably produce the same response; a tap below the kneecap of a bent leg will always cause the lower leg to jerk as the quadriceps muscle contracts. Reflex actions effectively allow the body to cruise on auto-pilot, reacting to stimuli without the need to think. Nonetheless, all except the simplest reflexes can usually be modified when the need arises. For example, sitting on an upturned drawing-pin might well provoke a leap to your feet and a yell—both reflex responses—but an anticipated injection in the same part of your anatomy results in a much less violent response. And most aspects of human behaviour are more like the response to the injection than to that of the drawing-pin, depending upon many factors in addition to the stimulus. Psychologists describe this by saying that a 'belief system' is interposed between stimulus and response (Figure 10.1). The belief system interprets the stimuli according to what is believed by the individual about the situation he or she is in. The belief system, which resides in the brain, involves the interplay of memory and reasoning plus the input from all the senses. The belief system is our 'psychological make-up', which is established by inheritance and moulded by all the environmental inputs ('experiences') we have ever received. It is this moulding which is so important in the present context for it implies that a belief system can be altered, i.e. trained!

As an example of how an athlete's belief system, or psychological make-up, might affect performance, let us consider our athlete as he or she is overtaken in the final lap of a 5000 m race. This is the stimulus: what will be the response? By this stage of the race, the athlete's muscles will be low in fuel, so that extra effort and consequent pain would have to be accepted in a 'fight for the tape'. The under-confident athlete will accept the situation, fail to kick back and, in the absence of a positive response, come second. But if our athlete has trained his or her mind for just this situation and can use the rehearsed mental cues for focusing attention only on the positive approach, the behavioural response should also be positive. This will be aided by a positive physiological approach—the athlete appreciates that preparation for the race has been good, that the pace has been below the anaerobic threshold, that the diet in preparation for the race will have boosted glycogen levels and that glycogen has been conserved during the race. Our athlete believes that an increase in pace

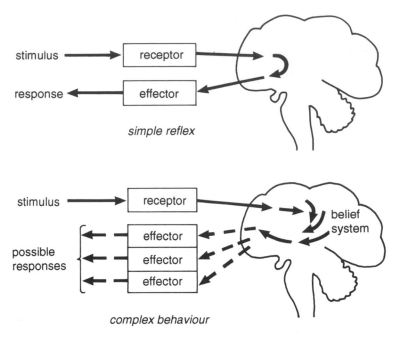

Figure 10.1. From simple reflex to complex behaviour

is not only possible but has been planned for and goes on to win the race! This functional link between physiology and psychology in sport is an area of increasing interest in relation to the stress of competition and providing for optimal performance.

In this chapter we will try to:

- Identify the desirable elements of an athlete's belief system.
- Show how an athlete can assess his or her own psychological make-up.
- Indicate how this might, if necessary, be modified, i.e. how the mind can be trained.
- Interrelate the physiology and psychology of stress.

Further practical details are given in Part II(C).

THE ATHLETE'S MIND

In other chapters of this book there are many statements of the kind: *performance* depends on a *physical parameter*; for example, *time* for the

10 000 m depends partially on $\dot{V}O_{2\ max}$; *anaerobic* performance depends partially on *buffering capacity*; *performance* in the marathon depends on *glycogen stores*. These may be over-simplifications—often small parts of a complex picture—but they provide models which can be tested, quantified and put back into the big picture. Ideally we should now extend this approach to psychological factors. It is not easy, and some might say impossibly difficult, but the approach has already benefited athletes in practice. We have to accept that the model will not be very precise because psychological parameters cannot be dissected out and quantified in the same way as physical ones. One consequence of this is the lack of adequate definitions of terms like stress, anxiety and arousal which would allow them to be used unambiguously.

But we have to start somewhere and a good place seems to be the inverted-U hypothesis first introduced by Yerkes and Dodson in 1908 (Figure 10.2). We have chosen to label the x coordinate 'arousal' and will attempt to describe the term, if not define it, below; others have used the terms 'stress' or 'anxiety'. It is important to note that all we are asking of the model is to describe the relationship; it would be quite another matter to claim that it explains the relationship.

We do not perform well in tasks we 'are not bothered about' because arousal level is too low. This produces the 'it will be alright on the night' phenomenon, because during the actual performance stress will

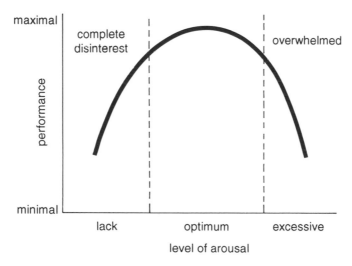

Figure 10.2. The inverted-U model of the relationship between performance and level of arousal

increase the arousal levels and the quality of the acting will rise accordingly. However, it is also possible for too much stress to increase the arousal levels too much, so the performance is poor, or even worse—we 'go to pieces'. So there is an optimum level of this easy-to-appreciate but difficult-to-define characteristic—arousal—at which performance is best. For some individuals, this optimum is a narrow peak from which it is easy to slide in either direction; for others it is broader.

In the athlete, low levels of arousal result in loss of interest in training and even in competition itself. The cause may be actual or impending illness, for example a cold or intestinal upset or, in the female athlete, pre-menstrual tension. Other causes of low arousal may lie outside athletics, emanating from anxieties of many kinds which may be unrelated to sport.

A particular danger of low arousal is positive feedback; performance falls and, as a result, arousal levels diminish further and in turn reduce performance even more. For the dedicated athlete the response might be different. He or she, with difficulty, increases the training effort but this, under certain conditions, can lead to overtraining—with a further decrease in performance as in the situation described above. A low level of arousal is, in fact, an early symptom of overtraining. An important job for the coach, therefore, is to identify the *basic* cause of the problem and take or suggest steps to overcome or remove it.

High arousal is equally detrimental to the athlete; it is, in this sense, synonymous with anxiety. Anxieties are irrational concerns which interfere with normal behaviour and performance. They are best viewed as entirely negative, but just how detrimental will depend on the nature and intensity of the anxiety.

It is now considered by sports psychologists that anxiety can usefully be divided into two components: cognitive anxiety, which is generated in the mind; and somatic anxiety, which is manifest in physiological ways such as increased heart rate, sweating hands and 'butterflies in the stomach'.

Improving the Inverted-U

Models such as the inverted-U are first approximations to be modified as understanding increases. In time, however, a balance must be struck between their accuracy (which often means complexity) and their usefulness.

The most obvious inadequacy of the inverted-U is already clear—

the fact that 'arousal' has a number, perhaps a very large number, of components. This had been apparent from the start; curves with optima usually result from an interacting blend of positive and negative factors. Psychologists accept that the relationship between performance and 'arousal' is multidimensional but such relationships are not easy to depict in graphs.

Another inadequacy of the inverted-U is that although it is justified by subjective experience it does not actually fit too well with the real world. Take an athlete, or anyone else in a stressful situation, and increase the pressure. There may well come a point when he or she 'goes over the top', and when it does the change is not gradual, as the curve would predict, but dramatic. In some contexts we would call it panic; we don't just slow down, we freeze. From this point, recovery is not just a matter of backing off and reversing the curve. The pressure will have to be reduced a long way and for a long time before performance returns to normal. The inverted-U in real life is neither symmetrical nor reversible but has a different shape depending on the direction it is traversed—a property known as hysteresis (Figure 10.3).

Recently the psychologist Lew Hardy has brought these ideas together by applying the mathematics of catastrophe theory to the subject. In catastrophe theory a number of continuously varying functions—and it can be as few as two or many more—interact to produce discontinuities. Hysteretic behaviour is one consequence of

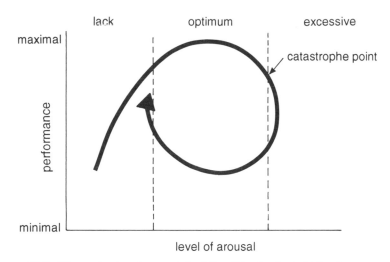

Figure 10.3. The catastrophe model. After Hardy, L. (1990). A catastrophe model of performance in sport. In *Stress and Performance in Sport* pp. 81–106 (Eds. Jones, S.G. and Hardy, L.) Wiley & Sons, Chichester

this. Nonetheless, however good the model, it will be appreciated by athletes if they can make use of it. Perhaps they can. It predicts that a high level of somatic anxiety will have little adverse effect on the athlete unless cognitive anxiety is also high. If cognitive anxiety is high, then a catastrophic fall in performance can be triggered by otherwise fairly harmless rise in somatic anxiety. A vital task of the coach (for the athlete will be too close to 'see') therefore is to identify indicators of high cognitive anxiety and help the athlete to deal with these before they cause a serious problem. Those that can arise for the track athlete include:

- *Distraction.* Concentration diminishes and tactical judgement is impaired. Strategic errors are made and races lost.
- *Avoidance.* The athlete may be worried about failure to reach a particular training goal, e.g. a 400 m interval in 60 s. So it is omitted from the schedules. But the athlete does not actually *forget* about it so the anxiety persists (and increases). Rather than fooling himself or herself, the athlete should, of course, adopt a positive approach and discuss the problem with the coach at an early stage.
- *Extension.* Even when caused by a specific problem, as in the example above, anxiety has a habit of mushrooming and, consequently, affecting all aspects of training.
- *Hypnotic effects.* These may occur when the runner focuses on the problem rather than its cause. If, for example, because of nervous tension, an 800 m runner starts too fast and fatigues early, the runner, overly conscious of this habit, may be quite unable to break it and so starts every race too fast!

If untreated, anxiety can lead to other illnesses, both real and 'imagined', with the latter often more difficult to treat than the former. Performance will deteriorate, training schedules will be broken, and the athlete may even give up the sport.

EXPLAINING AROUSAL

Roger Bannister considered, in 1955, that psychological states are 'totally beyond the ken of physiology' (and presumably biochemistry). This may still be true of cognitive anxiety but there are some areas where useful connections can be made and we can begin to understand how stress can influence performance. It is now just possible to put forward theories to account for some effects of stress in terms of the biochemistry and physiology described in previous chapters. For example, arousal could influence the motor centre of the brain so that, when arousal levels are high, more fibres are recruited, with the result that each individual fibre has less work to do and can obtain more of its energy from aerobic metabolism. Conversely, with low levels of arousal, fewer fibres may be working, so each will be more likely to exceed its anaerobic threshold and depend more on the fatigue-producing anaerobic metabolism. High levels of arousal are associated with a rise in the levels of the stress hormones—adrenaline in the blood, and noradrenaline in the tissues—which help to regulate the precise rate of glycogen degradation necessary to provide energy for the working muscle. Under-stimulation could result in too little glycogen being broken down, so increasing the use of glucose and hence increasing the risk of hypoglycaemia; over-stimulation (over-arousal) could result in too much glycogen breakdown, wasting this fuel and producing excess fatigue-inducing lactic acid.

The stress hormones also promote the mobilization of the fat stores in adipose tissue, increasing fatty acid release and raising the level of fatty acids in the blood. In this way, a high level of arousal could cause too great a rate of fatty acid mobilization and consequent oxidation, which could cause problems for two reasons:

- To generate the same amount of ATP, fatty acid oxidation requires more oxygen than glycogen oxidation. Since it is oxygen supply that limits performance in the middle distances, either the pace must slow or more energy must be provided anaerobically, with the result of early fatigue.
- High blood fatty acid levels increase the plasma level of free tryptophan and this influences the concentration of an important messenger—5-hydroxytryptamine—in the brain, causing central fatigue (see pp. 127–130). It is just possible that part of the effect on the brain of cognitive anxiety is via an increase in the effectiveness of 5-hydroxytryptamine. This then would be one mechanism by which cognitive and somatic anxiety could interact to cause a very large increase in the effectiveness of this messenger within the brain, the result then being a marked fall in performance.

The balance between under-stimulation and over-stimulation, essential for optimal performance, may be difficult to judge, especially as it may vary from athlete to athlete, and be quite narrow. The assessment of the psychological profile of an individual athlete can play an important part in attempting to achieve this balance.

FINDING OUT ABOUT ME

The first step in improving your mental approach to athletic competition is to discover your strengths and weaknesses. In one respect, psychological testing is simpler than physiological testing; it does not need complex instrumentation. This fact opens the way to self-assessment, and a variety of tests are available, including POMS (Profile of Mood States), SCAT (Sports Competition Anxiety Test) and SERP (Sport Emotional-Reaction Profile). In each, the complexities of personality are identified from a list of characteristics which are numerous enough to cover all important aspects but few enough to be handled practically. One of these (SERP) is described in more detail below, and instructions on how to determine your own SERP are presented in Part II. The advantage of this knowledge is that the training of the mind can be directed towards improving those traits

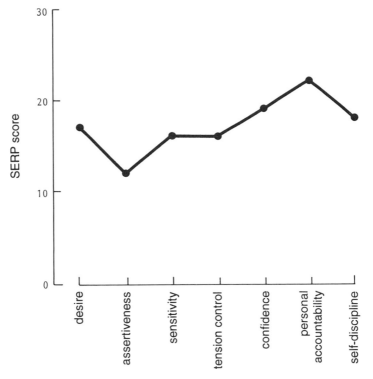

Figure 10.4. An example of a Sport Emotional-Reaction Profile. From Tutko, T. and Tosi, U. (1978) *Sports Psyching: Playing Your Best Game all the Time.* Tarcher, Los Angeles

which may be sufficiently abnormal to influence performance. But a word of warning; there is no ideal value for any psychological trait. Profiles only serve to indicate areas where an individual deviates markedly from those of successful athletes in general and where some remedial attention might prove beneficial.

The SERP was devised by Thomas Tutko and Umberto Tosi, and we have taken our approach from their book *Sports Psyching* (1978). The test involves answering (honestly) 42 questions (reproduced on p. 354) with one of the responses:

almost always/often/sometimes/seldom/almost never

Half the questions are positive in the sense that an 'almost always' answer scores highest, and half are negative. Analysis involves grouping the questions into seven categories representing seven psychological characteristics important in competition. The SERP is then the scores for each of these seven characteristics presented graphically (Figure 10.4). The 'normal' range for each trait is within the range 10–25; scores higher or lower than this could indicate problems, which are elaborated below under the headings of the seven psychological traits comprising the SERP in Part II(C).

ARE ATHLETES DIFFERENT?

Are athletes different from the normal population? The answer is a qualified yes. Just as particular physiological and biochemical characteristics are characteristic of élite athletes, so too are psychological traits. The use of the SERP cannot provide a comparison as it is not readily applicable to non-athletes, but the POMS is and has provided some interesting results. In this test, the prevailing mood of the subject is scored under six headings—*tension, depression/dejection, anger/ hostility, vigour/activity, fatigue/inertia* and *confusion/bewilderment*— on the bases of the response to a series of words or phrases which include unhappy, tense, careless, listless, cheerful, inability to concentrate, etc. For each of these, the subject expresses how he or she felt over the previous week, the previous few days, the previous day or right now, using the responses:

not at all/a little/moderately/quite a lot/extremely

The interesting result from studies, carried out by Dr W. P. Morgan of the University of Wisconsin, is that athletes have a distinctive

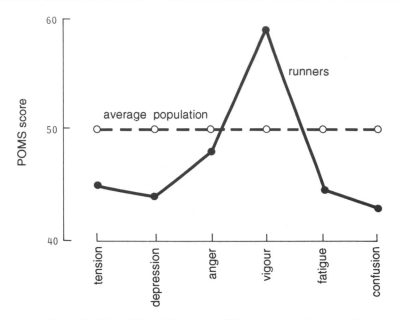

Figure 10.5. A Profile of Mood State for élite runners, showing the 'iceberg' profile characteristic of athletes. From Morgan, W.P. (1980). Test of the champions: the iceberg profile *Psychol. Today* 6th July, 92–108

POMS profile. Athletes score below average for tension, depression, fatigue and confusion, they score about average for anger, and they score well above average for vigour. When presented as a graph, the characteristic shape of the profile for athletes has given rise to the term 'iceberg' profile (Figure 10.5). Iceberg profiles are characteristic not only of runners but of other athletes, including rowers and wrestlers. Furthermore, the more élite the athlete, the more pronounced the 'iceberg'. Interestingly, the 'iceberg' profile becomes inverted in overtrained athletes, and the POMS test may be one of the best indicators of the overtrained state. Unfortunately, once the profile is disturbed it takes longer for athletes than non-athletes to restore it.

TRAINING TECHNIQUES

Behavioural modification has a long, and not entirely savoury, history. Its clinical benefit in correcting psychological problems is considerable but it has a darker side, exemplified by brainwashing. The fact is that it works; training the mind is possible. Indeed, those involved with the

Box 10.1 The mentality of success

The most direct way of finding out which mental attributes lead to athletic success is to ask successful athletes. Dr Brent Rushall did precisely that and came up with a list of important mental attributes for élite athletes. These are given below with our comments.

- *The ability to concentrate totally throughout the training period on the one major competition.*
  Concentration on a specific competition enables the coach and athlete to achieve peak physical and mental fitness for a particular event. There may well be a peak in fitness even when training is maintained or decreased, so that timing is of paramount importance. And timing may be different for different athletes.
- *The ability to put more effort and intensity into competition than into training.*
  Intensive training immediately before a competition will be counter-productive. A 'rest and repair' period of between 2 and 4 days (and in some cases even longer) before the event is needed. During this time, control of arousal levels by relaxation techniques and mental rehearsal rather than physical preparation should enable performance in competition to exceed that in training.
- *Confidence to perform up to expectation.*
- *The ability to judge accurately performance in competition.*
  Confidence comes from the knowledge that you have done everything right—training, peaking, rest, diet and mental approach—and knowing that you are not overtrained by careful measurements and diaries. Understanding what is happening to the body helps a great deal in training and competition and it should provide a great boost to confidence. Getting the pace right is vital; too rapid a start and anaerobic metabolism builds up problems which cannot be resolved at race speed. Only through appropriate training will the runner develop an accurate judgement of time and distance.
- *A detailed competitive strategy is prepared and learnt.*
- *The strategy includes what to do if things go wrong.*
- *Before competition, it is important to perform as many mental rehearsals of the event as is possible.*
  Strategy wins races but it must be the right one, it must be applied in 'the heat of the moment' and it must be amended if circumstances change. Applying the strategy involves extensive pre-race

continued

continued

mental rehearsals to avoid anxiety-making indecision during the race. Being able to modify the strategy involves not only the interpretation of the behaviour of other competitors but also the correct interpretation of metabolism and physiological signals that the athlete receives from his or her own body during the race.

- *Small distractions or problems that arise before competition do not upset the athlete.*
- *Knowledge of what to do to regain composure if lost prior to competition.*
- *Knowledge of how to overcome excessive excitement prior to competition.*
- *Knowledge of how to regain confidence if lost.*
- *Unfamiliar competitive arenas do not disturb the athlete.*
- *Ability to handle any unusual circumstance or distraction.*
  Being able to relax prior to and during the race prevents levels of stress hormones increasing too much and disturbing the balance between fat and carbohydrate metabolism, to the detriment of performance.
- *Other competitors do not worry the athlete before competition.*
  The best way of ignoring other competitors is to make sure you are well prepared and know how to relax and yet concentrate on the event.
- *Some athletes prefer to be alone immediately before competition and prefer to warm-up alone.*
  Warming up is a technique in itself which requires a rehearsed strategy and a minimum of interference. But if the athlete feels the presence of the coach is important, he or she should be there. Remember a short period of complete rest (10–15 min), after warm-up and before the event may be very important for some athletes.
- *Controlled levels of nervousness and tension at the start of the competition.*
  Keeping a low level of stress hormones is important for most athletes although less so for the sprinter.

It is interesting to note that many of these points were followed by Roger Bannister in his preparation for the attempt on the four-minute mile barrier in 1954. He trained minimally, so avoided overtraining; he had 5 days rest prior to the event; he decreased tension on the day by working and by visiting friends in Oxford; his coach was present on the day to provide confidence and even to order Bannister to relax

continued

continued

during the race. In contrast, in the 1952 Helsinki Olympic marathon, Jim Peters was beaten by Zatopek despite the fact that Peters had, 6 weeks before, broken the world record by more than 4½ min (2 h 20 min 42 s) and, prior to the marathon, Zatopek had raced in the 5 and 10 km races and won them! The British team had to travel to Helsinki not on a scheduled flight but on an old four-engine transport plane. The flight took 9 h and during the flight the plane was struck by lightning. Peters arrived feeling sick, stiff and with a headache—hardly a state to provide confidence or allow relaxation prior to his big event!

training of athletes from the former Eastern bloc countries have long recognized its potential. Sports psyching, as it is sometimes known, is both an art and a science but increasingly more of the latter; it certainly involves much more than a 'pep' talk given by the coach just before an event. To be effective, it must start early in the life of an athlete and be continued throughout his or her athletic career.

Most psychological training is directed toward adjusting the level of arousal to bring it into the 'zone of optimal functioning' and above all to prevent the catastrophe point being reached (Figure 10.3). Different sports benefit from different levels of arousal; for power and contact sports the levels need to be much higher than, for example, rifle shooting, where fine motor control is paramount.

One way of preventing arousal from reaching catastrophe point is to make use of relaxation and concentration training. These decrease the effect of stress either by training the individual to cope with it or to ignore stress-promoting stimuli, and they include *stress inoculation training, psychological stress management* and *cognitive behaviour therapy.*

Techniques devised to increase relaxation, including yoga, meditation and self-hypnosis, share a number of common elements. The first element is slow and controlled deep breathing, which itself reduces heart rate and blood pressure. Second is mental concentration, usually involving the elimination of extraneous (and disturbing) thoughts by concentration on a single word or part of the body. The third element is that of physical isolation from environmental distractions, achieved by assuming specific postures (as in yoga) and by putting aside a special time, usually at least 15–20 min, for relaxation. The techniques with the most appeal to athletes are probably those developed by

Jacobsen, in which successive muscle groups around the body are first tensed and then relaxed. Further details are given in Part II(C).

Learning to focus attention on essentials is achieved through concentration training, also described in Part II(C). The ability to ignore what is going on around and to concentrate on the task in hand is of enormous benefit in most of life's endeavours but especially in sport. In a competition, however, this presents severe problems. First, there are the normal distractions of any competition; secondly there are the 'one-upmanship' ploys by other competitors, with distracting rumours of remarkable training times; and thirdly there is the anxiety of performing well after all the hard work of the training and the work of the coach. With concentration training, the athlete should be able to switch off from the distractions and concentrate on the job in hand. The athlete's thoughts are directed along 'associative' lines, related to performance at that instant, rather than 'dissociative' lines which have nothing directly to do with the athletic endeavour in progress. This is effectively the acquisition of 'mental blinkers'—as important during training as they are during competition in order to establish concentration as a habit. Of course, care must be taken to ensure that the focusing is wide enough to include all relevant aspects; the runner concentrating on the tape must be aware of those behind.

Another means of focusing on essentials is mental rehearsal—planning ahead what should be done in any situation. It is as important in other aspects of life and may increase the chance of survival in an aircraft accident as much as that of winning the championship. The athlete must repeatedly go over, in his or her mind, all the details of an event, from warming-up to crossing the line. The rehearsal must include not only positive aspects but also what it will feel like to be overtaken in a race, to hear stories of new unofficial records before the competition and to cross the line fast—first in slow motion, then faster and faster until the mental rehearsal occurs at race speed. This can be done almost anywhere, in an armchair, stuck in a traffic jam or while waiting at the airport. Mental rehearsal is a psychological trick that allows you to take what you would *most like to do* and turn it into what you *will most likely do*.

The most important thing to remember is that psychological training takes time and is best integrated with physiological training. And just as our basic physiological and biochemical characteristics are determined genetically, so too are our basic psychological characteristics. We cannot choose our parents but we can make the best of what they have given us!

Chapter 11

Food for Fitness

*An animal diet alone is prescribed and beef and mutton are preferred ...
the legs of the fowl are highly esteemed ... biscuits and stale bread are
the only preparations of vegetable matter which are permitted.*
A. R. Downer, Scottish AAA 100, 220 and 440 yd champion, 1883, 1884
and 1885.

*Runners are now realizing the importance of nutrition. You shouldn't
become obsessed by it however, especially in the age of the professional
runner when everyone is looking for ways of improving performance. Your
diet is important but it should be looked at sensibly.*
Dr Sarah Rowell (marathon best of 2 h 28 min 6 s in London Marathon,
1985).

*Under normal circumstances, athletic performance improves as an athle-
te's state of training improves. However, it is sometimes observed that
athletic performance deteriorates even when indices of the state of training
are improved or unchanged. On the other hand, training capacity sometimes deteriorates without explanation. There are many theories about the
mechanisms underlying this deterioration in training and performance.
One of these theories is that the decreased performance is caused by an
acute depletion or chronic reduction in the bodily carbohydrate reserves.*
W. M. Sherman and G. S. Wimer

Athletes have always been concerned about their diet and there has
never been a shortage of advice. Food is something upon which we all
have an opinion, but what do the food scientists say? For many years
they have worked to establish the minimum requirements of the
different food components needed to sustain a healthy life. Such
studies are not easy. For example, feeding humans on synthetic diets
for any length of time is neither feasible nor ethical. And every
mouthful of real food contains hundreds of chemicals, each of which
may have a different nutritional effect. Furthermore, individuals will
differ in their requirements—and think how long it would take to
show whether cod-liver oil, taken as a child, reduced the incidence of
heart attacks in old age.

Box 11.1   Food of the gods

The Ancient Greek diet was an inherently sound one for the athlete, consisting mainly of fish (fresh and dried), bread, fruit (especially figs, grapes and dates), thick vegetable soups and a variety of cakes sweetened with honey (a modern-day equivalent is paklava). Olive oil was used in cooking, and wine, watered down, was the main beverage. The Greeks were not vegetarians but ate meat only on special occasions. Provided that the athlete could obtain enough of this food, especially the carbohydrate-rich components, his performance should not have been limited by diet. Ancient athletes, however, were just as likely to have had food fads as their present-day counterparts, as Harris, in his book on Greek athletics, informs us:

> There are, of course, reasons why an athlete must be careful about his food. Xenophon hints at this when he says that the man in training should avoid bread, clearly the Greeks knew the danger of too much starch.

From this statement, it appears that the author, writing in 1972, knew as little about the relationship between nutrition and exercise performance as did Xenophon writing nearly 2500 years earlier.

Surprisingly, it is only in recent years that a high-carbohydrate diet for athletic performance has been generally recommended. Fortunately, it would be just as likely that the depletion of muscle glycogen produced by an arduous training session in Ancient Greece would have produced the same craving for sweet foods in the ancient athlete as it does in modern-day athletes. If sweet foods were available, no doubt they would have been eaten, ensuring repletion of muscle glycogen and ability to train or compete effectively on the next day.

There are many references in Greek literature to the amount of food eaten by athletes, widely held to be too much. Galen, born in AD 180, writes:

> Neglecting the old advice of moderation in all things they spend their time over-exercising, in over-eating and over-sleeping like pigs.

Moderation in all things remains good advice to the athlete two millennia later—all things, that is, except for dietary carbohydrate.

Despite the difficulties, recommended dietary allowances (RDAs) for all nutrients have now been established for men, women and children. One problem is that they are slightly different for different countries since they are based on different experimental studies. But what about athletes? Little research has been done, but the common-sense approach is for the athlete to add on to general well-founded dietary advice the special requirements suggested by an understanding of the body's demands during intense periods of training and its needs during competition.

To complicate dietary considerations further, it is increasingly recognized that many diseases are exacerbated, and some would say caused, by a poorly balanced diet. In other words, a diet that contains enough of each individual component and lacks anything specifically harmful can still be unhealthy. Add to this the vested interests of food manufacturers and no wonder the general public—some athletes included—are confused about diet. So where do we start in an attempt to clarify the issue? A good place would be the report by the National Advisory Committee on Nutrition Education (NACNE) which was published in 1983 and which made five recommendations for healthy eating. We can then go on to consider how these recommendations might be modified for the special needs of athletes.

The NACNE recommendations are:

- No more than 30% of energy should come from fats.
- A high proportion of these should be unsaturated.
- Carbohydrate, preferably complex, should form 50–60% of the energy intake.
- Fibre intake should be higher.
- Salt intake should be moderate.

Even this short list indicates complexities; there are fats and fats, carbohydrates and carbohydrates, and, as we shall see, even proteins and proteins. There is no way around it—the athlete who wishes to be nutritionally informed has to know a little food chemistry in order to select the best foods for training and competition.

THE CARBOHYDRATES: SIMPLE AND COMPLEX

Carbohydrate is the collective term for both sugars and polysaccharides, which, despite their chemical relationship, have somewhat different dietary roles. Sugars are soluble and sweet. The most important sugar for the athlete to know something about is glucose, which is transported in the blood as a fuel for the tissues of the body. To fulfil this role, its concentration has to be maintained between fairly narrow limits. Relatively little glucose occurs in a natural diet, although it is present in fruits and honey and in some commercially available soft drinks. On average we consume about 16 g of glucose per day (Table 11.1). Much, much more glucose is, however, present in polymerized form in starch (see below).

Glucose is a monosaccharide—a single-unit sugar. Much more abundant in the diet are the disaccharide sugars, in which two simple sugar units are joined together. Disaccharides are also sweet and soluble, especially sucrose—a chemical association of glucose and fructose (a variant of glucose which also occurs free in honey and fruit). Sucrose is table sugar which is obtained either from sugar-cane or sugar-beet, in which it serves as a fuel store. It forms nearly 30% of the average daily intake of carbohydrate in Western man (Table 11.1). A second disaccharide, lactose—this time a combination of glucose and galactose—is the sugar present in milk.

Polysaccharides—the complex carbohydrates—are composed of monosaccharide units (mostly glucose) linked chemically into long, often very long chains. The main component of starch—the storage fuel of many plants and the most abundant complex carbohydrate in the diet—consists of chains containing over 5000 glucose units, which are linked end to end. A second component of starch is a branched polymer of glucose, much more like glycogen in molecular structure (see p. 73). Despite its similarity to glycogen, it still has to be digested to glucose in the intestine before it is absorbed into the body. Indeed all polysaccharides and all disaccharides must be hydrolysed to the monosaccharides before they can pass into the blood from the intestines and be put to use (Figure 11.1). This digestion means in general that glucose enters the body more slowly from polysaccharides than it would if free in the food. Just how fast depends on the type of food and how it has been cooked.

A rather different group of polysaccharides has hit the dietary headlines in recent years, namely those present in fibre. These are the complex carbohydrates that are not well digested in the human small intestine and do not contribute much to the energy of the body. Interest in fibre stems from the good correlation between a high-fibre diet and good health because fibre:

- Adds bulk to food, so promoting satiation and reducing the likelihood of overeating.

Table 11.1. Sugars and starch intake in various food by individuals in Britain. This is based on food recorded in the National Food Survey in 1987

	Intake (g per person per day)				
Total	Sucrose 57.2	Glucose 13.2	Fructose 10.4	Lactose 16.9	Starch 141.1

Food recorded in National Food Survey

	Sucrose	Glucose	Fructose	Lactose	Starch
Table sugar	31.8	0	0	0	0
Milk, cheese	0.8	0.2	0.1	15.5	0.1
Meat, fish	0.1	0.1	0	0.1	5.4
Potatoes	0.6	0.4	0.3	0	19.2
Fresh and processed vegetables	2.8	1.4	1.2	0	10.5
Fruit and fruit products	5.2	4.3	5.5	0	0.4
Bread and flour	0.7	2.5	0.2	0	67.0
Cakes, biscuits and cereal products	10.8	1.2	0.9	0.6	36.6
Other foods	4.4	3.1	2.2	0.7	1.9
Additional foods					
Chocolate and sugar confectionery	16.1	2.1	0.3	1.2	0
Alcoholic drinks	0.1	1.0	0.4	0	0
Totals	73.4	16.3	11.1	18.1	141.1

A total of 7.1 g other sugars, mainly galactose and maltose, were consumed each day.
From Lewis, J. and Buss, D. H. (1990). Intakes of individual sugars in Britain. *Proc. Nutr. Soc.*, **49**, 58A.

- Increases the retention of water in the faeces, keeping them soft and reducing the danger of bowel damage.
- Improves the elimination of certain toxic substances from the large intestine.

A further benefit of fibre may be that it provides nutrients for the cells lining the large intestine and improves their function. This possibility arises because bacteria in the large intestine do, in part, digest fibre and the products of digestion are used by the cells of the large intestine.

Plant products are generally high in fibre, unless this has been processed out, as with white flour. Some fibre, such as the very abundant cellulose, is only moderately good at bringing about the benefits. Rather better are the pectins and gums—not truly fibrous but nevertheless non-digestible—which are present in most fruits. The down-side of a high-fibre diet is that it can reduce the absorption of important nutrients, especially minerals (see below); bran, which is often added to foods to improve their fibre content, has a particularly bad reputation for this. Fibre will also decrease the amount of digestible carbohydrate in the diet which will restrict repletion of the glycogen stores. Fibre intake therefore should be kept to a minimum during intense training periods and prior to competition.

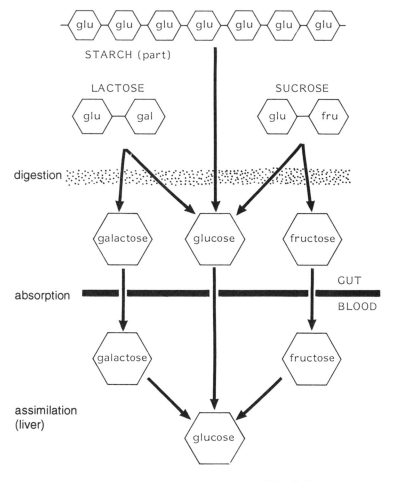

Figure 11.1. The dietary origins of blood glucose

The rationale behind advising the general public to eat more carbohydrate is that they will, as a result, eat less fat. This is deemed beneficial because a high-fat diet is a factor in the development of some of the more prevalent modern diseases, such as heart disease and obesity. Complex carbohydrates rather than sugars are recommended because of the propensity for the latter to promote tooth decay and because the large-scale ingestion produces undesirably rapid increases in blood glucose level. It is now appreciated that some complex carbohydrate in the diet, if cooked in certain ways, can also cause rapid elevation of blood glucose levels and can also promote tooth decay! This then emphasizes the importance of dental hygiene (brushing teeth frequently) and exercise, which helps to prevent large increases in the blood glucose level.

WHAT ABOUT THE ATHLETE?

The level of glycogen in the muscles is critically important for all athletes who run distances from 800 m upwards. It is moreover important for all athletes during hard training sessions when, for example, many sprints may be performed coupled with workouts with weights, etc. For middle-distance runners, the greater the glycogen store the greater the amount of fuel-depleting but oxygen-saving and ATP-producing anaerobic metabolism that can be allowed. In longer-distance events, a large muscle glycogen store prevents the runner, in the last stages of a race, from relying too heavily on fat as a fuel, which cannot provide energy for the muscle at the same rate as carbohydrate (p. 111).

Glucose, once it enters the bloodstream from whatever source, is preferentially directed towards filling the glycogen stores in muscle. This is particularly so soon after the stores have been decreased or emptied by training or competition (Figure 11.2). For 2–3 h after exercise, fatty acids are made available in the bloodstream and these, at rest, provide a fuel for most tissues, so that virtually all the glucose that enters the body is available for storage in muscle as glycogen. What is more, if the stores can be filled rapidly, the amount of glycogen that is actually stored may be increased above normal levels.

So how should the athlete go about replenishing his or her muscle glycogen after a long-distance run or a heavy training session? The problem is that many tempting convenience snacks (e.g. crisps, biscuits, cake, chocolate, ice-cream) are actually richer in fats than carbohydrates. And this may be a particular problem for the endur-

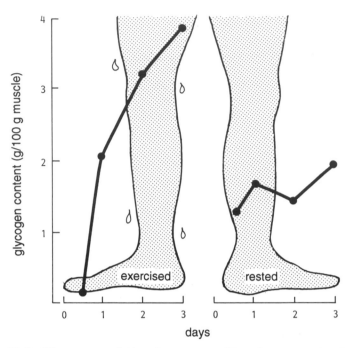

Figure 11.2. Glycogen repletion is more rapid and more extensive after exercise. In this experiment, subjects exercise one leg, but not the other, to exhaustion on a cycle ergometer. During the next few days the subjects consumed a high-carbohydrate diet and glycogen levels were measured in the quadriceps muscles of both legs (Bergström, J. and Hultman, E. 1966). The effect of exercise on muscle glycogen and electrolytes in normals. *Scand. J. Clin. Invest.* **18**, 16–20

ance athlete since recent evidence suggests that 30–35% of his or her daily energy intake arises from snacks. Not only do snacks provide only a small amount of carbohydrate but fats actually slow down digestion and absorption of carbohydrates, so that much of the glucose may enter the body late, missing the optimal post-exercise period for glycogen synthesis in the muscle. One solution to the problem is to consume carbohydrate-rich drinks which can be bought ready made. Some of the latter contain polymers of glucose which are broken down gradually over the whole two hour optimal period for glycogen synthesis immediately after exercise has finished. This may encourage more of the glucose that enters the body to be converted into muscle glycogen, but athletes need to be less worried than others about the dangers of excessive blood glucose 'highs' from ingesting large quantities of simple sugars since, with extreme glycogen depletion after heavy training sessions, resynthesis will take place so rapidly that the blood glucose level will not remain elevated for long.

It has been suggested that one way of satisfying the need for large amounts of carbohydrate without excessively elevating blood glucose levels is for the athlete to take fructose. This is a naturally occurring component of sucrose which is converted to glycogen in the liver without appearing as blood glucose. It looks like a good idea but a note of caution must be sounded. Fructose might be 'natural' but large quantities are not. Large-scale metabolism of fructose by the liver is known to deplete ATP levels in that organ and to produce a serious energy deficit which can damage the liver. Too much fructose or, indeed, too much sucrose, is probably best avoided.

Ideally, what is needed after training is a simple-to-prepare snack which is rich in carbohydrates and low in fats, such as a large bowl of cornflakes (or any other refined cereal) moistened either with skimmed milk or with the syrup from a can of fruit. The fruit itself will provide fibre, more carbohydrates and plenty of potassium to replace that lost during training. This can be washed down with a carbohydrate-rich drink. All this can be packed into the training bag with the rest of the kit, but don't forget the tin-opener! Post-exercise glycogen replenishment must be seen as an essential aspect of training, not a luxury to be indulged in if time allows.

So the athlete in training need not be shy of simple sugars and should benefit from them as a means of raising the total carbohydrate ingested to provide at least 60% of his or her energy requirements. This is probably sufficient for all but the most exceptional requirements. However, on the basis of studies of energy expenditure at levels experienced by top-class cyclists in, for example, the Tour de France race, Dr Fred Brouns recommends that a massive 80% of the energy content of the diet should be carbohydrate in order to permit adequate glycogen resynthesis (Table 11.2). To prepare and eat such a high-carbohydrate energy intake, providing 17 mJ per day, means eating 600 g digestible carbohydrate—almost twice that in a normal diet. Note that this is 600 g of pure, dry, carbohydrate, not 600 g of carbohydrate-containing food. The proportion of the energy provided by carbohydrates and other dietary components in some commonly eaten foods is given in Table 11.3, and suggestions for preparing carbohydrate-rich meals are offered in Part II.

It should be appreciated that just as proper training for competition is not easy, neither is proper eating. The difficulties of a very high

Table 11.2. Matching energy intake and expenditure in Tour de France cyclists

After two days spent acclimatizing in a large calorimeter each cyclist was allowed unlimited food and drink on demand and encouraged to eat as much as possible, especially carbohydrate. Day 3 was spent resting and, as expected, food intake exceeding energy expended. On days 4 and 5 the volunteers exercised on a cycle ergometer at levels corresponding to Tour de France cycling. On these days they consumed substantially less than they expended—7500 kJ, nearly as much as a normal female consumes in a day—and drew upon their fat reserves. These were partly repleted during a subsequent day of rest. In a separate experiment, it was found that the energy intake to match expenditure could only be maintained if drinks containing carbohydrate were taken frequently by the cyclists in addition to the normal high-carbohydrate meals and snacks.

Day of experiment	Condition of subject	Energy (kJ/day)		Difference (kJ/day)
		Intake	Expenditure	
3	Rested	19 400	16 100	+3300
4	Exercised	19 300	26 800	−7500
5	Exercised	19 500	25 200	−5700
6	Rested	21 200	16 100	+5100

From Brouns, F. (1991). Effect of diet manipulation on substrate availability and metabolism in trained cyclists. *Biochem. Soc. Trans.*, **19**, 363–367.

carbohydrate diet are considerable:

- The large bulk required may cause abdominal extension and interfere with subsequent exercise.
- Essential protein may be displaced from the diet.
- An intensive training programme may not leave enough time for preparation, consumption and digestion of such large amounts of carbohydrate-rich food.
- Unless carefully planned and prepared, a high-carbohydrate meal may not be very palatable.

In order to consume such large amounts of carbohydrate, carbohydrate-containing drinks must be taken together with the kind of high-carbohydrate meals and snacks suggested in Part II.

There is just one situation where an athlete ought not to consume carbohydrate—immediately before a race. Sugars are only 'instant' energy for the brain; muscles get almost all of their energy from glycogen and it takes several hours for ingested glucose to be assimilated into this store. The problem with sugars before a race is that they may increase the level of insulin in the blood, which can then decrease the rate of glycogen breakdown (and lower the blood glucose concentration), hence interfering with the metabolism of the major fuel for muscle.

In contrast, for the marathon runner, and particularly for the ultra-marathon runner, sugar-containing drinks are advantageous during the race. For the non-élite marathon runner, taking glucose- or carbohydrate-containing drinks during the race may help to conserve the muscle glycogen for the whole of the race but is more likely to restrict the mobilization of fatty acids from adipose tissue, so that muscle uses only carbohydrate-based fuels. This is advantageous for two reasons:

- Oxidation of fatty acid requires more oxygen to produce the same amount of ATP, so that it is less 'efficient' on the basis of oxygen consumption (pp. 78).
- High plasma levels of fatty acids may induce central fatigue (pp. 112).

In addition, in the marathon, the ultra-marathon and during very long training runs, glucose-containing drinks may prevent hypoglycaemia. In order to encourage rapid absorption into the body, drinks should not contain too much sugar; about 10% is recommended, i.e. 10 g/100 ml.

It may be even more advantageous for élite cyclists to consume carbohydrate-containing drinks since they can be more easily taken during a race and, since there is less jolting of the body, there is less discomfort due to movement of fluid in the stomach.

In burst activities such as soccer, rugby and hockey it has become fashionable to consume glucose-rich drinks before the event. For reasons given above, this is unlikely to have any benefit on performance. However, Dr B. Ekblom in Stockholm has discovered that soccer players frequently deplete their muscle glycogen stores before the end of the match. Thus glucose-containing drinks at half-time could be of value, and a high-carbohydrate diet consumed for the 2–3 days before a match might also reduce the avalanche of goals that occurs late in many soccer games!

Table 11.3. Percentage of energy as carbohydrate, fat and protein in some common foods

Food	Percentage energy		
	Carbohydrate	Fat	Protein
Chocolate bars			
Cadbury's Crunchie bar	60	37	3
Fry's chocolate cream	67	30	3
Cadbury's cream egg	57.5	38.5	4
Hershey milk chocolate bar	43	51	6
Hershey peanut milk chocolate bar	31	59	10
Mars bar	61	34	5
Cadbury's dairy milk	43	51	6
Bread			
Bread roll	80	13	7
White bread	72	14	14
Whole-wheat bread	68	16	16
Whole meal bread	73	11	16
Biscuits			
Jaffa cakes	76	20	4
Digestive sweetmeal	56	39	5
Rye wafer	83	4	13
Shortcake	52	43	5
Cream crackers	61.5	30.5	8
Rice			
Ground rice (for puddings)	90	3	7
White rice	91	1	8
Brown rice	86	5	9
Cow's milk			
Full cream (gold top)	24	56	20
Semi-skimmed	39	33	28
Skimmed	56	3	41
Normal (homogenized)	28	52	20
Whole milk (N. America)	29	49	22
2% low fat (N. America)	39	32	29
Milkshake	73	17	10
Cereals			
Cornflakes	89	2	9
Porridge oats	67	21	12
Shredded wheat	81	5	14
Weetabix	79	7	14
Pasta shells	81	15	4
Flour (plain white)	83	5	12
Macaroni	83	3	14

Table 11.3. (*continued*)

Food	Percentage energy		
	Carbohydrate	Fat	Protein
Vegetables			
Potato:			
baked	88	1	11
boiled	87	1	12
french-fried (chips)	51	43	6
Avocado	16	79	5
Broccoli	57	6.5	36.5
Brussels sprouts	61	5	34
Carrots (boiled)	84	5	11
Cauliflower (boiled, whole flower buds)	56	4	40
Celery	73.5	5.5	21
Chick-peas	68	9	23
Meals			
Bacon and egg McMuffin (McDonalds)	32	42	26
Macaroni cheese (baked in casserole)	37	47	16
Big Mac (McDonalds)	28	52	20
Egg salad sandwich	43	41	16
Tuna salad	10	53	37
Potato salad	63	25	12
Chef's salad	4	77	19
Fillet of fish (McDonalds)	38	42	20
Chicken McNuggets (McDonalds)	17	53	30
Cheeseburger (McDonalds)	38	40	22
Eggs (chicken, hard boiled)	3	64.5	32.5
Chicken (roasted, light meat, no skin)	0	23	77
Cakes			
Muffin blueberry	63	29	8
bran	54	36	10
Doughnut	36	58	6
Danish pastry	44	49	7
Chocolate cake (chocolate icing)	55	40	5
Doughnut (cake type)	46.5	48.5	5
Apple pie (McDonalds)	47	49	4
Fruit			
Apple	93	5.5	1.5
Apricot	82	11	7
Banana	91	5	4
Grapefruit	90	3	7
Grapes	89	4	7
Melon honeydew	92	3	5
water	84	8	8

Table 11.3. (*continued*)

| Food | Percentage energy | | |
	Carbohydrate	Fat	Protein
Fruit			
Orange	90	3	7
Pineapple	89	8	3
Plums	86	9	5
Dates (dried)	97	–	3
Figs (fresh)	93	3	4
Figs (dried)	92	3	5
Dairy produce			
Butter	0.4	99.2	0.4
Cream	4	94	2
Eggs (chicken, boiled)	3	64	33
Tinned foods			
Tomato soup	54	40	6
Sweetcorn	82	7	11
Baked beans	67	5	28
Spaghetti	86	4	10

GLYCOGEN LOADING

Endurance athletes were not slow to exploit the Scandinavian discovery, reported in 1967, that endurance performance depends on the size of muscle glycogen stores and that these can be increased by dietary manipulation. This information was probably first used by the British marathon runner Ron Hill, in preparation for the 1969 European Championship in Athens; Hill won the marathon.

In the original regime, followed by Hill, muscle glycogen levels were first depleted by a strenuous run 6 days prior to the competition. After 3 days on a low-carbohydrate diet, a second strenuous run was undertaken to completely exhaust muscle glycogen. For the final 3 days, a high-carbohydrate diet was consumed so that 'supercompensation' took place and more glycogen was laid down than was used up by the runs. In the original study, this procedure doubled glycogen levels in the untrained volunteers used. Élite marathon runners, however, experience less supercompensation because exhaustion of glycogen stores occurs frequently during their training and the effect diminishes with repetition. In fact many runners found that this regime interfered with normal training, caused gastrointestinal upsets and possibly increased their susceptibility to viral infection. Today, most marathon runners settle for a compromise regime with fewer difficulties. Since normal training will have drastically lowered their muscle glycogen level anyway, they just settle for the high-carbohydrate diet during the few days before a race. Some athletes precede this with a period of low-carbohydrate consumption but bodies differ and personal experimentation is necessary.

Timing, however, is crucial, for the overfilling persists for but a short time even in the absence of exercise. Pasta parties the night before an event may be fun but as far as glycogen loading is concerned just provide the 'icing on the cake'; the hard work has already been done. Athletes use a number of clues to monitor the progress of their glycogen-loading bouts, including:

- Diarrhoea occurs if so much carbohydrate is ingested that not all the glucose released by digestion can be absorbed in the small intestine, and some reaches the large intestine. This is the time to stop loading.
- Careful weighing at the same time each day can reveal progress, since a 'full load' of glycogen with its associated water adds around 5 pounds to body mass.
- Unloading is accompanied by a marked increase in urine flow as the water bound to glycogen is released. This can occur without exercise if loading was begun too early. A corollary of this is the importance of maintaining sufficient fluid intake during loading to avoid dehydration.

What began as a special dietary manipulation to benefit marathon runners is now seen as a slight extension of the general principle that all runners of middle distances and over will benefit from keeping muscle glycogen levels as high as possible. This can be achieved with the kind of high-carbohydrate meals advocated in Part II(D).

THE FATS: HIGH ENERGY BUT ...

Fat is an almost ideal long-term energy storage fuel, with its high energy content and its ability to be packed away with virtually no water (see Chapter 4). It is not, however, used to any significant extent in track events although it plays a role in the marathon and is particularly important in ultra-marathon events.

The food we eat is largely the energy reserves of other organisms, so inevitably these include fats. Fats are an economical source of energy in the diet and no bad thing unless consumed in excess, as they so often are in our 'soft Western world' where starvation is rare and over-indulgence the norm. With their ready availability, concentrated form and dietary appeal, it is all too easy to cram the fats in. Evolution, through harsher times, has adapted humans to store this excess energy so that today obesity rather than survival is the result. Nutritionists recommend that less than 30% of our energy intake should come from fats. In primitive societies, this figure is often less than 10% and during periods of intense training athletes, too, should aim towards this figure.

One problem with following this advice is that fats often increase the palatability of the diet and most food preparation, 'fast' or otherwise, adds fat. Very special efforts with our meals are necessary to get the fat content down to 10%; for example, skimmed milk (0.4% fat) must be substituted for full milk (3.4% fat) and cottage cheese (19% fat) for Cheddar (65% fat).

At least as important as keeping the fat low in the diet is the kind of fat consumed: saturated or unsaturated. These terms have nothing to do with water content but refer to the presence of double bonds in

---

Box 11.2   What do athletes really eat?

Finding out what people actually eat is fraught with difficulties. It is tedious to have to record everything eaten with exact portion sizes, and the nutrient composition of actual meals will often only be known imperfectly. Subjects may also, consciously or subconsciously, be fooling themselves or the investigator by recording what they ought to have eaten rather than what they did.

In 1985 Dr William Haskell and his associates carried out a most revealing study on 13 members of the US Nordic ski team. They recorded their food intake for a 3-day period on four separate occasions during a training year, two of which were at training camps when food was prepared for the skiers. The following points of interest emerged:

continued

continued

- Energy consumption was high (205–318 kJ/kg body weight per day for men and 176–297 kJ/kg body weight per day for women) but probably not high enough to support their total energy expenditure under these circumstances.
- The proportion of energy consumed as carbohydrate (about 45%) was well below the 60% recommended as a conservative minimum for intensively training athletes. The proportion taken as fat (38–39%) was correspondingly high.
- The proportion of energy consumed as carbohydrate was lower at training camps than it was when athletes planned and ate their own food at home. Whether this reflected the inappropriate choices available at camp or whether decisions were made on the basis of palatability rather than nutritional value is not clear. Certainly there will always be the temptation to take a second piece of fried chicken rather than another helping of potato.
- The iron intake of the female athletes was consistently, albeit slightly, below the recommended daily allowance for non-athletic women.

Van Eng-Baart and colleagues (1992) have carried out a detailed study over several years on the eating habits of top athletes, many of whom competed at an international level. The athletes were asked to complete detailed food diaries for a minimum of four consecutive days and, if possible, for seven. A total of 419 athletes, who trained at least 1–2 h per day, were studied. The major findings were:

- Protein intake was sufficient to satisfy requirements.
- The contribution of carbohydrate to energy intake varied between 40% and 63%. Although the highest values for carbohydrate intake were found in the endurance athletes (50–60% of total energy), even these appear to be low when compared with the 70% recommended (see p. 221).
- Thirty-five per cent of the total energy intake was taken in the form of snacks, i.e. food taken in at times other than during the three main meals. It appeared that athletes eat frequently throughout the whole day, possibly because bulky meals can affect performance whether in training or competition. The carbohydrate content of snacks for athletes is therefore particularly important.
- The food most preferred by the athletes was bread.

the fatty acids composing the fats (Figure 11.3). Although this may seem an abstruse chemical point, it is one with considerable dietary significance for there is much evidence that a diet high in saturated fats and low in unsaturated fats predisposes towards heart attacks and strokes, not to mention gallstones, diabetes and certain forms of cancer. To keep things simple, it can be assumed that oils derived from fish and plants are rich in unsaturated fatty acids and that fats

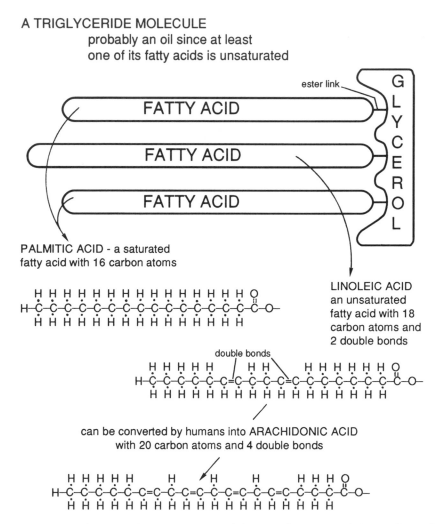

Figure 11.3. Saturated and unsaturated fatty acids as part of the triglyceride molecule

Table 11.4. Percentage fatty acid composition of some fats, oils and meats

	Approximate fatty composition (%)		
	Saturated	Mono-unsaturated	Polyunsaturated
Butter	67	30	3
Corn oil	14	31	55
Chicken	35	45	20
Fish	23	27	50
Margarine (hard)	54	33	13
Margarine (soft)	25	22	53
Olive oil	15	73	12
Sunflower seed oil	19	21	60
Safflower seed oil	19	21	60

obtained from other animals and animal products are rich in saturated fatty acids (Table 11.4).

DOWN TO ESSENTIALS

The story so far is that fatty foods are rich in energy and must be eaten in moderation to avoid weight gain, and that increasing the proportion of unsaturated fatty acids in the diet has long-term health benefits. In fact, fats can be made in the body quite readily from carbohydrate, although it is not possible to convert fat into carbohydrate. This means that any carbohydrate consumed in excess of that required for immediate energy demands, or to replenish glycogen stores, will be converted into fat and stored in adipose tissue. So is fat needed in the diet at all? It most certainly is, because supplying energy is not the only role of dietary fats; the fat of the plant oils and also fish oils contains essential fatty acids. What makes them essential is that they are needed by the body but cannot be made from any other food component. Chemically they possess more than one double bond (Figure 11.3)—the sign of unsaturation—so are known as polyunsaturated fatty acids, or PUFAs for short. Although the human liver can carry out an immense number of chemical transformations, one thing it cannot do is introduce double bonds into the correct positions in a fatty acid to produce PUFAs, which must therefore be supplied ready made, and in this modern age that means taken from the supermarket shelf.

PUFAs have two special roles in the body. The first involves the structure of the membranes which isolate cells from their surroundings and form structures, such as mitochondria, within them. A major component of all membranes is phospholipid—a fat-like molecule bearing two fatty acid chains, one of which is almost invariably polyunsaturated. PUFAs are needed to provide the right kind of phospholipids not only as the body grows but also for the repair of damaged cells. The cycle of damage and repair to the cell membranes is massively speeded up during training and, although some of the PUFAs in these membranes will be recycled, many will have been damaged and are then broken down. The only source of new PUFAs to replace the damaged ones is the diet, so it is particularly important for the athlete during peak training to be provided with a good supply of PUFAs.

The second role of PUFAs is in the synthesis of prostaglandins, which act as chemical messengers controlling many processes within tissues. One of these is the control of repair after training damage. Prostaglandins are also involved in the inflammation process and in sensitizing tissues to pain—responses that are diminished by drugs such as aspirin which inhibit prostaglandin synthesis.

So from where can the athlete get PUFAs? The answer is from plant or fish oils. Oils are simply fats with low melting points so that at normal room temperature they are liquid. Since the low melting point is conferred on oils by unsaturated fatty acids, oils are bound to be rich in PUFAs. The best sources of PUFAs are vegetable seed oils (especially sunflower and safflower), fish oils (e.g. cod-liver) and the 'meat' of fatty fish (e.g. mackerel, salmon, herring). It is especially important for the athlete that these oils should be substituted for animal fats whenever possible so that the intake of PUFAs is maintained while that of total fat in the diet is kept low. One way of doing this is to replace butter with margarines which are rich in polyunsaturated fatty acids, and another is to use only oils in food preparation. Polyunsaturated oils, however, should not be used for frying since heating them produces free radicals—very reactive chemicals which may be harmful.

Whether all PUFAs are equally beneficial is controversial at the present time. One PUFA that is known to be important in the body is *arachidonic acid*, which can be formed in our livers from other PUFAs normally present at high levels in seed oils. But there may be a problem. This conversion involves enzymes and there is some evidence that the catalytic activity of at least one enzyme involved in the formation of arachidonic acid can be rather sluggish in some people. For this reason, it may be beneficial to consume γ-linolenic acid, enabling the slow step en route to arachidonic acid to be bypassed. For

Box 11.3   Spreading confusion

With the recognition that butter is not a good thing to eat, at least not in large amounts, came the proliferation of 'spreads', known collectively as margarines. Margarines, however, were originally developed not as health foods but as less costly alternatives to butter. Plant oils are, in general, much cheaper than animal fats but it is not easy to spread a plant oil on, for example, a piece of toast—try it! The chemical solution is drastic but effective—heat them with gaseous hydrogen in the presence of powdered nickel as a catalyst. This treatment adds hydrogen atoms to double bonds, so converting unsaturated fats to saturated ones. This provides a material physically similar to butter (but not of course tasting the same), namely margarine. Such hard margarines spread well at room temperature but as domestic refrigerators became commonplace this was no longer an advantage; indeed they were difficult to spread 'straight from the fridge'. Soft margarines were therefore produced, with a higher content of unsaturated fats. Their higher PUFA content conferred additional health benefits and sales took off.

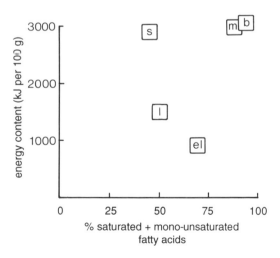

Figure 11.4. Energy content and percentage of fat which is not polyunsaturated in spreads. Key: b, butter; m, hard margarine; s, soft margarine; l, low-fat margarine; el, extra-low-fat margarine

continued

┌─ *continued* ───┐

A further aspect of spread marketing has been the advent of 'low-calorie spreads' devised to help the consumer who wishes to reduce the energy consumed. To produce them polyunsaturated fats are homogenized with a large amount of water, so the same amount of spread contains less energy. Yet another line of products has originated from the combination of butter, with its very popular flavour, with cheaper, healthier and more spreadable vegetable oils.

Manufacturers of margarine products have undoubtedly benefited from health concern over butter and, whilst they have to avoid false claims, many of their advertisements do little to resolve the confusion about health benefits of margarines. Perhaps Figure 11.4 will help.

the athlete who during peak training periods wishes to supplement his or her diet in this way, γ-linolenic acid is present in oil of the evening primrose (now commercially available, for example, as *Effamol* capsules). Although this has not been tested with athletes there is evidence that it is beneficial in some pathological conditions such as premenstrual tension, atopic eczema and diabetic neuropathy.

THE PROTEINS: VARIATIONS ON AN AMINO ACID THEME

One way of producing large molecules is to connect together a whole lot of smaller ones. The process is called polymerization and is used by chemists to produce plastics. If small identical units (monomers) link head to tail you end up with polymer molecules which are also identical except for the number of monomer units they contain. However, if you start with several different monomers and allow them to connect in pre-determined sequences, a great many different polymers can be produced. In the case of proteins, 20 different amino acid monomers are available and can be linked into defined sequences usually containing from 50 to several hundred amino acids (Figure 11.5). An astronomical number of proteins are therefore possible and, from them, evolution has selected a few thousand which carry out such diverse functions as catalysing reactions (the enzymes), transporting oxygen (haemoglobin) and forming hair (keratin).

Almost every cell in the human body has the apparatus to synthesize proteins, but can only do so when supplied with amino acids. Half of the 20 amino acids needed can be made from components which are

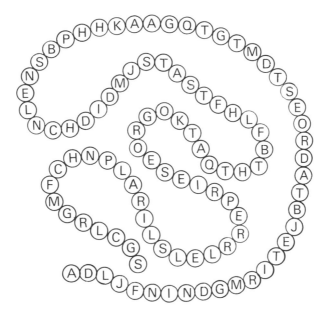

Figure 11.5. The structure of a small hypothetical protein. Each circle represents an amino acid

readily available in the body; in contrast, the other half—the *essential* amino acids—must be provided in the diet. Digestion of protein in the intestine releases individual amino acids which are absorbed into the bloodstream and then taken up by the tissues that need them.

Because cells are always being replaced, and proteins within cells are continuously being broken down and resynthesized, the demand for protein continues even after growth has ceased. The World Health Organization recommends that the daily intake of protein should be at least 0.8 g for each kilogram of body weight, i.e. about 56 g for the average adult weighing 70 kg. Growing children need much more (2.4 g/kg body weight for the first few months and 1.5 g/kg at 6 months); sadly in many parts of the world they do not get it. It is widely accepted that during periods of intense training athletes also need more, but just how much more is debated. For very active people in the age range 18–34 the UK Department of Health recommends 1.2 g/kg body weight per day for males and 1.0 g/kg for females. The 84 g needed by a 70 kg male in this category could be provided by about 1 lb of best steak each day, but of course protein is supplied by many foods other than steak.There have been suggestions that in athletes who are training intensively protein intake should be as high as 1.5–1.8 g/kg body weight per day.

Athletes have long accepted the need for a high-protein diet; after all, muscles are made of protein, but those who follow the traditional 'red meat and eggs' diet or even Downer's idiosyncratic version of 'beef, mutton and legs of fowl' undoubtedly ingest much more protein than they need. This is unlikely to be beneficial, but could it be disadvantageous or even harmful? There are several reasons why it may be:

- Protein-rich foods are generally expensive.
- Diets rich in protein usually contain mainly animal protein, which is often associated with large amounts of saturated fat.
- Satiation with excessive amounts of protein-rich foods usually means that less carbohydrate is consumed, which would have provided much-needed glucose for repletion of glycogen stores in the muscles.
- The nitrogen present in amino acids is converted into urea for excretion in the urine and the water needed for this could increase the danger of dehydration during subsequent exercise.

So, although protein is important, the athlete must avoid the temptation to follow the old-fashioned advice that a very high-protein diet is essential. Particularly during intensive training periods and in preparation for competition, meals must be carbohydrate rich and protein adequate.

Consideration of daily protein requirements is complicated by the fact that not all proteins in the diet have the same nutritional value, since they contain different amounts of essential amino acids. Proteins present in foods such as eggs, milk and meat, contain enough of each essential amino acid to allow protein synthesis to occur without the need to eat extra protein (Figure 11.6).

Proteins of plant origin, by contrast, may be deficient in particular essential amino acids. Fortunately, not all plants are deficient in the same amino acids, so that by eating a range of plant foods, for example cereals and legumes, adequate amounts of each of the essential amino acids can be obtained from a vegetarian diet. A vegan athlete has to plan his or her diet carefully for recovery after peak training. This, however, probably poses no problems since vegans normally give considerable thought to their diet. Recent research suggests that a vegan diet can be quite adequate for maintaining intense training and performance.

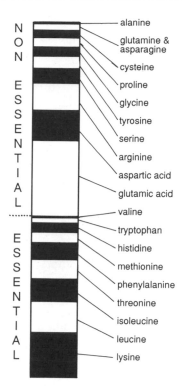

Figure 11.6. The amino acid composition of myosin, one of the two major proteins in muscle and therefore in lean meat

So the athlete must seek a balance. Too much protein and the diet is distorted; too little and recovery after intense training might be slowed. This problem leads to a consideration of supplementation of the diet with essential amino acids, especially during peak training. But should just the amino acids known to be essential be provided? Help has perhaps arrived from an unexpected direction. Very small and very premature babies can be kept alive in incubators; the question of protein nutrition has arisen for these babies since amino acids can no longer be provided by the mother and feeding by mouth is not possible. It is now apparent that to maintain growth and development of these premature babies some of the amino acids that we have previously considered as non-essential are in fact essential for these infants. Although their liver can make non-essential amino acids, it cannot make them fast enough to satisfy the premature baby's requirements for protein synthesis, so they must be provided.

The amino acid requirements for these infants *suggest* that the athlete in peak training might consider supplementation with the following amino acids: glycine, arginine, glutamine, serine, taurine, methionine, branched-chain amino acids and cysteine, of which only the last three are generally considered to be essential. A number of points arise from this list of amino acids:

- *Methionine* in the body is converted to both cysteine and taurine, so that if enough methionine is taken it can ensure sufficient levels of the other two amino acids. Taurine is not a component of proteins but is probably used for repair and recovery after damage such as that caused by training.
- A small family of amino acids, the *branched-chain amino acids* (valine, leucine and isoleucine), may be particularly important in promoting muscle growth during recovery after prolonged exercise or after very hard training sessions, and also in reducing tiredness (Box 11.4).
- *Glutamine* is not yet available commercially in sports drinks since it can, during storage, be converted spontaneously into a toxic chemical. In the future it may be made available in a powder form to be sprinkled on food or dissolved in water and consumed soon after it is dissolved.

Box 11.4   A branched-chain solution?

The branched-chain amino acids (BCAAs) are rather special, being the only ones used to generate energy in exercising muscle. As glycogen levels fall towards the end of a middle- or long-distance race, these BCAAs begin to make a contribution to energy supply. Although this contribution is likely to be small, its consequences may be much more significant.

In Chapter 6 it was explained that the BCAAs are transported into brain cells via the same carrier which transports tryptophan. In the brain, tryptophan is used as a precursor for the synthesis of 5-hydroxytryptamine (5-HT), which could play a role in 'central fatigue', i.e. fatigue initiated in the brain rather than the muscle. Too high a concentration of 5-HT in certain parts of the brain could make it more difficult to maintain a given pace, so the athlete either has to apply greater mental effort or slow down. As BCAAs are used to provide

continued

continued

energy, their concentration in blood will fall, so they no longer compete so effectively with tryptophan for entry into the brain. Consequently, more tryptophan enters and more 5-HT is made, which increases central fatigue. By maintaining the BCAA level in the blood it should be possible to prevent this increased 5-HT production.

So much for the theory; how about the practice? Half of the 193 participants in the Stockholm Marathon who had volunteered for this experiment were given drinks containing BCAAs four times during the race. The remaining half, selected at random, received a placebo drink. The experiment was carried out double-blind: neither runners nor scientists knew who was receiving BCAAs and who was receiving the placebo.

On the face of it, the results were disappointing; the BCAA group, on the whole, did not perform significantly better than the others, but closer examination did reveal a difference. If only the slower competitors were considered (i.e. those taking from 3 h 5 min to 3 h 30 min) the experimental group did do better than the control—by around 5–6 min. Why should the better runners not have benefited in this way? Possibly because they were less susceptible to central fatigue or because their glycogen stores supported them for longer and they were able to run with much lower levels of fatty acids in the blood (pp. 127–130).

In other studies of a similar kind, no improvement in performance could be attributed to the consumption of BCAA drinks, but questionnaires showed the perceived effort to be significantly lower—it made the run that much easier! Studies in other sports such as soccer, tennis, squash and rowing are in progress and the product is now commercially available.

Athletes should be aware that, although some of the claims made for individual amino acid supplementation are founded on sound biochemical knowledge, the benefits are untested. Human metabolism is very complex and there may be no simple solutions to problems faced by athletes during intense training and competition. In summary, the best advice that can be given at present to the athlete training intensively is:

- Eat an adequate but not excessive amount of protein.
- Avoid protein sources which are also rich in saturated fats (such as red meats, hamburgers and sausages).

- Consider supplementation, after intensive training sessions, with a mixture of amino acids.

VITAMINS: THE ESSENTIAL ALPHABET

Something about vitamins catches the imagination. Perhaps it is the way they were discovered—seemingly magical cures for diseases like scurvy, rickets and beri-beri; or amazement at their effectiveness in such small doses or because they can be cheaply synthesized and formulated into pills so that everyone can 'treat' his or her own dietary imbalance.

The definition of vitamins, as organic substances needed in small amounts but not capable of being manufactured by the body in adequate quantities, seems straightforward enough. It implies that if particular vitamins are not present in the diet, some problem—a deficiency disease—will arise. But vitamin nutrition is still plagued by uncertainties. To begin with, many substances were falsely identified as vitamins; the B series reached vitamin B_{20}! This is not surprising considering the small quantities involved and how difficult it is to carry out nutritional experiments on humans (not all species have the same vitamin requirements). Some of these non-vitamins were, and perhaps still are, commercially exploited long after being discredited.

In some cases the body can synthesize a vital compound but may not be able to do so at an adequate rate under all circumstances. Vitamin D is a good example; the action of sunlight on skin can generate all the vitamin D the human body needs but, in northern latitudes, not much skin is exposed to not much sunlight, so that dietary sources of vitamin D are essential. It is also possible that a certain compound can be made fast enough to supply normal needs but increased demand pushes it into the 'vitamin' category. Athletic training increases the demand for virtually all nutrients and may well be responsible for elevating choline to the status of a vitamin.

The real difficulty with vitamins is knowing whether a shortage is responsible for *slight* effects: occasional headaches; increased incidence of colds; a small percentage decrease in performance; soreness after a particular training session. The problem is that there are always other explanations, but dietary supplementation is positive action that can easily be taken.

About a dozen chemicals are widely recognized as vitamins (Table 11.5) although some are actually families of interconvertible chemical forms. A further group, including choline, inositol and bioflavinoids,

Box 11.5 Food for the brain—and the athlete

Nature is parsimonious. A relatively small repertoire of molecules is pressed into a wide range of services. Choline, for example—a small nitrogen-rich alcohol—forms not only part of the neurotransmitter *acetylcholine*, which is vitally important in the brain and the neuro-muscular junctions, but also part of the phospholipid *lecithin*—an essential component of cell membranes. Phospholipids resemble trig-lycerides (Figure 11.3) in that they contain a glycerol unit, but this is linked to two rather than three fatty acids. The remaining position on the glycerol is occupied by a phosphate group and one of a small range of bases—including choline. Membranes are formed by phos-pholipid molecules aligning in a double layer with their fatty acid groups projecting inwards and their phosphate–base groups outwards. Unlike fatty acids, these groups are hydrophilic, i.e. they form a stable association with water—an ideal arrangement for a membrane which has to separate two aqueous compartments. The phospholipid which contains choline is known as phosphatidylcholine, or lecithin.

There is no doubt that enough choline can be made in the body to satisfy normal demands, but those of an athlete during peak training are hardly normal. Choline levels in the blood fall markedly after a marathon race, possibly because of the amount needed to repair the membranes in tissues damaged by the intense exercise. Under these circumstances a shortage of choline may limit repair and recovery, so that additional dietary choline may be of value in the diet. For the athlete during intense training, choline may actually be a vitamin, although there is no scientific evidence for this as yet.

If the prudent athlete wishes to consume a choline-rich diet, one of the best ways of doing this is to eat plenty of fish—long considered to be good for the brain. At peak training, additional choline may be needed and can be taken as such or in the form of lecithin granules, which can be sprinkled on that carbohydrate-rich snack consumed as soon as training is over.

Table 11.5. Some vitamins: their roles and sources

Vitamin	Role of vitamin	Sources of vitamin
Water-soluble vitamins		
B_1 (thiamine)	Involved in aerobic metabolism, so important for middle-distance and endurance runners	Fresh vegetables, husk of cereal grains, meats, especially liver
B_2 (riboflavin)	As above, and also in growth, so may be particularly important in intensive training	Milk and meat products
Nicotinic acid (niacin)	Involved in all energy metabolism	Liver, lean meats, cereals, legumes
B_6 (pyridoxine)	Important in the function of the nervous system and in amino acid metabolism so important in recovery after intensive training	Meats, cereals, lentils, nuts, some fruits and vegetables
Pantothenic acid	Widely involved in metabolic processes, so important both for energy provision and in training	Liver, meats, cereals, milk, egg yolk, vegetables
Folates	Involved in growth and repair, especially nucleic acid metabolism	Yeast, liver, fresh green vegetables
B_{12} (cobalamin)	Needed for red cell formation, etc.; may be lacking in vegetarians	Meat, fish, poultry, milk and milk products; produced also by bacteria in the large intestine

Biotin	Involved in many aspects of amino acid metabolism	Yeast, organ meats, muscle meats, dairy products, grains, fruits; produced by microorganisms
Choline	A component of neurotransmitter and phospholipid in cell membranes. Some is made in the body	Meat, egg yolk, legumes, cereals
Vitamin C ascorbic acid	Plays a role in synthesis of connective tissue and hence repair of tissue damaged by hard training. Also plays a role as an antioxidant together with vitamin E	Fresh fruits and vegetables
Fat-soluble vitamins Vitamin A retinol	A component of the pigment used for low-light vision	Animal tissue, liver, green plants
Vitamin D cholecalciferol	Controls uptake and mobilization of calcium in the body, so needed for bone strength	Produced in skin during summer; added to some foods, e.g. margarine
Vitamin E tocopherol	An antioxidant which may help prevent damage to membranes caused by oxygen free radicals	Vegetable seed oils, milk, eggs, meat
Vitamin K phylloquinone	Involved in synthesis and activation of blood-clotting factors	Green leafy vegetables, meats, dairy produce

are in the 'possible' category—at least in the eyes of some experts. (The essential fatty acids and essential amino acids are excluded as vitamins for historical reasons and because they are needed in rather larger amounts than the true vitamins.) The recommended dietary allowances of vitamins per day for adults range from 3 μg (0.000003 g) for vitamin B_{12} to 60 mg (0.06 g) for vitamin C.

Four vitamins—A, D, E and K—are *fat soluble* and the rest are *water soluble*. This distinction partly explains their different dietary sources (Table 11.5) and, if supplementation is being carried out, fat-soluble vitamins must be taken during, or immediately after, a meal that contains some fat for effective absorption.

The advice on vitamins for the general population is that supplementation is unnecessary except where the diet is abnormal. This may occur in the elderly or the very young, when food absorption problems exist, or when there is an exceptional demand for vitamins, as in pregnancy. The relevant question is whether the intensively training athlete is also a special case. Some scientists answer this question with a definite no and others with a qualified yes! Dr W. Saris concluded from his study of cyclists in the 1986 Tour de France that their vitamin B (especially vitamin B_1) and C intakes, although 'normal', were inadequate under these circumstances. And other athletes who are training hard but restricting food intake in an attempt to lose weight may have an inadequate intake of some vitamins. Furthermore, an understanding of how vitamin E, vitamin C and choline are used by the body strongly suggests that an athlete will need much more of each during really intensive training.

In a study on trained mountaineers, participants were divided into two groups. Each climber in the first group was given 400 mg of vitamin E per day for 4 weeks, while those in the control group received no supplement. Both groups then carried out a strenuous 5000 m ascent. Halfway up, and again at the top, the anaerobic threshold of each climber was measured using an ergometer and muscle damage was assessed. The group receiving the vitamin E supplement showed an improved anaerobic threshold and less muscle damage. This suggests that vitamin E supplementation may have a beneficial effect on athletic performance during what is equivalent to hard training.

There is increasing evidence that damage can occur to the sensitive absorptive cells that line the small intestine when blood flow to the intestine is reduced for any length of time, as it is during intense exercise. This can cause diarrhoea and increase the incidence of bacterial and viral attacks as the immunological barrier provided by the absorptive cells is more readily breached. An interesting point is that

Table 11.6. Recommended dietary allowances for some vitamins and other substances, together with supplementation level reported by athletes. Data are given for the intake for one day

Group	Vitamin	US RDA (mg) Male	US RDA (mg) Female	British RNI (mg) Male	British RNI (mg) Female	Ranges reported to be supplemented by some athletes (mg)
A	Retinol	1.0	0.8	0.7	0.6	1–9
B	Thiamine (B$_1$)	1.4	1.0	1.0	0.8	40–600
B	Riboflavin (B$_2$)	1.6	1.2	1.3	1.1	30–250
B	Niacin (nicotinic acid)	18	13	17	13	100–1000
B	Pantothenic acid	4–7	4–7	–	–	50–1000
B	Pyridoxine (B$_6$)	2.2	2.0	1.4	1.2	40–300
B	Cobalamins (B$_{12}$)	0.003	0.003	0.0015	0.0115	0.1–0.3
B	Folates	0.4	0.4	0.2	0.2	2–30
B	Biotin	0.1–0.2	0.1–0.2	–	–	2–100
B	Inositol	–	–	–	–	100–1000
C	Ascorbate	60	60	40	40	2000–16000
D	Cholecalciferol	5	5	–	–	5–62
E	Tocopherols	10	8	–	–	200–1600
K	Phylloquinone	0.07–0.14	0.07–0.14	–	–	–
	p-Amino-benzoic acid	–	–	–	–	100–500
	Lecithin	–	–	–	–	200–2000

RDA stands for recommended dietary allowance (US) and RNI is the recommended nutritional intake.
It should be noted that for some vitamins (especially A) intakes several times above the RDA value may be toxic.
From Bloch, A. S. and Shils, M. E. (1988). Appendix. In *Modern Nutrition in Health and Disease*, pp. 1488–1489 (eds Shills, M. E. and Young, V. R.). Lea & Febiger, Philadelphia, and Report of the Panel on Dietary Reference Values of the Committee on Medical Aspects of Food Policy, Vol. 41. *Dietary Reference Values for Food, Energy and Nutrients for the United Kingdom*. HMSO, London.

this damage may occur not so much during the period when the blood flow is reduced, but after the exercise is over, when blood flow increases towards normal. Vitamin C will help to protect against this damage and should be consumed with the carbohydrate-rich drink immediately after the training session. Vitamin E will also protect but has to be taken with meals during the days prior to the intense training period and during this training period.

Surveys have shown that between 30% and 80% of athletes do feel the need to supplement their diet with additional vitamins (Table 11.6). Factors they should bear in mind include the following:

- The water-soluble vitamins (B and C) are not stored to any large extent in the body, so any effects caused by their deficiency will become apparent very quickly. Supplementation should therefore be carried out during the intense training period.
- The fat-soluble vitamins (A, D, E and K) are stored in the body, so there may be an advantage in supplementing *prior* to the peak training programme.
- There is no firm evidence that very high doses of any vitamin produce beneficial effects unrelated to their normal vitamin function.
- Very large doses of vitamins can be harmful and in the case of vitamin A fatal (a risk which is reduced if the vitamin is taken in the form of β-carotene). Even vitamin C, if taken in massive amounts (e.g. in an attempt to reduce the chance of catching a cold), can cause gastrointestinal problems.
- Excessive consumption of alcohol may impair the uptake of some water-soluble vitamins.
- Some drugs, including oral contraceptives, and smoking, increase the body's demand for vitamins B, C and E.

In view of the doubts that exist in this area we would suggest that supplementation be at the level of the recommended dietary allowances (RDA) in Table 11.6 for vitamins A and D but that somewhat larger amounts of vitamins B, C and E can be usefully taken.

MINERALS: LIFE'S ADDITIONAL ELEMENTS

Out of the 92 naturally occurring chemical elements, only 21 are needed to build the human body and to allow it to function. Only four of them—*carbon, hydrogen, oxygen* and *nitrogen*—come from the organic compounds on which we have already placed considerable emphasis (carbohydrate, fat and protein) and two more—sulphur and phosphorus—occur in combination with these organic compounds. The remaining 15 elements, known as the minerals, fulfil a wide range of functions and are required in very different amounts, from grams of sodium and potassium to milligrams, or less, of the so-called *trace elements* like chromium and molybdenum (Table 11.7).

Shortage of some minerals in the diet causes well-known and well-defined deficiency diseases such as anaemia, due to lack of iron, and goitre, due to lack of iodine. Many suspect, however, that a number of other aspects of poor health are also attributable to mineral deficiencies. For example, it has been suggested that a deficiency of zinc can lead to a decreased response of the immune system and so to an increased susceptibility to colds, coughs and throat infections. Although scientific evidence for these effects is lacking, we do know that severe exercise increases the elimination of some minerals, presumably as a consequence of the increased turnover of body constituents that are involved in tissue repair. Athletes undergoing intensive training might consider published RDAs (Table 11.7) to be conservative and so consider moderate supplementation, for example with multi-mineral capsules, but must take care not to consume excessive amounts of any one since this can impair the uptake of others. Excessive iron intake can, for example, reduce uptake of zinc, copper and chromium.

Some of the minerals that have been discussed in the scientific literature in relation to athletic performance are considered below, in alphabetical order. This discussion should not be taken to imply that athletes will necessarily lack sufficient in their diets.

Calcium

Salts of calcium, especially calcium phosphate, are responsible for the rigidity of bone, but this rigidity does not mean that bone is biochemically inert. Far from it, for cells within the bone are continuously taking up and releasing calcium and phosphate, and the small amounts that are inevitably lost from the body must be replaced. This turnover increases with exercise, especially in young athletes, and enables a rapid response to be made if damage to the bone occurs.

Many of the other functions of calcium involve the control of chemical reactions within cells. For example, calcium ions are released from reservoirs within muscle fibres to switch on contraction in the myofibrils (see Chapter 2). Although the amounts of calcium needed for

Table 11.7.   Recommended dietary allowances for some minerals and supplementation levels reported by athletes

Mineral	US RDA (mg)		British RNI (mg)		Ranges reported to be supplemented by some athletes (mg)
	Male	Female	Male	Female	
Calcium	800	800	700	700	1000–3500
Chromium[a]	0.05–0.2	0.05–0.2	–	–	50–500
Copper	2.3	2.3	1.2	1.2	0–5
Iron	10	18	8.7	14.8	30–60
Iodine	0.15	0.15	0.14	0.14	0.15–1.0
Manganese[a]	2.5–5.0	2.5–5.0	–	–	20–100
Magnesium	350	300	300	270	1000–2000
Molybdenum[a]	0.15–0.5	0.15–0.5	1.2	1.2	0–5
Phosphorus	800	800	550	550	200–2000
Potassium[a]	1525–4575	1525–4575	3500	3500	198–5000
Selenium[a]	0.05–0.2	0.05–0.2	0.075	0.060	0.2–1.0
Sodium[a]	900–2700	900–2700	1600	1600	–
Zinc	15	15	9.5	7.0	50–150

It should be noted that in some cases ingestion of several times more than the RDA values for some minerals could be dangerous.

[a]It is considered in the USA that there is insufficient information for this mineral on which to base an allowance, so that a range is given.

From Report of the Panel on Dietary Reference Values of the Committee on Medical Aspects of Food Policy, Vol. 41. *Dietary Reference Values of Food, Energy and Nutrients for the United Kingdom*. HMSO, London (1991) and Bloch, A. S. and Shils, M. (1988). Appendix. In *Modern Nutrition in Health and Disease*, pp. 1488–1489 (eds Shills, M. E. and Young, V. R.). Lea & Febiger, Philadelphia.

control are small compared with that needed in bone, the requirement is literally vital, so that if the diet supplies too little calcium it will be released from bones. In time, this will weaken them, making fractures more likely and slowing the healing of bone damage.

Dairy products are the main source of calcium in the diet, so the athlete may run into trouble if he or she decreases intake of foods such as milk on the grounds of its high fat content. The answer is to go for low-fat forms, such as skimmed milk and cottage cheese. Some adults, however, are unable to enjoy milk in any form as it causes flatulence and diarrhoea. Their problem, and it is one which is more prevalent amongst Africans and Asians, is that they have not retained the ability to produce the enzyme lactase. This enzyme is produced in the intestine, where it breaks down the milk sugar—lactose—into glucose and galactose, which are absorbed into the bloodstream. In the absence of the enzyme, the lactose, which cannot be absorbed, remains undigested and once it enters the large intestine hinders the uptake of water and is fermented by gas-producing bacteria. The obvious solution to this problem is to avoid milk altogether but take calcium tablets. Alternatively, eating yogurt that contains live bacteria at the same time as drinking the milk may overcome the problem, for the bacteria in the yogurt contain the enzyme that is missing.

Copper

This metal plays a part in the immune system which defends the body against disease, in collagen formation (see pp. 261), in the formation of red blood cells, and in protection against the damage caused by stresses such as vigorous exercise. A deficiency of copper results in poor control of the blood glucose level, increased fat levels in the blood and cardiovascular problems. Indeed, one study into a low copper-containing diet in man had to be abandoned since four out of 23 participants developed cardiac abnormalities.

The plasma level of copper increases with exercise but very little is lost in the urine. More is lost in sweat, so that care should be taken to ensure adequacy of copper intake when training occurs in the heat or indoors.

Chromium

Although there has been controversy over whether this element is in fact essential, the current view is that it does have a natural role (probably as part of an organic complex) in regulating the use of glucose in the body. Athletes have been shown to lose twice as much chromium in their urine on an exercise day than on a non-exercise day so may benefit from taking additional chromium. A small anabolic effect has also been claimed as a result of chromium supplementation.

Iron

In contrast to the other metals discussed, iron deficiency in athletes is well documented and reasonably common. Iron is a component of haemoglobin and its deficiency causes anaemia—a lowering of the red blood cell count. Since the function of red blood cells is to carry oxygen, anaemia results in a decrease in oxygen supply to muscle and hence a greater dependence on anaerobic metabolism. For the athlete this will manifest itself as a lowering of the anaerobic threshold and the $VO_{2\,max}$, so for the same pace there will be a faster rate of lactic acid accumulation in the muscle—the so-called 'anaemic fatigue'. In passing it should be noted that a reduced haematocrit in athletes does not necessarily indicate an iron problem. Endurance training often elevates total blood volume more than it increases the number of red cells, reducing the haematocrit by 1–4%. That such pseudo-anaemia or 'sports anaemia' should occur reminds us that oxygen transport is not the only function of blood.

Anaemia can arise from an inadequate supply of iron in the diet, excessive loss through bleeding, impaired absorption of iron from the gut or from a defect in the synthesis of haem. It has long been recognized as a potential problem for female athletes as a consequence of heavy and prolonged menstrual bleeding, especially if they follow a vegetarian diet. There is also evidence that iron deficiency in male athletes is increasing, possibly as a result of greater intensity of training and a decrease in the intake of red meat. Furthermore it appears that impact damage during running can actually harm red blood cells, so that they are destroyed in the body at an increased rate. Although most of the iron that is released from the red blood cells is salvaged and is therefore used in the synthesis of new red blood cells, there are inevitable losses, so if dietary iron intake is marginal anaemia can result.

The dietary solution is to eat more red meat and more green vegetables but these may bring other dietary disadvantages; red meat is associated with saturated fat and vegetables are bulky. In any case, iron absorption from vegetables is relatively poor because of their phytic acid content. Liver is a good source of iron, as it is of other minerals, but it is not to every athlete's taste. Supplementation must be carried out with care since excesses of iron can be dangerous, and anyone suspecting they suffer from anaemia should consult a general practitioner or sports physician.

Magnesium

Magnesium is the mineral most directly associated with energy metabolism since every molecule of ATP must complex with a magnesium ion before it can undergo any enzyme-catalysed reaction. In normal circumstances magnesium deficiency never occurs for the element is widespread in food; green plants are an important source, since the chlorophyll molecule itself contains a magnesium atom. Despite this, blood magnesium levels can fall dramatically after intensive exercise and athletes might consider magnesium supplementation, despite the absence of scientific evidence for its benefit.

Selenium

Selenium is required in extremely small amounts but plays a role in the body which is particularly relevant to the athlete. It provides an essential part of the enzyme *glutathione peroxidase*, which is involved in the repair of damage to membranes that is caused by intense physical activity. Despite the absence of scientific evidence for its effectiveness, selenium supplementation is often recommended but the dangers of consuming an excess should not be ignored.

Zinc

Zinc atoms are a vital part of more than 100 enzymes which carry out a wide range of cellular functions, including ATP generation in muscle; indeed, 50–60% of the body's zinc is present in this tissue. A deficiency of zinc in humans results in growth retardation, delay of sexual maturity, slow wound healing, decreased appetite, loss of taste and smell and decreased immune function. Plasma levels increase after vigorous short-term exercise, presumably as a result of muscle damage which releases zinc into the plasma, from where some of it is lost in the urine and in sweat. More prolonged exercise (e.g. a 10-mile run) results in a decrease in the plasma level of zinc, probably due to redistribution into tissues like the liver and immune cells. If zinc supplementation is used it should be started just before peak training and continued throughout, but as yet there is no consistent scientific finding to support the view that taking additional zinc benefits performance.

ELECTROLYTES: TOPPING UP THE BATTERY

Because they are present in relatively high concentration, sodium, potassium and chloride ions make the largest contribution to the electrical conductivity of body fluids and are known as electrolytes. Their ability to maintain total solute concentration prevents excessive movement of water into or out of cells through osmosis, but they have a more specific role too. The electrical impulses which carry information along nerves are generated and propagated by the controlled movement of these ions across cell membranes. Severe disruption of sodium or potassium levels in the body interferes with this signalling, just as a fall in electrolyte level in a car battery impairs its function.

Virtually all of the dissolved material in sweat, forming 2–3% of its total volume, are these electrolytes, so that exercise on a hot day can cause considerable loss. Nonetheless, at least as far as sodium and chloride is concerned, a normal diet contains plenty, so that the loss is soon made up. In the meantime, the kidney reduces its excretion of sodium and chloride ions in the urine. Unless the exercise is really severe, say an ultra-marathon or a triathlon on a hot day, salt tablets are not normally recommended.

But potassium is a different matter. For one thing there is less in the normal diet and, for another, sweat actually contains more potassium than does the blood, although this difference disappears with training. After training or severe competition, the first priority must be to consume water plus carbohydrate, but then some thought should be given to restoring the body's potassium levels. Fruit and fruit juices are good natural sources of this mineral. Beer also contains potassium but athletes should be aware that this is not its *only* constituent; alcohol is a diuretic and can promote an inappropriate loss of water.

Chapter 12

When Training Goes Wrong

For a few months after my first Comrades Marathon in 1973, I developed a persistent injury that resisted all conventional medical advice. Only when I attended the 1976 New York Academy of Sciences Conference on the Marathon ... and heard the presentation by doctors George Sheehan, Richard Schuster and Steven Sabotrick did I begin to appreciate that attention to my running shoes and use of an orthotic might cure my injury. These measures worked and since then I have not suffered any further running injuries.

T. Noakes (1992).

At many Sports Injury Clinics, the largest single category of injuries is those caused by running—even greater than those caused by soccer or rugby in which player–player contact is frequent. This does not mean that running is a dangerous sport; in part, these figures reflect its popularity, but the fact remains that athletes not only push their bodies to physiological and biochemical limits but they also push them to their mechanical limits—and beyond. The good news is that few of these injuries are in any way serious and that most can be completely cured. Nonetheless, knowledge and understanding of what can go wrong, and why, may help the injured athlete to recover more quickly or, even better, may help to prevent injury in the first place.

Acute injuries are caused by a single event—an impact or some other force which exceeds the strength of our mechanical components. Other injuries result from stresses that are individually quite small but, when they are repeated frequently, the accumulated damage can be serious; these are known as chronic or stress injuries. The fact that they are also known as 'over-use' injuries should not imply that they are caused simply by excessive exercise. There is likely to be an underlying mechanical problem, and this will have to be resolved if the problem is not to recur. One problem with this epidemic of running injuries is that most doctors asked to treat them are inexperienced in this field and may not be able to identify the cause of the problem. The specialist sports physician can be of enormous help but it is equally important for the injured athlete (and his or her coach) to have some understanding of the injury and its treatment. Cooperation between all those involved should result in a speedy return to the track.

It is an aim of this chapter to help athletes and their coaches towards a better understanding of injuries and their treatment. We have been particularly impressed with the detailed advice on injuries given by Dr Tim Noakes—not only a physician but a runner and a scientist— and we reproduce some of his specific advice on running injuries and their treatment in Part IIE.

STRUCTURAL DAMAGE

The human locomotion system involves bones, cartilages, ligaments, tendons and muscles, all of which are susceptible to damage and injury.

Bone Injuries

Actual fractures are rare in running, although they may result from a fall. After a fracture, the bone must be immobilized to allow cells within the bone to produce new protein fibres and new mineral components within the damaged area. Other cells re-organize the protein and mineral and provide the precise structure which gives bone its rigidity.

A much commoner bone injury, especially among younger athletes, is the stress fracture, in which there is no actual break but a disruption of the highly ordered mineral structure which gives limb bones their strength (Figure 12.1). Repeated impacts during running, especially on hard surfaces, are responsible and the bones most often affected are the tibia and metatarsals. In female athletes, changes in the levels of hormones associated with disturbances in the menstrual cycle, due to prolonged sessions of exercise, can impair the deposition of calcium salts in the bones so that the rate of the normal repair processes, which take place after every training session, may not be adequate. The immediate treatment for a stress fracture is rest but the runner may need to change his or her style or intensity of running to prevent recurrence. Supplementation of the diet with calcium may also be important (see Chapter 11) but hormone replacement therapy should be considered in conjunction with the sports physician.

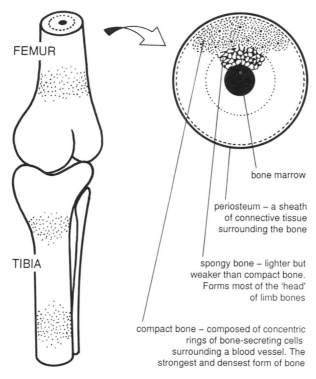

FEMUR

TIBIA

bone marrow

periosteum – a sheath
of connective tissue
surrounding the bone

spongy bone – lighter but
weaker than compact bone.
Forms most of the 'head'
of limb bones

compact bone – composed of concentric
rings of bone-secreting cells
surrounding a blood vessel. The
strongest and densest form of bone

Figure 12.1. Structure of limb bones showing common sites of stress fracture
(shaded)

Cartilage Problems

Joints are complex pieces of biological engineering which enable the
ends of bones to slide smoothly over each other to allow movement
(Figure 12.2). The articulating surfaces are cushioned with a resilient
pad of cartilage which in many joints is thin and virtually without
fibres, but in others, such as the knee, it is more extensive and contains
collagen fibres (Figure 12.3). Unfortunately, these do not always provide sufficient strength and, in response to a large stress, the cartilage
tears. Damage to the knee usually occurs when it is twisted while
bearing weight, and soccer players are most at risk. Displaced parts of
the cartilage can get between the articulating surfaces and 'lock' the
joint. This is a particularly serious injury and the only treatment is
surgery, followed by a long period of rest while the slowly healing
cartilage repairs itself.

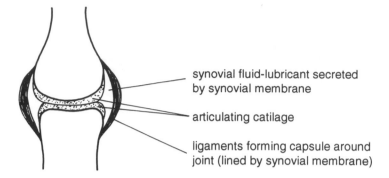

synovial fluid-lubricant secreted
by synovial membrane

articulating catilage

ligaments forming capsule around
joint (lined by synovial membrane)

Figure 12.2. Section through a synovial joint

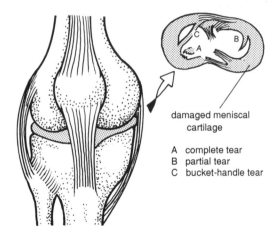

damaged meniscal
cartilage

A complete tear
B partial tear
C bucket-handle tear

Figure 12.3. Front view of right knee and damaged cartilage. After Lachmann, S. (1988). *Soft Tissue Injuries in Sport*, p. 76. Blackwell Scientific
Publications, Oxford

Ligament Injuries

Ligaments connect bone to bone, holding them together at a joint
(Figure 12.2). Some ligaments form part of the capsule that surrounds
a joint and retains the synovial fluid which lubricates it, while other
ligaments are outside the capsule. All are composed of tough inexten-
sible collagen fibres embedded in a matrix. Awkward strain on the
joint can 'sprain' the ligaments, i.e. cause them to tear partially. Only
rarely does a ligament rupture completely, in which case surgery is
necessary.

Muscle Injuries

A blow can cause bruising due to blood leaking from burst capillaries. If the blow is severe, sufficient blood may leak out to form a blood clot within the muscle and in so doing cause a specific localized and painful swelling—a haematoma. If large, this can take a long time to heal because the clot has to disperse before the surrounding tissue can repair.

By far the commonest muscle injury is the 'pull' or 'strain', which occurs when a small number of fibres have been torn and some bleeding occurs into the muscle. Only rarely does a muscle actually tear apart, in which case surgery is needed to re-join the severed ends. Muscles tear most easily when they are cold and unstretched; the importance of an adequate warm-up, which includes stretching exercises prior to any training or competition, cannot be over-emphasized.

Tendon Injuries

Tendons are bundles of fibres, mostly collagen but with some elastic fibres, which connect muscle fibres to each other and to bone. The cells producing these collagen fibres are embedded in the matrix of the tendon. Healthy tendons are very tough and are rarely damaged but the bone-to-tendon and the tendon-to-muscle attachments may be disrupted by excessive force. The Achilles tendon—the longest in the body (Figure 12.4)—is particularly prone to damage and will rupture

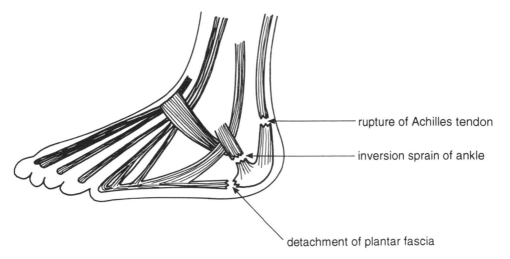

Figure 12.4. Tendons of the foot showing common sites of injury

relatively easily, especially as it weakens as part of the natural ageing process.

In the course of their natural action, tendons move past stationary objects, such as a bone projection. If this friction causes damage, then inflammation results and a vicious circle will have begun in which the enlarged tissue rubs more firmly against its surroundings and this further increases the inflammation. Rest, physiotherapy (physical therapy) and drugs may be necessary to break the circle. Tennis elbow (pain in the outside of the elbow, especially when gripping and twisting), housemaid's knee and Achilles tendinitis are all manifestations of this condition.

Skin Injuries

Skin has evolved to tolerate a great deal of abrasion, but rubbing can all too readily produce blisters (Figure 12.5). In a blister, friction has caused the epidermis to separate from the underlying dermis and the gap between becomes filled with extracellular fluid. Blisters are one consequence of a mismatch between foot shape and shoe shape. Treatment involves piercing the blister with a sterile needle and draining it before applying a dressing.

The skin responds to extra pressure by thickening the epidermis at that site. This is often beneficial but on the feet a corn can be formed and the thickened skin can press painfully on the underlying tissues. In such cases the services of a chiropodist may be needed.

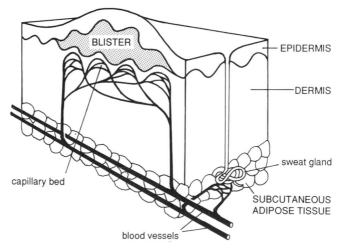

Figure 12.5. Diagrammatic section through skin showing blister

Cramp and Stitch

Although not true injuries, cramp and stitch are discomforts experienced by most athletes at some time. Despite their common occurrence there is no satisfactory explanation for either. They are not caused by lactic acid build-up, although damage resulting from acidity may be partly responsible for a cramp. One theory is that cramps occur because damaged muscle membranes allow a large quantity of calcium to 'leak' into the muscle fibre which is sufficient to initiate a strong contraction. This strong local contraction results in pain and, since the response of muscle to pain is to contract, more motor units are recruited and the pain increases—an uncomfortable example of positive feedback. The cure is to generate tension in the antagonistic muscles so that by reciprocal inhibition the nervous stimulation to the cramping muscle will be decreased. It is most unlikely that the condition has anything to do with lack of salt, despite popular opinion.

A stitch is a sharp pain or spasm in the side of the abdomen. There are many theories concerning its cause and, indeed, there may be many causes. One suggestion is that it may be caused by food in the small intestine which could pull on the connective tissue in this region of the abdominal cavity and cause pain by activation of stretch receptors. The affected runner has a choice; either stop the exercise causing the stitch or continue and ignore the pain. In both cases the stitch goes.

INJURY AND HEALING

Swelling and pain are the almost invariable consequences of mechanical injury and, since much of the early treatment is directed towards ameliorating these symptoms, it is helpful to understand their nature. Damaged cells release a number of chemical signals, which initiate a series of biochemical events that result in inflammation—a complex response to injury characterized by heat, swelling, redness, pain and loss of function. The initial response is vasoconstriction (decreased blood flow) which reduces blood loss from damaged vessels. But, as soon as the damaged vessels have been plugged by a blood clot, there is a massive local vasodilation, which can increase the blood flow up to 10-fold. This extra blood brings oxygen, nutrients and white blood cells to the region, and increased capillary permeability allows them access to the site of injury and accounts for the swelling. These changes are orchestrated by local hormone-like chemicals, which include bradykinin, leucotrienes and prostaglandins, which also stimulate

pain receptors. The resulting pain, exacerbated by any pressure at the
site of injury, prevents the patient from using the damaged part. This
pain has evolved to provide rest for the damaged part of the anatomy.
Blood clots that form during the first response to the injury are
gradually dispersed by white blood cells, which will also remove
harmful chemicals that accumulate at these injury sites and, of course,
bacteria.

All this activity can be likened to a house damaged by fire. Once a
peaceful abode but, as soon as repair starts, it becomes anything but
quiet; traffic increases and people with different jobs to do come and
go with considerable noise and activity. The occupants are pained and
disturbed by all this activity but it is essential for the ultimate repair
of the house.

Joints are not simply passive mechanical structures but are bristling
with sensors, known as proprioceptors, which relay information from
the joint back to the spinal cord and brain. This information includes
the forces within the joint and the relative position of its parts, and is
used by the central nervous system to adjust the tension in the muscles
which move the bones at that joint. Inflammation at a joint will
interfere with the function of these sensors and will reduce the amount
of information concerning the state of the joint that passes to the brain.
Consequently, if the joint is used, lack of adequate feedback information can lead to further damage. An athlete who continues to run on
a recently damaged joint can, therefore, compound the problem. It is
the job of the physiotherapist to assess the damage and its rate of
recovery, and inform the athlete and coach just how much exercise can
be taken during recovery. The physiotherapist can help to re-educate
the joint in relation to its proprioceptive function so that once again
it provides useful information to the central nervous system. This may
be equivalent to 'training' for the joint and can, for example, best be
done for ankle injuries by using a wobble board under supervision of
a physiotherapist.

The Healing Process

The healing process does not replace original tissue in the same way
that a broken light-bulb is fixed but is a very gradual process which
may take months to complete. Damage to a tissue causes activation of
cells that have been lying dormant, and these now begin to produce
the proteins and other large molecules characteristic of the tissue
which has been damaged. Some of these proteins will be secreted to

form fibres, mostly of collagen, outside the cells. On the third day after the injury, new capillaries will have begun to form but it will take several more days before they are complete. By about day 7, the continuity of the damaged area will have been restored but it will take a further two weeks of intensive repair activity before the collagen content has become maximal. Even then, this repairing tissue has much less tensile strength than normal, so that it is more susceptible to tearing if undue tension or movement occurs. Further, any tearing will result in extensive bleeding, since the blood supply to the damaged area is still increased above normal, and may well result in additional inflammation which will set back recovery even further.

As repair progresses, strength will gradually increase but it may take three months before the athlete is back to normal, and, even then, scar tissue will be present. For tendons and ligaments, this is not very different from normal tissue and will achieve a tensile strength of up to 95% of the original. In muscle, however, the scar tissue itself will not contribute much power and, more significantly, will be less elastic, bringing the danger that it will tear again more readily than previously. In this way, a progressively deteriorating injury problem can occur. This does not, however, mean that complete rest of an injured limb is recommended. Stretching exercises, ideally done under advice of a physiotherapist, during recovery, will ensure that the new fibres in the scar tissue are aligned with the direction of normal pull and so decrease the risk of a further tear during normal activity once the damaged area has repaired.

The ability to train the mind to work positively in situations such as competition and peak training is discussed in Chapter 10. The means for providing positive and focused attention to physical performance may also apply to the healing process. Positive preparation, mental imagery of the healing process, the achievement of recovery goals and emphasis on the positive side of recovery are suggested as a means of improving the rate of recovery. There is considerable current interest in the way in which the mind can influence the immune system, which plays a fundamental role in the healing process.

RICE (ICER) FOR FIRST AID

Either way this mnemonic summarizes the first aid treatment that can ease the athlete's pain and speed recovery after injury; the letters stand for rest, ice, compression and elevation.

- Rest is obvious and may well be unavoidable if the pain is intense—in which case the pain is doing its job!
- Ice is the magic weapon in the first aider's armoury. Rapid application, maintained for about 5 min, will dramatically reduce swelling. But is this desirable? Since swelling is the manifestation of an increased blood supply and capillary permeability that initiate healing, should it be reduced by the ice bag? The answer is yes! It will slow down the rate of internal bleeding, so that the size of the clot formed as a result of capillary damage is smaller than it otherwise would be.
- Compression, via a compression bandage, applied to the injured region should provide gentle and even pressure to prevent excessive swelling and provide some relief.
- Elevation—raising the injured region—if possible, so that it is above the level of the heart, will reduce local blood pressure and reduce bleeding. This should be carried out at the same time as the remainder of the treatment, so perhaps ICER is the better mnemonic.

Killing the Pain

Chemicals called prostaglandins are in part responsible for causing both pain and inflammation at the site of injury. A number of drugs have been found which interfere with the synthesis of these prostaglandins and so reduce their concentration at the site of injury, decreasing pain and inflammation. Aspirin is just such a drug and has the advantage of ready availability. (Note that paracetamol, although also a prostaglandin synthesis inhibitor, only acts within the brain, so that it is not effective in reducing inflammation.) In recommended doses, aspirin, particularly soluble aspirin, has an excellent safety record, although it can cause problems if taken for long periods. If something 'stronger' is needed, the non-steroidal anti-inflammatory drugs (NSAIDS) such as *ibuprofen*, *indomethacin* and *fenbufen* may be prescribed; indeed some of these are available without prescription. The 'non-steroidal' description distinguishes them from the corticosteroids (including cortisone), which have remarkable anti-inflammatory powers but have to be used with some caution because of the side-effects that can occur if administration is prolonged.

It would appear that pain-killing drugs do not delay the healing process despite reducing the inflammatory response. However, pain-killers turn off the normal warning signals of the body, and this must not imply that normal activity can now be resumed. Chronic pain that does not respond to drugs is sometimes a major problem; acupuncture has in some cases been successful but the advice of a sports physician should be sought before this treatment is undertaken.

CALL IN THE PHYSIO!

Physiotherapy is the practice of aiding recovery of the muscular and skeletal systems after injury or operation. The role of the physiotherapist is to return the athlete to full functional fitness in the shortest and safest possible time. Any reasonably serious injury to an athlete will require the attention of a trained physiotherapist, and even minor injury may benefit from their advice and treatment. Some knowledge of the techniques used may help the athlete seek and accept treatment from the physiotherapist more readily and even, in the case of minor injury, duplicate it at home. The physiotherapist is, for most such injuries, far more important than the physician and should carry out a clinical examination and take a full history of the injury.

This means that the best physiotherapists will spend a lot of time with their patients, attempting to assess the extent of the damage, its cause and then its proper treatment. If your physiotherapist is not providing you with such a service, change your physio! Finally, during recovery, the physiotherapist should work hand in hand with the coach towards a gradual return to full fitness, using some of the following techniques.

Massage

Some athletes use massage to relax their muscles as a routine prior to competition, and this may be particularly important for previously damaged areas of muscle. During recovery, the main benefit from massage is the increased flow of blood to the muscles, which promotes healing. Massage may also help to improve the orientation of collagen fibres in scar tissue so that subsequent stretching is less likely to cause damage, and for this purpose a vibrator is often used. Massage may not be of much benefit immediately after finishing a training session, except to improve relaxation, and is not recommended immediately after injury.

Whether embrocations or liniments assist healing is a matter of debate. They certainly cause vasodilation in the skin, with accompanying feelings of warmth, but this effect is superficial and any influence on blood flow through deeper tissues is more questionable. Their main benefit may be as lubricants to facilitate massage.

Stretching

Regular and frequent stretching is important during the healing of muscle fibres for, like massage, it assists in the correct orientation of fibres and counteracts the normal tendency for scar tissues to shorten and pucker. Even after healing is complete, stretching exercises remain of value to dissuade scar tissue from contracting and so becoming more vulnerable to tearing.

Exercise

The development of tension in injured muscles themselves, and consequently in associated tendons and ligaments, might not at first be thought to be conducive to healing but, like passive stretching, movement of the muscles promotes good orientation of the fibres in soft-tissue scars.

Initially, the exercise must be light but it can progressively increase in intensity as healing progresses. The professional training of the physiotherapist or the long experience of the veteran coach is invaluable in encouraging a safe but effective level of exercise. In the early stages of recovery, they may well advise isometric exercises in which tension is developed without producing movement at joints. The assessment of strength on isometric machines and the range of movement possible can be used quantitatively and objectively to assess the benefit and progress of the treatment.

Strapping and Support

Like exercising damaged tissues, the use of strapping, or other means of reducing mobility, is a matter of fine judgement. Light support may be desirable in some cases as a preventive measure or as a slight protection, but it must be borne in mind that immobilization is the opposite of exercise! Not only is there a danger of it reducing the rate of healing but also the possibility that it might put additional strain on hitherto undamaged parts of the anatomy.

Heat

The rationale behind heat therapy is that the raised temperature induces better blood flow to the damaged area and so speeds healing.

The heat can be applied by immersion in hot water, electrical heating pads, hot towels or infra-red lamps. However, the degree of penetration of such superficially applied sources of heat is questionable and the benefits may be of a more generally comforting nature. Heat should not be used within 48 h of the injury since it might encourage bleeding.

Electrotherapy

Deeper-reaching, and thus more effective, heating can be achieved using more sophisticated devices which need expert knowledge for their safe application. These are collectively known as *electrotherapy* and include ultrasound, short-wave diathermy and, more recently, lasers. The physics behind each of these treatments is different but they all warm deep tissues. So far, however, there are no scientific studies to show that they differ significantly in their effects. Short-wave diathermy is perhaps the most widely used of these techniques and relies on the fact that short-wavelength electromagnetic radiation penetrates tissues and is absorbed by the molecules in the tissues. The absorbed energy causes the molecules to vibrate, converting this energy into heat just as in a domestic microwave oven.

Ultrasound is a second technique in which molecules within the tissues are induced to vibrate. This time the movement is generated by sound waves of a very high frequency which are produced by an oscillating crystal applied to the skin. Sound waves pass readily into soft, wet tissues but not through bones or air. Benefits, which are not directly related to the heating effect of ultrasound, have also been claimed, including an analgesic effect, a direct stimulation of protein fibre-producing cells and an enhanced absorption of extracellular fluid into blood vessels to reduce swelling. Further scientific work is needed to test these claims.

Cold Therapy

The use of ice in the first aid treatment of sports injuries has already been advocated but it also has a part to play in the healing process. Somewhat paradoxically, it works because it increases blood flow in the deep tissues. When ice is first applied there is a vasoconstriction, which reduces blood flow and lessens the immediate discomfort, but after 5–10 min this is replaced by a vasodilation in both the skin and, more importantly, in the deeper tissues. If the low temperature is maintained, vasodilation and vasoconstriction tend to oscillate, apparently due to imperfect functioning of the feedback control mechanisms regulating blood flow. In practice, the skin is oiled to prevent surface tissue damage and a pack of melting ice (no colder) is applied for about 10 min. The treatment can be repeated several times each day and, although it is uncomfortable, it actually induces deeper heating than if external heat itself were applied.

It is possible for several of these treatments to be used sequentially; for example, ice pack followed by ultrasonics followed by short-wave diathermy.

Prevention is Better than Cure

Although injuries heal, they are always bad news to the athlete. If nothing else, valuable time is lost during recovery and it can prevent the appearance of the athlete in a major competition for which he or she may have been preparing for many months or even years. The golden rules in an attempt to prevent serious injury are as follows:

- Carry out stretching exercises to reduce the danger of damage.
- Treat minor injuries early so that they do not develop into major ones.
- Allow for a full recovery before returning to full training schedules.

The track athlete should also remember that exercise other than running is possible and, for example, swimming, cycling and skiing avoid the impact problems of running, while maintaining cardiovascular fitness and producing the general feeling of improved mood and well-being normally obtained from running.

OVERTRAINING: TOO MUCH OF A GOOD THING

Alberto Salazar, an élite North American marathon runner during the 1980s, is reputed to have said:

> The last couple of years I thought that if 110 [miles a week] got me a 2:08 [marathon], if I went to 130 I could run 2:07. That didn't happen. It seems so obvious; training is a good thing so harder training must be better. But life is not so simple ... You cross the borderline between proper training and overtraining.

So what is overtraining? It is the phenomenon that occurs when an increase in apparently appropriate training results in a decrease in performance (Figure 12.6). Athletes know it by other names too:

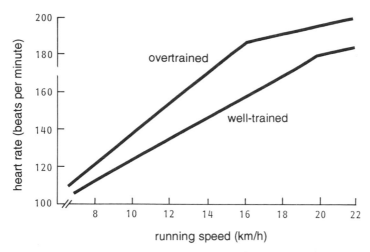

Figure 12.6. An idealized plot to show the effect of overtraining on heart rate inflection point. From Conconi, F., Ferrari, M., Ziglio, P. G. *et al.* (1982). Determination of the anaerobic threshold by a non-invasive field test in runners. *J. Appl. Physiol.*, **52**, 869–873

overwork, overload, burnout, staleness and *chronic fatigue*—simple terms for a complex phenomenon.

A syndrome is a set of symptoms which occur together, usually, it is assumed, as a consequence of one underlying cause. The term is legitimately applied to the overtraining situation because overtraining manifests itself in many ways other than simply decreased athletic performance (Table 12.1). Tim Noakes wrote in 1992 of those present-

Table 12.1. Some of the more quantifiable characteristics that may occur in the overtrained state

Increased early-morning heart rate
Retarded recovery of heart rate after exercise
Postural hypotension
Fall in haematocrit
Decreased performance
Amenorrhoea
Decreased $\dot{V}O_{2\,max}$
Weight loss
Increased incidence of infections
Poor healing of wounds
Inverted iceberg POMS profile (see Figures 10.5 and 12.8)

From Budgett, R. (1990). Overtraining syndrome. *Br. J. Sports Med.*, **24**, 231–236.

ing with the overtraining syndrome:

> The casualties of just this approach [overtraining] were making their daily appearance. There were visitations from runners whose training greed had reduced them to the walking wounded. Some suffered generalized fatigue and recurrent headaches, diarrhoea and weight loss, sexual disinterest and little appetite for food or work. Others were unable to sleep properly, complained they were troubled by early-morning waking, an inability to relax and a general listless attitude to life. Generalized swelling of lymph glands suddenly appeared, allergies had inexplicably worsened; colds, 'flu and other respiratory infections resisted all conventional therapy.

Training is all about stressing the system so that it responds and then functions in an improved way, but there is a limit—the overtraining limit. It is interesting to speculate that the overtraining syndrome is perhaps the manifestation in the athlete of what, in the businessman, raises blood pressure, causes duodenal ulcers and precipitates nervous breakdowns: *executive stress*. And, as with businessmen, if the early symptoms are ignored (itself a manifestation of the stress syndrome) the condition progresses to a less easily reversible state.

At first with training, the athlete is rewarded by moderately increased performance; then comes a stage when additional training effort (peak training) carries the athlete into a 'super-adaptive phase' where performance increases dramatically. It is at this crucial stage that the élite athlete is on the knife-edge between peak performance and overtraining and should keep a wary eye out for the symptoms described below.

The overtraining syndrome is something that particularly affects middle- and long-distance runners, and it has been reported that at least 60% of élite distance runners have experienced it. It also occurs in other sports, including cycling, rowing, swimming and wrestling. In contrast, the overtraining syndrome appears to occur much less frequently in athletes who participate in 'explosive' sports lasting for less than 2 min, perhaps because it is more difficult during training for these events to do too much; fatigue does its job.

One of the difficulties, especially for the coach, is to separate over-reaching from overtraining. Over-reaching is doing too much on one or two days so that tiredness and fatigue set in but 2 or 3 days of rest cures the problem. The condition is aptly described by Noakes (1992) as the 'plods'! The problem for many athletes is that poor performance during training causes anger and frustration at the apparent 'feebleness' of his or her body, so that the next training sessions are planned to be even harder. This in turn causes further stress and a vicious

---

Box 12.1 The unexpected result

Jet lag is a familiar but unwelcome consequence of flying through several time zones and most travellers find it more of a problem when flying west-to-east than in the opposite direction. Potentially it poses a serious problem for the athlete in peak form who has to travel halfway round the world for a competition. Perhaps he or she should choose to fly east-to-west when there is an alternative. However, when Dr W. P. Morgan investigated the problem he found no significant differences between the way the two directions of travel affected athletes.

What did surprise him was that athletes on long flights, in whatever direction, reported improved mental health and decreased muscle soreness. When an experiment does not support a hypothesis (see Chapter 1) the hypothesis must be abandoned and a new one proposed. The most likely explanation is that athletes benefit from pre-competition rest and the long flight ensures that they get just that precisely when they need it. Perhaps rest without the travel would have even greater benefits!

---

circle develops, with the athlete well on the way to the overtrained state or, as Noakes has it, 'the superplods'.

The athlete who is chronically overtrained may never fulfil his or her potential. In a marathon run at Harlow, England, in 1973, the hot favourite was Ron Hill but he was beaten—well beaten—by Ian Thompson. At that stage Thompson was unknown and was training for no more than 70 miles a week. But he went on to become known by winning the Commonwealth and European titles and was advised that he would never be really good unless he ran at least 120–130 miles each week. He took this advice and never again repeated his successes of 1974! Was this a case of the overtraining syndrome?

Diagnosis

Some of the more quantifiable signs of overtraining are listed in Table 12.1. In addition the athlete may suffer:

- Intestinal disturbance, loss of appetite, diarrhoea.
- Increased perception of effort for a fixed level of exercise.

Table 12.2.   The fatigue rating scale of Rose/Noakes
To use this scale, record the number which best corresponds to your feeling
after training or competition. If the number falls below 5 Noakes would
recognize a case of 'the plods'; below 3 and the 'superplods' has struck. Rest is
then essential.

How did you feel during the training?	Score
Sluggish, exhausted. Unable to run	0
Sluggish with muscle soreness at start.	1
Worsened as run progressed. Quite unable to run any faster than a jog	
Sluggish with muscle soreness all the way	2
Sluggish with muscle soreness at start. Felt better as run progressed	3
No muscle soreness but legs and body still sluggish. Required great effort to run fast or uphill	4
Mildly tired but required less effort to run faster or uphill	5
Relaxed, enjoyable run. Effortless up hills or during short speed bursts	6
Moderate to hard effort. Fatigued at finish	7
Strong, hard effort. Fatigued at finish	8
Very strong hard effort. Only mild fatigue at finish	9
Best ever	10

From Noakes (1992).

- Muscle soreness.
- Decreased vigour.
- Disturbance of normal sleep pattern.
- Increased anxiety and depression.
- Decreased libido.

Noakes has devised a questionnaire to enable the runner to convert such subjective assessments into a fatigue scale (Table 12.2).

Three more specific tests may be helpful for detecting the over-trained state:

- *Resting heart rate.* The pulse should be taken on waking first thing in the morning. If it is increased by more than 5 beats/min for 7–10 days consecutively, this is an indication of the overtraining syndrome (Figure 12.7).
- *Resting body weight* . The body weight should be measured on the bathroom scales first thing in the morning after evacuating the

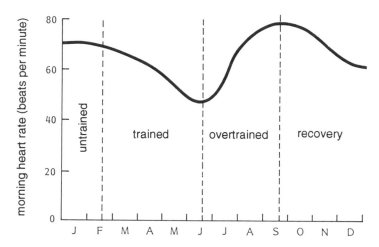

Figure 12.7. Changes recorded in the heart rate of skiers experiencing overtraining. Rates were measured 20 seconds after getting out of bed. From Czajkowski, W. (1982). A simple method to control fatigue in endurance training. In *Exercise and Sport Biology*, Vol. 10, pp. 207–212 (ed. Komi, P. V.). Human Kinetic Publishers, Champaign, IL

bladder and bowels. A decrease in weight of 2–3 pounds may be an indication of the overtraining syndrome.
- *Inversion of the iceberg profile.* The POMS (Profile of Mood States) test indicates a characteristic 'iceberg' profile for élite athletes (Chapter 10), which becomes inverted if overtraining occurs (Figure 12.8). Judicious use of this test can help to detect problems early and so prevent the 'plods' from developing into the 'superplods'. Use of this most helpful tool requires the assistance of a sports psychologist or at least for the coach to be trained in the use of the POMS test.

Although élite athletes may hit the headlines when they have to withdraw from a major event due to the overtraining syndrome (usually referred to as a 'virus'), it can equally easily affect the jogger or the club athlete who increases the intensity or the duration of training too quickly.

The overtraining syndrome can be precipitated by an event outside athletics which, during the stress of intense or peak training, simply adds another stress; the 'straw that breaks the camel's back'. Increased

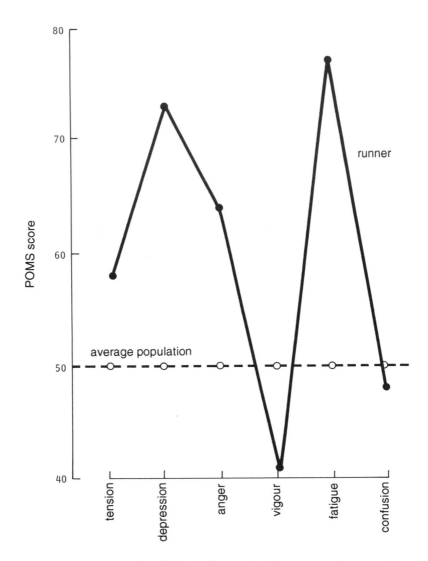

Figure 12.8. The Profile of Mood States for the same athlete as shown in Figure 10.5 after overtraining, showing an 'inverted iceberg' profile. From Morgan, W. P., Brown, D. R., Raglin, J. S. *et al.* (1987). Psychological monitoring of overtraining and staleness. *Br. J. Sports Med.*, **21**, 107–114

pressure at work, losing a job, domestic problems, financial problems or illness of a close relative can all push the hard-training athlete into the overtrained state. An alert coach should be aware of these influences. However, it must be appreciated, especially by coaches, that some athletes will succumb more readily than others to the overtraining syndrome. The reason, at present, is no more apparent than the variation in susceptibility to other stress-related conditions. Genetic factors, previous training patterns and intensity, frustrations, general lifestyle and even diet probably all play a part.

Treatment

If the athlete suffers from a case of full-blown overtraining syndrome a period of at least 6 weeks' rest or partial rest may be necessary to restore normality. During such long rest and recovery periods, particularly in response to overtraining, psychological problems, particularly depression, may occur which can further delay recovery. A suggested programme for recovery over 6 weeks is as follows:

- 1–2 weeks almost complete rest, only very light exercise.
- 2–4 weeks—a very slow increase in training volume.
- 4–6 weeks—increase training towards a normal volume, but high-intensity training should be completely avoided.

It takes a brave athlete to recognize overtraining at its early and readily reversible stage and agree to rest for a few days. Occasionally, however, circumstances conspire to prevent an athlete from training as intensively as he or she otherwise would. As Seb Coe recounts in his book *Running Free*, the consequences may be pleasantly unexpected:

> My previous aim in 1979 was to get a degree, everything else was subordinate to that ... A reduction in training from March onwards, exams in June and then a build-up of training again afterwards ... I'd withdrawn from a couple of international matches because I knew I wasn't in the right frame of mind after a month of revising until two or three in the morning for my finals, and only a handful of training runs. But out in Malmo I found my strength suddenly flooding back, and expending physical energy instead of mental energy was very relaxing. I found I was full of running in the 800 metres, kicking with 200 metres to go and getting home with plenty to spare.

On 3rd July 1979, Seb Coe ran the world's fastest 800 m (1 min 42.33 s), on 17th July he ran the world's fastest mile (3 min 48.95 s) and on 15th August he ran the world's fastest 1500 m (3 min 32.03 s). Three world records within 6 weeks from a man who had trained minimally for 4 months!

Chapter 13

Dying to Win: Drugs and the Athlete

When religion was strong and science weak, men looked to magic for medicine; now, when science is strong and religion weak, men look to medicine for magic.

Thomas Saaz.

Training is hard work; anything that can increase its effectiveness or can improve performance over and above that resulting from hard training is bound to tempt the athlete. In recent years, this temptation has been increased by the high financial rewards for success. Magic potions are out of fashion but the pharmaceutical industry has provided alternatives. In 1967, Tom Simpson collapsed just 2 km from the end of a very long climb (1828 m) in the Tour de France cycle race. He was dead on arrival at hospital and autopsy revealed a high concentration of amphetamine in his blood which had almost certainly precipitated his death from heat-stroke. This focused public attention on a practice that, despite the dangers and official disapproval, had been gathering momentum since the 1950s.

Although drug abuse in sport has mirrored drug abuse in the wider community, the aim is different; when athletes use drugs they generally do so in an attempt to boost performance and improve competitive ability. In 1986, laboratories accredited by the International Olympic Committee (IOC) Medical Commission detected banned substances in 623 urine samples, nearly 2% of all samples tested, and taken mostly from athletes competing in major championships. In the 1988 Olympic Games, drug incidents created more headlines and more interest than the performances themselves, but the taking of drugs in an attempt to improve performance is not a recent phenomenon. In the 1904 Olympic Games in St Louis, Thomas Hicks was given strychnine, which although a powerful poison may act as a stimulant at low doses, together with brandy, during the last 12 km of the marathon. Compounds that may improve performance have, in fact, been used since the earliest documented athletic competition and probably before. According to the Greek physician, Galen, the athletes of Ancient Greece used stimulants as early as the third century BC. Whether their favoured brew of asses' hooves, ground and boiled in oil with roses, would be banned by the IOC is not clear! And the Aztecs, too, used stimulants obtained from cacti, now known to contain a chemical which resembles strychnine, in an attempt to improve their performance in runs that lasted up to 72 h.

Drugs are chemicals introduced into the body generally for one of three purposes: to cure or ameliorate disease; to produce an altered state of mind; or to improve performance in sport. The last two are generally considered to be drug abuse but it is not always easy to draw a clear distinction between drug use and drug abuse in sport. Why should it be necessary to draw such a distinction? If athletes are permitted to use different training regimes, different coaches, different shoes, train at altitude, eat different foods, etc., why should they not take different chemical compounds? No doubt such philosophical questions have been much discussed at meetings of sports governing bodies throughout the world and at least four reasons have been put forward for banning the use of drugs in sport:

- Drugs may give athletes an unfair advantage over other competitors. Professor A. H. Beckett expressed this succinctly by stating that 'competition should be between athletes, not pharmacologists or physicians' (Figure 13.1).
- Competitors who use drugs risk dependency, serious damage to their health and possibly death. Responding to the immense pressure of success, athletes will be tempted to do anything, or take

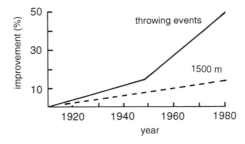

Figure 13.1. Increases in best performances for 1500 m and for throwing events. Differences between the curves have led to the suggestion that anabolic steroids have played a part in improving throwing performance

anything, to improve their performance—especially if they believe other competitors are doing the same.

- Some drugs impair judgement and could pose dangers to other competitors.
- And, perhaps most importantly, athletes are undoubtedly role models for very many young people and their influence is therefore highly significant.

Recreational drug use now occurs on an enormous scale (an estimated 4 million North Americans use cocaine regularly) and probably brings much more unhappiness than pleasure. President Ronald Reagan, in his address to the nation on drug abuse and its prevention, had a special message for athletes: 'On the athletic field you men and women are among the most beloved citizens of our country . . . Few of us can give youngsters something as special and strong to look up to as you. Please do not let them down.'

Box 13.1   A legal loophole?

As with any set of rules, those drawn up by the IOC Medical Commission covering the use of drugs in sport must be unambiguous. But with so much at stake, ambiguity becomes a relative term. Take, for example, the case of clenbuterol—a drug introduced to treat asthma but which also acts both as a stimulant and an anabolic agent (despite not being a steroid). It seems ideal for the pharmacologically inclined athlete and a number have used it.

In the 1992 Barcelona Olympics, the British weight-lifters Andrew Saxton and Andrew Davies were sent home in disgrace after testing positive for clenbuterol. They admitted using the drug during preparation for the Games, but had they contravened IOC regulations? These stated clearly that, like other stimulants, clenbuterol was banned during competition but not out of competition. This makes sense as the effect of stimulants is an immediate one. Anabolic steroids are equally clearly banned in and out of competition since their effects are long-term. Clenbuterol is not listed under the drugs in this category and the catch-all phrase 'and related substances' cannot refer to clenbuterol, it is argued, because it is most certainly not related chemically to steroids.

Saxton and Davies were subsequently cleared but not before their reputations, and perhaps that of the IOC Medical Commission, had been tarnished.

To oppose the use of drugs in sport is simple; to draw up a set of practical rules is much more difficult. Some of the problems are implicit in the four-point declaration produced by the IOC Medical Commission:

- To prevent in sport the use of those drugs which are dangerous to other competitors and the health of the athletes themselves.
- To prevent drug abuse but with minimum interference with the correct therapeutic use of drugs.
- To ban only those drugs for which suitable analytical techniques exist for their unambiguous detection in urine (or blood) samples. (Since modern drug-testing procedures are extremely sensitive, great care has to be taken to ensure that the procedures are reliable and that no possibility of error can arise.)
- To ban classes of drugs (based on pharmacological activity) rather than individual drugs. (This is to avoid use of so-called 'designer drugs' in which trivial chemical modifications produce a 'new' drug without significantly altering its effect on the body. (Despite this careful wording, ambiguities do exist.) A list of some of the substances banned by the IOC is given in Part II(F).

So much for legislation—undoubtedly important but unlikely to eliminate the problem unless it gets support from the athletes. This requires education, and the remainder of this chapter is an attempt to provide information on how the different classes of drug used in sport affect the human body.

Box 13.2   Catching the culprits

Whether the athlete is under suspicion or a random check is being carried out, the following procedure must be followed:

- The athlete is summoned to the Doping Control Centre, and may be accompanied by a team assistant and, if necessary, an interpreter.
- Only one athlete at a time is permitted in the waiting room.
- The athlete must be clearly identified by the Director of the Control Centre.
- The athlete then chooses a collecting vessel and accompanies the official in charge of taking samples to the room where a urine sample of at least 70 ml has to be given. The fact that a urine sample

continued

— *continued* —

is taken in front of an official has led to the suggestion that 'sex tests' are no longer required (see pp. 163–165).

- The sample of urine is then divided into two bottles, chosen by the athlete.
- A code is selected by the athlete for the samples and the two bottles are sealed.
- The Control Centre establishes from the athlete or team assistant what drugs, if any, have been prescribed and taken by the athlete within the preceding 48 h.
- The athlete must sign that all procedures have been carried out according to the Doping Control Regulations.
- One bottle is placed in a sealed container for transportation to the laboratories. The other bottle is placed in a container for reserve samples.
- If a positive result is obtained with the first sample a similar analysis is repeated on the second sample.

At present, most tests are carried out at major meetings but, increasingly, random testing at any time of the year is becoming the norm in most countries. Athletes need to give their permission in advance for such random samples to be taken.

The problem faced by the analytical chemist is that human urine contains thousands of chemical compounds—most in extremely small quantities. Detection of banned substances depends firstly on the separation of these compounds, usually achieved by gas chromatography or high-performance liquid chromatography. In these techniques, the mixture in the original urine is passed along a tube containing adsorbent material which adsorbs different compounds to different extents. The compounds can be detached from the adsorbent material by the flow of a solvent and they emerge from the column in order according to how firmly they are bound to the column, i.e. they are separated. Much can be deduced from the order of appearance but unambiguous identification often depends on mass spectrometry—a sophisticated technique in which molecules of the compound are shattered by a beam of electrons and the pattern of sizes of the fragments determined. The power and precision of modern analytical techniques are awesome—it is even possible to detect traces of steroids in the urine several weeks after the athlete has stopped taking them. Strict monitoring of laboratory performance, including the analysis of standard test samples prepared independently, is, however, essential since an athlete's future may depend on a laboratory's report.

STIMULANTS

Drugs in this class, as their name suggests, increase purposeful movement, mental activity and, usually, elevate mood. The best-known
members are the amphetamine drugs, known on the street as 'speed'.
Their main benefit to the athlete is considered to be the delay in the
onset of fatigue but almost certainly the effect is on the central nervous
system, so that it is perceived fatigue which is reduced, rather than
any process which actually limits muscle power output. Whatever
their mode of action, the athlete should remember that fatigue is
nature's safety valve and that interfering with safety valves can be
dangerous.

Amphetamines probably cause their effects by interfering with the
action in the brain of an important group of substances known as
catecholamines. These include adrenaline (known in the USA as
epinephrine) and noradrenaline (norepinephrine). These, together
with a number of other substances, act as neurotransmitters in the
brain (and in some other parts of the nervous system). Neurotransmitters are chemicals which are released from the tips of excited
neurones (nerve fibres) and affect other neurones in the same area.
The very small gap between adjacent neurones is known as a synapse,
and neurotransmitters released into a synapse either stimulate electrical activity in the next neurone or inhibit further electrical activity
(Figure 13.2). In this way, synapses act as switches, thrown by bursts
of neurotransmitters, that provide the basis for information processing
by networks of neurones. From this, it is believed, arises our capability
not only to control our bodies but also to achieve higher functions such
as rational thought.

So what have amphetamines got to do with the catecholamine
neurotransmitters? The answer is that they are rather similar in
chemical structure. Chemists use structural formulae to show the
arrangement of atoms in space, which determines the properties of the
compound and how it will react with other compounds. But you do not
have to be a chemist to see from Figure 13.3 that there is considerable
resemblance between amphetamines and the naturally occurring
neurotransmitters. Amphetamines increase the amounts of catecholamines, probably in quite specific parts of the brain, either by releasing
stores of the neurotransmitters or by interfering with their uptake
back into neurones after they have done their job. In this way, the
effectiveness of the neurotransmitter is increased and, depending on
which part of the brain the increase occurs in, some aspect of behaviour
will be altered.

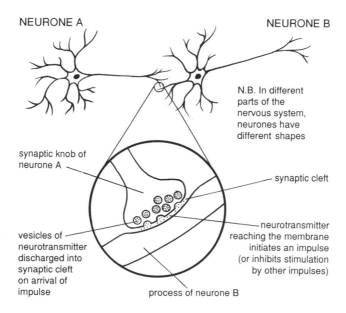

Figure 13.2. Transmission of nerve impulses from one neurone to the next at a synapse. These diagrams are not drawn to scale—the synaptic cleft is only 0.00002 mm across

The information in Figure 13.3 also throws light on Linford Christie's problems in the 1988 Olympic Games. The British runner came third in the 100 m but was promoted to the silver medal position when the winner (Ben Johnson of Canada) was disqualified after anabolic steroids were found in his urine. Christie's urine was then found to contain ephedrine, which is similar in chemical structure to amphetamine and is a banned substance. Ephedrine occurs naturally in plants of the genus *Ephedra* and has long been used in Asia as a herbal remedy, and in modern medicine as a useful drug to simulate the effects of adrenaline and widen the bronchial passages into the lung in the relief of asthmatic attacks, in other allergic conditions and in chronic bronchitis. It is also a stimulant of the central nervous system but has a much weaker effect than amphetamine. Problems for athletes can arise because extracts of these plants are included in many off-prescription formulations used to alleviate colds, hay fever and asthma. But this was not the cause of Linford Christie's problem. The 1988 Olympics were held in Korea, where ginseng tea was available as a matter of course, along with other beverages, in the canteen in the Olympic Village. Christie enjoyed a cup on the day before his race

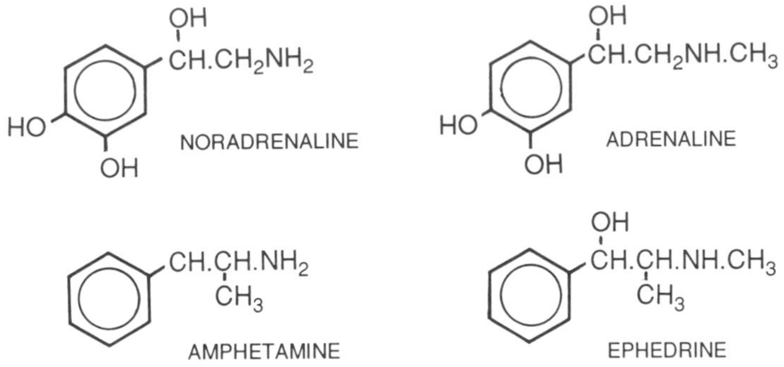

OH
│
CH.CH₂NH₂

HO   NORADRENALINE

OH

OH
│
CH.CH₂NH.CH₃

HO   ADRENALINE

OH

CH.CH.NH₂
    CH₃

AMPHETAMINE

OH
│
CH.CH.NH.CH₃
    CH₃

EPHEDRINE

Figure 13.3. Comparison of molecular structures of stimulant drugs and catecholamines occurring in the brain

without realizing that ginseng contains small amounts of ephedrine. Once this had been established by the Committee he was allowed to retain his silver medal, but this unfortunate episode underlines the important responsibility shared by athletes and their coaches for ensuring that no banned chemicals are consumed in medicaments, food or beverages.

An even more widely used stimulant is caffeine. It, too, appears on the IOC banned list but coffee drinkers can take comfort from the fact that in this case a limit is set (12 μg/ml urine) and only if this is exceeded is action taken. At least six large cups of strong coffee would need to be drunk over a period of a few hours to achieve this level, but caffeine is a component of readily available 'stimulant' tablets.

Also on the list of banned stimulants is cocaine, a widely used 'recreational' drug with serious dependency consequences. Although it does not share a close chemical resemblance with amphetamine, it too exerts its effect by increasing the concentration of catecholamines in the synapses in some parts of the brain. Its mood-enhancing effect is more short lived than that of amphetamine; 20–30 min as opposed to 6–9 h. Perhaps because of this rapid and large effect, it is known as the 'champagne of psychostimulants', but it can also have rapid effects on the heart, resulting in sudden cardiac arrest. It quickly produces physical dependence and, even worse, larger and larger doses are required to produce the same effect. Until 1906 Coca-Cola, advertised as 'the brain tonic and intellectual soda-fountain beverage', contained cocaine but this was replaced by caffeine. Again, athletes are not likely to consume enough to give a positive urine test and in any case a caffeine-free form of this popular beverage is now available.

Box 13.3 The scientific approach

It sounds simple—take two groups of athletes, give the drug to one group but not to the other, monitor their performance and find out whether the drug is effective. Unfortunately, such experiments are not so simple in practice. The first step is to establish whether the experiment is ethically sound. Is it appropriate to administer drugs which could cause harm, especially when there is no medical benefit? Ethical committees ponder such questions; they are not easy to answer.

Humans vary in response to drugs, as they do in other ways. This means that large experimental groups are needed, especially if the effects of the drug are small. Results have to be analysed mathematically to demonstrate that the results are statistically significant, i.e. any differences are due to the drug rather than to chance. The group not taking the drug is called the control group; its role is to show that any effect seen in the drug-users is due to the drugs alone. The control and experimental groups must be as similar as possible in all respects apart from actual drug-taking, including gender, body composition, age, athletic ability and training experience. Then there is the possibility that receiving the drug will affect performance not because of any direct effect but because of expectations—positive or negative—on the part of the subject. To eliminate this effect a placebo is used; members of the control group are given the 'drug' without its active ingredient. Participants are 'blind' in the sense that they do not know whether they have been given the drug or not. But this is not the only source of bias. The experimenters themselves can unwittingly affect the outcome of the experiment by treating the experimental and control groups differently. For this reason they are also 'blind', not knowing which subject is taking the placebo and which is taking the drug, until this is revealed after the experimental results have been obtained. Such 'double-blind' tests are now considered essential in any experiment devised to test the effectiveness of a drug.

One of the most frequently asked questions about drugs in sport is 'do they work?' Subjective impressions are that stimulants can improve performance but scientific experiments are needed to establish the point conclusively. Such experiments are very difficult to do and to our knowledge few have been carried out. One study showed that amphetamines do indeed improve swimming performance (Table 13.1).

Table 13.1. Effect of amphetamines on swimming performance

A dose of 14 mg *dl*-amphetamine sulphate per 70 kg weight was given 2–3 h before the event. Each time represents the average of three swimmers on four separate occasions. Although the overall effect was small, 14 out of the 15 swimmers showed improvement. The authors later went on to show that with highly trained swimmers variation was even less. In a similar test on runners, 19 out of 26 showed improvement but the effects were more variable.

Event	Time (s) Placebo	Amphetamine	% improvement
100 yd free-style	57.47	56.87	1.04
100 yd butterfly	70.96	69.36	2.25
200 yd free-style	136.88	135.94	0.69
200 yd back-stroke	159.80	158.32	0.93
200 yd breast-stroke	171.87	170.22	0.96

Data from Laties, V. G. and Weiss, B. (1981). The amphetamine margin in sports. *Fed. Proc.* **40**, 2689–2692.

Our knowledge of biochemistry tells us that middle-distance runners are unlikely to benefit from stimulants because these would increase the rate of release of free fatty acids from adipose tissue. The fatty acids released would be used by muscles in preference to glycogen, but less ATP is generated per litre of oxygen from fatty acids than from glycogen (see pp. 74–80) so, when oxygen supply is limiting, performance will suffer.

The real problem with amphetamines, apart from considerations of unfair competitive advantage, is the serious harm they can do to the athlete. Both performance and judgement may suffer. As tolerance sets in, higher and higher doses need to be taken to produce the same effect, and the undesirable side-effects of amphetamine, such as anxiety and depression, become disproportionately more troublesome. The stimulating effect of amphetamines on the heart increases blood pressure and with it the risk of stroke; heart beat can become irregular and on rare occasions the heart may stop beating. In practice, the most serious problem has been the dangerous increased susceptibility to hyperthermia—overheating of the body. Catecholamines function as the neurotransmitters for nerves that regulate the diameter of blood vessels and hence control the rates of blood flow through different organs. An increased rate of blood flow through the skin enables the large quantities of heat generated during exercise to be dissipated to the environment, so keeping the athlete's temperature stable. Amphetamines reduce the flow of blood through the skin and so interfere with this normally very effective cooling mechanism. It is no coincidence that Tom Simpson died in the Tour de France race when the ambient temperature was 90 °F. In the 1960 Olympic Games in Rome, three Danish cyclists suffered severe heat-stroke during the 100 km road race and one subsequently died. All three had taken nicotinyl alcohol, a stimulant. It has been estimated that over the past 10 years more than 100 athletes have died due to misuse of such compounds.

BETA-BLOCKERS

The catecholamines, which act as neurotransmitters within the central nervous system, also play a role as hormones outside of it. Adrenaline, with some noradrenaline, is released from the adrenal glands when the body is under threat or stress. It brings about many changes, including increased heart rate, diversion of blood supply to muscles and mobilization of energy reserves, all of which prepare the body for action. Noradrenaline is the neurotransmitter in that part of the peripheral nervous system (the nervous system outside the brain) which controls the basic functioning of the body—the part we cannot directly influence and which we take for granted. Hormones and the nervous system then interact and complement each other.

To exert an effect on cellular processes, chemicals, whether they be neurotransmitters or hormones, must combine with specific receptors either in, or on the surface of, cells. Two types of receptor, known as alpha- and beta-receptors, differ in their ability to bind different catecholamines, including the ones produced synthetically by chemists in the laboratory (Figure 13.4). The binding of catecholamines to alpha- or beta-receptors produces different effects. Some tissues, like the muscles of the uterus, possess both types; here stimulation of the alpha-receptors causes contraction, while stimulation of the beta-receptors causes relaxation. The response of the organ then depends upon the balance of the number of these two types of receptor.

If a certain chemical combines with a receptor without producing a response but prevents the binding of the normal stimulator, it is called a 'blocker' (Figure 13.5). The discovery that some agents blocked only beta-receptors was made by Sir James Black in the laboratories of ICI in Britain, and this discovery has been of great medical consequence. The point is that the receptors in the heart are of the beta type and their blockage prevents adrenaline increasing both heart rate and the force with which the heart contracts (Figure 13.5). Beta-blockers, such as propranolol (Figure 13.6), therefore, slow the heart without affect-

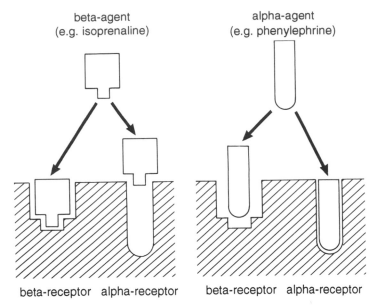

Figure 13.4. Alpha-agents (α-agonists) fit alpha-receptors and beta-agents (β-agonists) fit beta-receptors. Only if a cell possesses the appropriate receptor on its membrane can it respond to the presence of the chemical

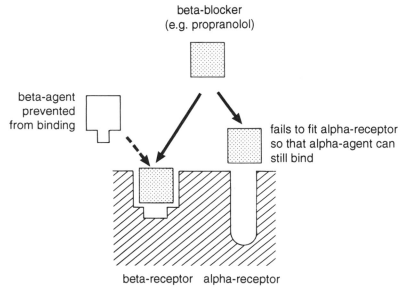

Figure 13.5. Action of a beta-blocking drug on a cell with both alpha- and beta-receptors

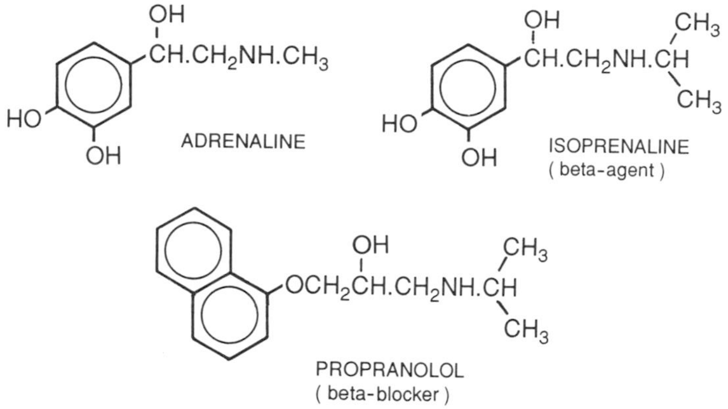

Figure 13.6. Molecular structures of alpha- and beta-agents and of a beta-blocker

ing the functions controlled by alpha-receptors. Such drugs have been outstandingly successful in the treatment of high blood pressure, angina and heart beat irregularities. In recognition of this work (and also his work on histamine receptors), Sir James was one of the recipients of the 1988 Nobel prize for physiology and medicine.

A reduction in cardiac output is not, in general, likely to benefit the athlete! There are, however, sports in which excessive heart activity does cause problems. Pounding of the heart can cause sufficient movement of the shoulders, arm and hands to disturb the aim of rifle and pistol shooters, archers and even snooker players. Indeed, top-class marksmen subconsciously squeeze the trigger, and archers release the arrow, at a stage in the cardiac cycle when the heart is most relaxed. The problem is exacerbated by the additional adrenaline released in response to the tension of competition. Further, adrenaline can cause tremor, which would clearly be a major problem in these sports. What beta-blockers do for such athletes (or would, if they were permitted) is to steady their upper limb muscles. Another 'application' of beta-blockers in sport is to reduce the effects of adrenaline released in massive amounts in 'scary' sports such as ski-jumping and bob-sleighing, in which fine control is still essential.

The big practical problem faced in this area by governing bodies is how to respond to a competitor who claims, perhaps with justification, that he or she has a genuine medical condition which necessitates the use of beta-blockers. To find alternative drugs that are not banned by the IOC for the treatment of the patient's condition is a problem for the sports physician.

NARCOTIC ANALGESICS

Analgesics are drugs which relieve pain and some of the most effective are also narcotics, i.e. sleep-inducers. These include morphine and the more widely used codeine, both of which are obtained from opium, the dried latex of the poppy *Papaver somniferum*, and both of which are banned by the IOC Medical Commission.

There is evidence that drugs of this class are used by athletes, although not widely, to improve athletic performance. Of the 623 urine tests in 1986 showing positive for banned substances, only 23 contained narcotic analgesics. It is possible that some were taken for 'recreational' reasons unconnected with sport, but the euphoria they can induce and their analgesic properties serve to dull the athlete's sensitivity and could decrease the response to fatigue signals. As with stimulants, drugs of this class, especially codeine, occur in non-prescription medications such as pain-killers and cough medicines. It is vital that athletes, their coaches and medical advisers, are scrupulous in their avoidance of such preparations and are familiar with 'safe' alternative analgesics, anti-inflammatory agents and cough suppressants.

The danger with narcotic analgesics is their depressant effect on the respiratory centre in the brain. Indeed, they can so seriously reduce breathing that death results from a shortage of oxygen as effectively as if the windpipe is compressed by force. In addition, the danger of physical and psychological dependence is a very real one for many of these drugs.

ANABOLIC STEROIDS

Anabolic means growth promoting, so that anabolic steroids are those steroids that increase the muscle bulk of the body. Chemically, these drugs are related to the male sex hormone, testosterone. An increase in the concentration of this hormone in boys at puberty is responsible for the development of the male secondary sexual characteristics, including deepening of the voice, increased size of the genitalia and changes in the amount and distribution of body hair. Of course, these are not the effects sought after by users of anabolic steroids, although their development in female athletes, together with suppression of normal ovarian function, can cause problems. The desired effect is one which is also seen in adolescent males, namely an increase in skeletal

---

Box 13.4   It's not natural

The testosterone that some athletes choose to inject or take by mouth is chemically identical to the hormone that males normally produce. There is natural variation in the amount of hormone in different individuals, so the athlete might claim that the high level found in his sample simply reflects a naturally high concentration in his blood. Who is to contradict him? Biochemists will, by pointing out that his testes will be producing not only testosterone but also a second hormone, dihydrotestosterone. Although chemically similar, these two compounds can be detected and separately measured in the laboratory. Normally the amount of these hormones circulating in the blood is controlled by negative feedback; as their concentration rises so release is reduced and conversely as their concentration falls so more hormone is released from the testes. This mechanism keeps the concentration of hormone constant despite fluctuations in the rate of their excretion. In the case of the athlete taking testosterone as a drug, the same mechanism will cause his testes to release less hormone after the drug has been injected or taken orally. However, his testes will produce not only less testosterone but also less dihydrotestosterone, so that the ratio of the concentration of dihydrotestosterone to testosterone in his urine will fall to an unusually low level, and it is this that will attract the attention of the stewards.

---

muscle mass, and hence in strength. They have also been used by the physician to restore muscle in females, for example, after self-inflicted starvation (anorexia nervosa). However, for the mature athlete, very large doses are needed for these steroids to be effective, and this raises the possibility that this particular effect of the anabolic steroid in these subjects is the result of a mechanism that does not play a part in normal development.

It has been suggested that anabolic steroids achieve their muscle-building reputation not so much by a direct effect on muscle but by allowing more frequent and more vigorous training; certainly their effect is only seen when steroids are taken during hard training. This could be because they have an effect on the brain which allows training sessions to be longer and harder—an extension perhaps of their established ability to increase aggressive behaviour. Another possibility is that these drugs somehow overcome a normal limiting factor for muscle protein production. It is an area where science lags behind the results obtained by the athlete.

Whatever the mode of action, there seems little doubt that the effects are real, and the resultant increased muscle mass means increased anaerobic power, hence better performance in sprints and other events requiring explosive bursts of activity. Sprinting, throwing and weight-lifting are events which have long been associated with a high level of anabolic steroid abuse. Anabolic steroids were responsible for two-thirds of the positive drug tests carried out on athletes in 1986.

Testosterone itself, taken by mouth, unless in very large quantities, has little effect on the body, mainly because of the speed with which it is destroyed by the liver. Injection, however, can get the drug into the blood faster than it can be destroyed. Since sex hormones have legitimate clinical uses, chemists soon got to work modifying the structure of testosterone to reduce its rate of degradation by the liver. Other modifications substantially reduced its effect on sexual develop-ment whilst maintaining or enhancing its anabolic (growth-promoting) properties. Nevertheless, users of anabolic steroids for 'muscle-building' find that they need to take between 10 and 40 times the therapeutic dose and at this level side-effects, many of which are irreversible, do occur, including acne, impotence, sterility, diabetes, heart disease and cancer of the liver. Evidence has been obtained which indicates that for athletes on steroids the sperm count is very low and size of the testicles is decreased by almost 40%. There is evidence that athletes may become dependent upon these drugs, so that withdrawal symptoms result when the steroid use is stopped. Athletes must not be expected, or even allowed, to sacrifice their health for competitive success.

DIURETICS

Do you avoid late evening cups of tea or coffee in case your sleep is disturbed by a call of nature? The problem arises because of the diuretic properties of the xanthines in these beverages which cause you to excrete more water in the urine than you consumed in the drink. Medically, diuretics are used to treat patients with high blood pressure because they reduce the volume of the blood. Athletes use, or misuse, them for one of two reasons. First, rapid loss of water will cause a corresponding decrease in body mass—a consideration for, say, the boxer who will gain an advantage by competing in a lower weight category. A second application is to expand the volume of urine by excreting more water, so that other banned substances are diluted and their concentration in the urine falls below those capable of being detected by the analytical chemist. Athletes who have this in mind clearly under-estimate the remarkable sensitivity of modern analytical techniques.

GROWTH HORMONE

Dwarfism is a rare and, for suffers, often tragic condition in which the limb bones fail to grow to their expected adult length. Affected individuals therefore have not only an exceptionally short stature but a disproportionately large head and body. The condition is usually caused by failure of the pituitary gland at the base of the brain to produce enough of a hormone—*growth hormone*—which controls growth during normal development. Dwarfism is much more rarely seen now that pure growth hormone is available and can be injected into young children who show this condition. Even more rarely, an over-production of growth hormone by the pituitary gland (usually due to a tumour in this gland) leads to gigantism. This condition is characterized by disproportionate length of the long bones (long arms and legs) and has led to the suggestion that administration of additional growth hormone to athletes of normal stature will turn them into giants, with correspondingly improved athletic prowess! However, once the limb bones have stopped growing (usually by the age of 18), they cannot be hormonally stimulated to grow any further and growth hormone is ineffective in stimulating further growth. Any 'benefit' of growth hormone to the mature athlete arises from its ability to promote an increase in the amount of muscle.

Increased muscle mass is not, however, the only consequence of growth hormone injection. *Some* bones in the adult can enlarge in response to growth hormone, including those in the lower jaw, feet and hands, to produce a condition known as acromegaly. Even the 'Underground Steroid Handbook' recognizes this danger:

> This is the only drug that can remedy bad genetics as it will make everybody grow. A few side-effects can occur, however. It may elongate your chin, feet and hands but this is arrested with cessation of the drug ... Growth hormone use is the biggest gamble an athlete can take as the side-effects are irreversible. Even with all that, we love the stuff.

Other serious side-effects include an increased risk of acquiring diabetes and the possibility of contracting the fatal Creutzfeldt–Jakob disease (transmitted from the human sources of pituitary glands from which the hormone was formerly extracted). With the advent of genetic engineering techniques, human growth hormone is now produced by living cells in culture. Medically this must be good news since it dramatically increases the safety of the hormone and brings down its price, but it will, however, make it more available to the gullible athlete. The danger of disease transmission will not have been totally eliminated because its use requires injection and with it the possibility that diseases such as hepatitis and AIDS will be passed on if needles and syringes are shared; there is evidence that at least one athlete has contracted AIDS through sharing needles for steroid injections.

The problem of banning growth hormone is one of detection. To date there is no means of detecting it or its breakdown products in the urine. It is possible, however, to detect its presence, or a chemical change as a result of a large amount, in the blood, and blood sampling has now been approved by the IOC.

BLOOD-DOPING

Although blood-doping does not involve the use of banned substances, the nature of the manipulation has led the IOC to declare it an illegal practice, hence its inclusion in this chapter. Its benefit depends on the assumption that oxygen availability in muscles limits aerobic performance and for most track events this may well be the case; it would also be of advantage in the marathon.

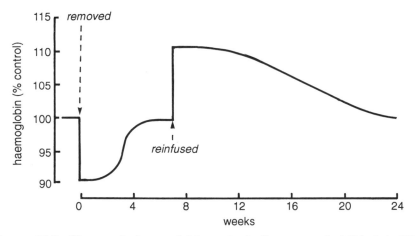

Figure 13.7. Changes in haemoglobin content after removal of 1½ pints (900 ml) of blood and subsequent re-infusion of red blood cells.

Some weeks before competition, the athlete has 1 litre of blood withdrawn from a vein and the blood is put into storage. This withdrawal means that the athlete has fewer red blood cells circulating in the bloodstream. This decrease in the number of red cells is somehow detected by the body and, as a result, the rate of their production in the bone marrow is speeded up so that, after a month or so, the number of red cells in the blood has returned to normal. At this point, the blood that was previously removed is re-infused and this increases the athlete's haemoglobin content by about 10%. Although this reverts to normal it is a slow process, so that the haemoglobin level will remain elevated for several weeks and possibly several months (Figure 13.7).

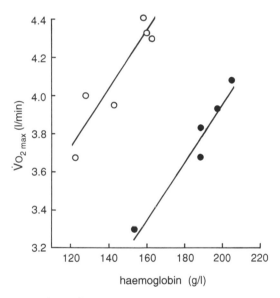

Figure 13.8. Changes in $\dot{V}_{O_2\,max}$ after several re-infusions of red cells in an individual with a low initial level of haemoglobin and one with a high level. In healthy adults there is a large variation in the haemoglobin level in the blood (approximately 120–170 g/l); the level is often low in athletes (pp. 147–148). It seemed possible that benefits from re-infusion would only occur in those individuals who had low initial levels of haemoglobin. This study showed that the increase in $\dot{V}_{O_2\,max}$ was similar after several re-infusions, whether the initial haemoglobin level was high or low. The data demonstrate an increase in $\dot{V}_{O_2\,max}$ of about 19 ml/min for every 1 g increase in haemoglobin. From Celsing, F., Svedenhag, J., Pihlstedt, P. *et al*, (1987). Effects of anaemia and stepwise-induced polycythaemia on maximal aerobic power in individuals with high and low haemoglobin concentrations. *Acta Physiol. Scand.*, **129**, 47–54

Experimental studies have shown that this procedure can raise $\dot{V}O_2$ max by 5% or more—quite enough to 'justify' its use by the athlete who is anxious to improve his or her competitive performance.

Indeed it is possible to carry out successive withdrawals and re-infusions of blood over a short period. These re-infusions have additive effects on the haemoglobin content and the $\dot{V}O_{2\,max}$, which was proportional to haemoglobin content over the range investigated in a Scandinavian study (Figure 13.8).

Although outlawed by the IOC, blood-doping is difficult to detect. One possible approach is to detect changes in blood chemistry which reflect the artificial increase in the number of red cells in the blood.

BLOOD-DOPING WITHOUT THE BLOOD

When a litre of blood is removed from the body for blood-doping, the body responds to a lower haematocrit by increasing the level of a hormone in the blood—a hormone that is produced by the kidney and is known as erythropoietin (EPO). EPO stimulates the rate of production of new red cells in the bone marrow which results, in a few days, in the restoration of the normal number of red cells in the blood. Therefore on re-infusion of the original cells, the haematocrit increases.

The same 'benefit' should result, therefore, from injecting EPO into a person from whom blood has not been removed. Indeed it does. Genetic engineering has made possible the commercial production of large quantities of EPO for the treatment of patients, such as those with defective kidneys, unable to produce enough of their own EPO or who are suffering from certain forms of anaemia. It has also made EPO available to athletes.

Part II

Principles into Action

Tulloh's Training Schedules

The implication through the first part of this book has been that by understanding more about how athletes perform at the limits of their capacity we will be in a better position to train our bodies to do likewise—or better. We firmly believe this to be so and would like, at this stage, to recommend training schedules, devised by Bruce Tulloh, which put these principles into practice. However, when we attempt to do so we run against some insuperable difficulties, the most serious of which is the lack of testing. As scientists we can only accept the benefits of a technique if trials with adequate control groups and proper statistical procedures have been carried out. Since they haven't, we could stop here, but we are going to press on and present a series of schedules which *seem* to us soundly based and ask you to accept subjective judgement in the absence of proof. It is the best we can offer, but we express the hope that members of sports science departments in universities and institutes might be induced to tackle such research.

The second difficulty is one which you, the reader, must solve. A schedule ideal for one person may not be right for another; one that improves the performance of an élite athlete will not necessarily help the fun runner. Only you know you, so we begin with some general advice.

EXAMINING YOURSELF

- *Body build*. Targets for performance should be set according to what is achievable with a particular body build. Body fat should be measured regularly (as skinfold thickness—the experts will use callipers but a qualitative indication can be obtained by pinching the skin just above the hip). Any excess hinders the runner and plays no part in providing fuel even for the longest track race. Even in the marathon, where fat is used, its amount never limits performance since the leanest runner has enough fat for 2 or 3 days of marathon running. And any sudden gain or loss of weight, which is not related to storage or use of glycogen, should be investigated.

- *Joint strength and mobility.* An experienced coach should check out the runner's action to pick up excessive movements of the main joints (hip, knee and ankle) which would render them susceptible to injury. Training intensity should be increased gradually to reduce the likelihood of injury.
- *Age and running background.* Sudden changes in the volume and type of training are to be avoided. If training has lapsed, an initial 4-week period of 30 miles a week should be established and thereafter an increase in total mileage of 10% per week is acceptable. Young runners will, in general, accept a more intense training load and recover rapidly from injury but can be harmed mentally by prolonged training. Older runners, however, recover more slowly from the intense training but are more likely to accept a prolonged training load. In general, it is safer to build up the volume first and then increase the intensity.

PLANNING YOUR STRATEGY

- *Clarify objectives.* Training can only be planned if it is known how many meets there will be in a season and how many races per meet. The élite middle-distance runner must be prepared to run three high-class races in as many days; the club sprinter trains for an explosive effort but the explosion may have to occur several times in the same evening if he or she, for example, is doing the relay and long jump as well.
- *Plan for the long term.* It may not be just the next season that matters but the gradual progression over several years. Not all the athlete's 'well-wishers' might appreciate this.
- *Set targets.* Decide by how much it is realistic to improve in a given year. Accept that this will decrease in absolute terms as you improve and that, as this improvement becomes smaller, performance is likely to be affected to a greater extent by other variables such as tactics in races, proper rest, proper diet, injury, viral infections and luck.
- *Keep records.* Either the coach or the athlete should keep a detailed daily diary on all aspects of the athlete's life including performances, subjective assessments, perceived effort, illnesses, injuries, changes in diet, etc. Looking back on this information may well reveal relationships, unnoticed at the time, which will help future

athletic development. It could also reveal early signs of overtraining (Table 12.1).

CONSTRUCTING THE SCHEDULES

- *Diversity*. A deliberate attempt should be made to stress all the potentially limiting factors for the event under consideration, and this is where the scientific approach should help. Training off the track (e.g. joint flexibility training, mental training) must also receive attention.
- *Timing and duration*. The aim of training is to produce the best performance when it matters. Ideally, the training athlete should put in as many hard sessions per week as other commitments permit, but without causing overtraining or injury. For most runners, most of the time, this might mean three hard sessions and one time trial each week, increasing this only in the final stages of peak training.
- *Sequence of training*. The traditional approach of middle- and long-distance runners is to have a build-up period of 4 weeks in which all running is done at a slow and easy pace. In general, however, out-of-season training should be of the same general type as the more intensive training of the competitive season but of much lower volume and intensity and with longer rest periods.
- *Volume*. The total volume must be dictated by the amount the athlete can handle, bearing in mind factors such as age, previous running experience, resistance to injury, psychological make-up and other demands on time. A hard session might be defined as around 3 miles of the appropriate intervals and should be completed about three times a week, interspersed with lighter flexibility or 'bounding' sessions.
- *Speed*. Speed and distance considerations are critical because they determine the way in which fuel utilization pathways are trained (see Chapter 9). Some guidance for the interpretation of the schedules is offered in Table A.1. For middle- and long-distance runners relatively little time, especially in later stages of training, should be devoted to short sprints at 100% speed since anaerobic capacity is maintained with little training and sprint-training can suppress aerobic capacity.
- *Length of recovery*. As a general rule, for short intervals, the recovery period should be twice as long as the interval and for longer intervals approximately equal to the duration of the run (see Box

Table A.1.

Training element	Equivalent race speed
150–200 m sprint	full speed (100% effort)
30 s intervals	½ mile (90–95% effort)
60–90 s intervals	2 miles (80% effort)
2–3 min intervals	3 miles
4–6 min intervals	6 miles

9.3). In the early part of the programme it may be acceptable to allow a longer period for recovery. One guide is to use pulse rate, starting the next interval when it falls to 120 per minute. If this produces too lengthy recovery periods the intensity of the interval should be reduced.

THE SCHEDULES IN GENERAL

These schedules can be considered as models to be modified according to the factors outlined above. For each event, sample schedules are shown for two athletes: an élite-level and a club-level athlete. Separate schedules are offered for the conditioning, pre-competition and competition phases of training. With the provisos outlined above, all the schedules are equally suitable for male and female athletes.

Each schedule involves two or three training sessions per day. In general the early sessions are the same day after day but the late sessions cycle through a series of seven (occasionally 10) exercises. The schedules are presented as complete weeks but the same number of 'hard' sessions can be spread over a 2-week period, interspersed with 'lighter' sessions, for those who cannot cope with the intensive programme. Details of exercises followed by a letter (e.g. [A]) will be found at the end of the schedules p. 346.

| 1 | 100 m/200 m | CLUB | CONDITIONING |

Target times: 10.7/21.8 s

SESSION 1   20–30 min; 4 or 5 days a week

5 min jogging or skipping
2 min loosening exercises [A]
5 min stretching exercises [B]
10–20 min all-round strengthening exercises with light weights [C]

SESSION 2   at least 3 h after session 1

Daily warm-up   5 min jogging or skipping
10 min loosening or stretching
5 min hopping, bounding or high-knee stepping

MONDAY   10 × 60 m hill run (12–15% slope) or 10 × 60 m
    resistance run [D]
60 s walk-back recovery
30–40 min weight-training [E]

TUESDAY   Rest or recuperation exercise [F]

WEDNESDAY   8–10 × 100–150 m hill run (10–12% slope)
2 min recovery
6 × 50 m acceleration run
1½–3 km (1–2 miles) warm-down

THURSDAY   30–40 min weight-training [E]
5 km (3 miles) run (4.00 min/km; 6.20 min mile)

FRIDAY   Rest

SATURDAY   8 km (5-mile) run
80 m, 160 m, 240 m, 320 m intervals at 10.00 s
    80 m with 2 min recovery
2–3 km (1½–2 miles) warm-down

SUNDAY   6 × 100 m hill run (10–12% slope) or 6 × 100 m
    resistance run [D]
2 min recovery
5 × 30 m high-knee stepping
5 min rest
6 × 100 m hill run (10–12% slope) or 6 × 100 m
    resistance run [D]
warm-down

| 2 | 100 m/200 m | CLUB | PRE-COMPETITION |

Target times: 10.7/21.8 s

SESSION 1   20–30 min; 4 or 5 days a week

5 min jogging or skipping
2 min loosening exercises [A]
5 min stretching exercises [B]
10–20 min all-round strengthening exercises with light weights [C]

SESSION 2   at least 3 h after session 1

Daily warm-up   5 min jogging or skipping
10 min loosening or stretching
5 min hopping, bounding or high-knee stepping
5–10 min jogging and striding over 50–80 m

MONDAY   Speed endurance runs at 90–95% effort:
150 m, 2 min rest – 250 m, 4 min rest – 150 m,
2 min rest – 300 m, 5 min rest – 150 m, 2 min
rest – 250 m, 3 min rest
1½ km (1 mile) warm-down

TUESDAY   30–40 min weight-training [E]

WEDNESDAY   5 × 60 m hill run (15% slope)
60 s walk-back recovery
5 × 50 m sprint drill (e.g. 'pulling' with front leg)
5 × 60 m hill run (15% slope)
60 s walk-back recovery
5 × 50 m sprint drill (e.g. picking up back leg)
1½ km (1 mile) warm-down

THURSDAY   6 × 60 m sprints at 95–100% effort from running
start with 2 min rest between
20–30 min light weight-training [C]
4 × 60 m sprints at 90–100% effort
1½–3 km (1–2 miles) warm-down

FRIDAY   Rest

SATURDAY   4 × 100 m round the bend, at 95% effort; 2 min
                recovery between
                6 × 30 m starting practice from blocks
                5 min rest
                110 m – 90 m – 70 m from running start, timed
                over final 50 m, 3 min rest between

SUNDAY   10 × 60 m resistance run
                20–30 min light weight-training [C]
                3 km (2 miles) steady running

3	100 m/200 m	CLUB	COMPETITION

Target times: 10.7/21.8 s

SESSION 1   20–30 min; 4 or 5 days a week

5 min jogging
5 min stretching exercises [B]
10 min run
10 min all-round strengthening exercise with light weights [C]

SESSION 2   at least 3 h after session 1

Daily warm-up   5 min jogging or skipping
10 min loosening or stretching
5 min hopping, bounding or high-knee stepping
5–10 min jogging and striding over 50–80 m

MONDAY   1 × 300 m, at 95% effort
5 min recovery
4 × 200 m 'differentials' [G]; 3 min recovery
    between
6 × 30 m starting practice from blocks
warm-down

TUESDAY   20 min light weight-training [C]

WEDNESDAY   Club competition, or
6 × 60 m at 95–100% effort; 2 min recovery
    between

THURSDAY   10 min additional flexibility exercises [A]
3 × 5 × 30 m sprint drills (high-knee stepping,
    pulling with front leg, picking up back leg)
4 × 50 m at 80% effort
1½ km (1 mile) warm-down

FRIDAY   Rest

SATURDAY   Race

SUNDAY   20 min light weight-training [C]
8 × 50 m acceleration runs
1½ km (1 mile) warm-down

4	100 m/200 m	ÉLITE	CONDITIONING

Target times: 10.0/19.9 s

SESSION 1

Daily warm-up   10 min slow jogging
15 min loosening exercises [A]
10 min jogging and striding at gradually increasing speed

MONDAY   Drills, e.g. 5 × 50 m high-knee lift; 5 × 50 m bounding; 5 × 40 m against a belt with slow walk-back recovery after each
10 min warm-down jogging

TUESDAY   Weight-training. Set of eight exercises covering all major muscle groups: × 10 at moderate weight; × 6 at higher weight; × 3 at highest weight
3 km (2 miles) warm-down (or massage)

WEDNESDAY   Indoor sport, e.g. basketball, or practice on another event

THURSDAY   Weight-training. Set of eight exercises covering all major muscle groups: × 10 at moderate weight; × 6 at higher weight; × 3 at highest weight

FRIDAY   Warm-up only

SATURDAY   Warm-up only

SUNDAY   Circuit training in gymnasium, including two-foot jumping, hopping and all-round body exercises

SESSION 2   at least 5 h after session 1

Daily warm-up   10 min slow jogging
15 min loosening exercises [A]
10 min jogging and striding at gradually increasing speed

MONDAY   6–8 × 80 m hill-training, fast (10% slope)
2 min recovery

TUESDAY	Untimed fast striding: 180 m, 160 m, 140 m, 130 m, 120 m, 110 m 2 min recovery 10 min warm-down jogging
WEDNESDAY	Resistance work, e.g. 10 × 30 m sand-dune sprints or 6 × 100 m in boots pulling tyre
THURSDAY	Untimed speed work 100 m, 90 m, 80 m, 70 m, 60 m, 50 m 2 min recovery 10 min warm-down jogging
FRIDAY	Drills, e.g. 5 × 50 m leg speed; 5 × 50 m ankle drive; 5 × 50 m back lift, with slow walk-back recovery after each 5 min jogging *after each set*
SATURDAY	10 × 60 m hill training (15% slope) or resistance work (see Wednesday)
SUNDAY	Rest

| 5 | 100 m/200 m | ÉLITE | PRE-COMPETITION |

Target times: 10.0/19.9 s

SESSION 1

Daily warm-up	10 min slow jogging 15 min loosening exercises [A] 10 min jogging and striding at gradually increasing speed
MONDAY	2 × (5 × 60 m) bounding on grass with slow walk-back recovery after each 60 m and 5 min jog after each set
TUESDAY	Weight-training. Set of eight exercises covering all major muscle groups: × 10 at moderate weight; × 6 at higher weight
WEDNESDAY	Warm-up only
THURSDAY	Circuit training in gymnasium, including two-foot jumping, hopping and all-round body exercises
FRIDAY	2 × (5 × 60 m) bounding on grass with slow walk-back recovery after each 60 m and 5 min jog after each set
SATURDAY	Warm-up only
SUNDAY	4 × 120 m hill run (5% slope) 2 min recovery after each 5 min jog 4 × 120 m down the slope—all on grass, fast but untimed

SESSION 2   at least 5 h after session 1

Daily warm-up	10 min slow jogging 15 min loosening exercises [A] 10 min jogging and striding at gradually increasing speed

MONDAY	6 × 60 m resistance work, through sand or against a belt
TUESDAY	Drills, e.g. 5 × 50 m high-knee lift; 5 × 50 m bounding; 5 × 40 m against a belt with slow walk-back recovery after each 10 min warm-down jogging
WEDNESDAY	'Speed–endurance' session at close to maximum effort over 120 m – 150 m – 180 m – 150 m – 120 m with 5–6 min recovery after each, timed and recorded
THURSDAY	5 × 60 m sprint drill—'knee lift' and 'arm drive' 10 min rest 6 × 40 m acceleration from blocks (filmed and reviewed by coach after each run)
FRIDAY	Rest
SATURDAY	Warm-up only
SUNDAY	3 km jog; 15 min loosening exercises [A]

| 6 | 100 m/200 m | ÉLITE | COMPETITION |

Target times: 10.0/19.9 s

SESSION 1

Daily warm-up	10 min slow jogging 15 min loosening exercises [A] 10 min jogging and striding at gradually increasing speed
MONDAY	Drills, e.g. 5 × 50 m high-knee lift; 5 × 50 m bounding; 5 × 40 m against a belt with slow walk-back recovery after each 10 min warm-down jogging
TUESDAY	Warm-up only
WEDNESDAY	Warm-up only
THURSDAY	Warm-up only
FRIDAY	Rest
SATURDAY	Semi-finals or relay heats of championship event Warm-down followed by massage
SUNDAY	Rest

SESSION 2   at least 5 h after session 1

Daily warm-up	10 min slow jogging 15 min loosening exercises [A] 10 min jogging and striding at gradually increasing speed
MONDAY	2 × 150 m + 2 × 110 m from running start, untimed, working on stride length and 'relaxation at speed' 5–10 min recovery after each
TUESDAY	6 × 60 m at 100% effort—timed (filmed and reviewed by coach) 5 min recovery after each 10 min warm-down jog

WEDNESDAY   Relay practice
Warm-down followed by massage

THURSDAY   Rest

FRIDAY   Long warm-up
Heats of championship event
Warm-down

SATURDAY   Long warm-up
Finals of championship event
Warm-down

SUNDAY   Untimed striding on grass, including 4 × 80 m up
5% slope
2 min recovery after each

7	400 m	CLUB	CONDITIONING

Target time: 48 s

SESSION 1   20–30 min; 4 or 5 days a week

5 min jogging or skipping
2 min loosening exercises [A]
5 min stretching exercises [B]
10–20 min strengthening exercises with light weights [C]

SESSION 2   at least 3 h after session 1

Daily warm-up   5 min jogging
10 min loosening and stretching exercises [A] [B]
5 min hopping, bounding or high-knee stepping

MONDAY   6–10 × 100 m hill run (12–15% slope) or 8–10 × 80–100 m resistance run [D]
30–40 min weight-training. 3–4 sets of 8 exercises: 2 for upper trunk, 2 for trunk and abdomen, 4 for legs. All done at medium load except for 2 leg exercises at high

TUESDAY   Rest or recuperation exercise [F]

WEDNESDAY   8–10 × 150 m hill run (10–12% slope); 2 min recovery
2–3 km (1–2 miles) warm-down including several 50 m strides

THURSDAY   30–40 min weight training, as Monday
5–8 km (3–5 miles) run (4.00 min/km; 6.20 min/mile)

FRIDAY   Rest

SATURDAY   5–8 km (3–5-mile) run (4.00 min/km; 6.20 min/mile)
Timed 80 m – 160 m – 240 m – 320 m with 2 min recovery, at 10–11 s/80 m
1½ km (1 mile) warm-down

SUNDAY   (Omit early session)
8–10 km (5–6 miles) run on grass including 4 × 60–90 s hard run, with 5 min jog recovery

8	400 m	CLUB	PRE-COMPETITION

Target time: 48 s

SESSION 1   daily

5 min jogging
5 min stretching exercises [B]
10 min continuous run (3.45 min/km; 6.00 min/mile)
10 min strengthening exercises [C]

SESSION 2   at least 3 h after session 1

Daily warm-up   10 min jogging
10 min loosening and stretching [A] [B]
5–10 min jogging and striding

MONDAY   600 m (84–86 s)
10 min rest
4 × 300 m (approx. 36 s)
5 min rest
2–3 km (1–2 miles) warm-down

TUESDAY   20 min light weight-training chiefly for legs (e.g.
step-ups, squat-jumps, heel-raising, skipping,
jumping)
6 × 60 m bounding
1½ km (1 mile) warm-down

WEDNESDAY   6–8 × 150 m hill run (10–12% slope); 2 min recovery
ery
2 × 5 × 30 m sprint drills
1½ km (1 mile) warm-down

THURSDAY   Fast running round bend at race speed: 130 m –
150 m – 170 m – 190 m – 190 m – 170 m – 150
m – 130 m, with 2–3 min recovery
1½ km (1 mile) warm-down

FRIDAY   Rest

SATURDAY	4–5 × 400 m differential runs with first 200 m in 28–29 s then maximum effort for second 200 m; 5 min recovery 1½ km (1 mile) jogging 3 × 5 × 30 m sprint drills
SUNDAY	7–10 km (4–6 miles) easy running on grass, including striding 20 min light weight-training, as on Tuesday

9	400 m	CLUB	COMPETITION

Target time: 48 s

SESSION 1   daily

5 min jogging
10 min stretching and loosening exercises [A] [B]
5 min abdomen and back-strengthening exercises
3 km (2 miles) at 3.45 min/km; 6 min/mile

SESSION 2   at least 3 h after session 1

Daily warm-up   10 min jogging
10 min stretching and loosening exercises [A] [B]
10 min jogging and striding

MONDAY   500–600 m (55 s/400 m)
6 min rest
250 m – 300 m – 250 m – 300 m (48 s/400 m) with
6 min rest after each; 2–3 km (1–2 miles) warm-
down

TUESDAY   20 min light weight-training chiefly for legs (e.g.
step-ups, squat-jumps, heel-raising, skipping,
jumping)

WEDNESDAY   4 × 400 m differential runs with first 200 m in
28–29 s then maximum effort for second 200 m;
6 min recovery
or 3 × 200 m at race speed (6 min recovery) *plus* 3
× 100 m at race speed (3 min recovery)
2–3 km (1–2 miles) warm-down

THURSDAY   3 × 5 × 40 m sprint drills
4–6 × 150 m 'race rehearsal' with 50 m acceleration, 50 m coasting, 50 m drive to finish
Warm-down

FRIDAY   Early session only

SATURDAY   Omit early session
                      Warm-up
                      Race
                      Warm-down

SUNDAY   Omit early session
                      8 km (5 miles) easy running with some short
                          strides

| 10 | 400 m | ÉLITE | CONDITIONING |

Target time: 44 s

SESSION 1   daily (7.00 a.m. approx.)

5 min jogging
10 min loosening and stretching [A] [B]
15 min steady run (3.45–4.05 min/km; 6.00–6.30 min/mile)

SESSION 2   daily (12.00 noon approx.)

Daily warm-up   5 min jogging
10 min loosening exercises [A]
10 min jogging and striding

MONDAY   6 × 60 m bounding; 6 × 60 m hopping on each leg;
6 × 60 m acceleration runs working up to sprint
speed

TUESDAY   30 min weight-training for all major muscle groups

WEDNESDAY   6–8 × 400 m (64–66 s); 2 min recovery
1½ km (1 mile) warm-down

THURSDAY   30 min weight-training for all major muscle groups

FRIDAY   5 km (3 miles) run (below 3.45 min/km; 6.00 min/
mile)

SATURDAY   8 × 200 m (28 s speed); 1 min recovery
1½ km (1 mile) warm-down

SUNDAY   5 km (3 miles) easy jogging

SESSION 3   daily, at least 5 h after session 2

Daily warm-up   5 min jogging
10 min flexibility work
10 min jogging and striding

MONDAY   8 × 30–40 s hill run (12½% slope); 2 min recovery
2–3 km (1–2 miles) warm-down

TUESDAY	6½–8 km (4–5 miles) steady run (below 3.45 min/ km; 6.00 min/mile)
WEDNESDAY	4 × 60 s hard effort through sand; 3 min rest 4 × 30 s hard effort through sand; 2 min rest 1½ km (1 mile) warm-down
THURSDAY	6 × 60 m bounding; 6 × 60 m hopping on each leg: 3 × 5 × 40 m sprint drills. 1½ km (1 mile) warm down
FRIDAY	Rest
SATURDAY	4 × 90 s hill run; 6 min recovery 3 km (2 miles) warm-down
SUNDAY	30 min weight-training for all major muscle groups

| 11 | 400 m | ÉLITE | PRE-COMPETITION |

Target time: 44 s

SESSION 1   daily (7.00 a.m. approx.)

5 min jogging
10 min loosening and stretching [A] [B]
3 km (2 miles) run (3.45 min/km; 6.00 min/mile)

SESSION 2   daily (12.00 noon approx.)

Daily warm-up   5 min jogging
10 min loosening exercises [A]
5 min abdominal and back-strengthening exercises
10 min jogging and striding

MONDAY   1 × 500 m (50 s/400 m)
10 min rest
6 × 60 m bounding; 10 × 60 m hopping
1½ km (1 mile) slow run

TUESDAY   3 × 5 × 40 m sprint drills
1½ km (1 mile) slow run

WEDNESDAY   5 km (3 miles) brisk run (3.45 min/km; 6.00 min/
mile)

THURSDAY   30 min weight-training
6 × 60 m bounding; 10 × 60 m hopping
1½–5 km (1–3 miles) slow run

FRIDAY   3 × 5 × 40 m sprint drills
1½ km (1 mile) slow run

SATURDAY   Omit session 1; warm-up only

SUNDAY   Omit session 1; 30 min weight-training

SESSION 3   daily at least 5 h after session 2

Daily warm-up   5 min jogging
10 min loosening exercises [A]
5 min abdominal and back-strengthening exercises
10 min jogging and striding

MONDAY   4 × 60 s hard effort through sand or uphill; 3 min
rest
4 × 30 s hard effort through sand or uphill; 2 min
rest

TUESDAY   4 × 'differential' 400 m with first 200 m in 28–29 s
then accelerating
1½–3 km (1–2 miles) warm-down

WEDNESDAY   6 × 400 m (60–62 s); 2 min jog recovery
1½–3 km (1–2 miles) warm-down

THURSDAY   100 m – 200 m – 100 m – 250 m – 150 m – 300
m – 200 m – 200 m (11–12 s/100 m, with rolling
starts); 2 min recovery/100 m
1½ km (1 mile) warm-down

FRIDAY   Rest

SATURDAY   3–4 × 300 m; 10 min recovery (with blood lactate
tests)
3–5 km (2–3 miles) warm-down

SUNDAY   6 × 150 m sprint–coast–sprint
Warm-down

12	400 m	ÉLITE	COMPETITION

Target time: 44 s

SESSION 1   daily

5 min jogging
10 min strengthening exercises for abdominal and back muscles
10 min *either* leg strength exercises *or* sprint drills
1½–3 km (1–2 miles) slow

SESSION 2   daily, at least 4 h after session 1

10-day pre-race programme:

Daily warm-up   5 min jogging
10 min loosening exercises [A]
10–15 min jogging and striding

DAY 1   200 m – 300 m – 300 m – 200 m (race speed, untimed); 8–10 min recovery
3 km (2 miles) slow jog

DAY 2   3 × 150 m; 3 × 100 m (sub-11 s/100 m, rolling start, timed); 5 min recovery
3 km (2 miles) warm-down

DAY 3   6 × 120 m fast relaxed running round bend, untimed
1½ km (1 mile) warm-down

DAY 4   3 × 400 m differentials (200 m in 25–26 s then maximum effort to finish); 12 min recovery
3 km (2 miles) slow jog

DAY 5   Warm-up only

DAY 6   200 m – 300 m – 300 m – 200 m (race speed, untimed) 8–10 min recovery
3 km (2 miles) warm-down

DAY 7   5–6 × 150 m tactical running, changing pace every 50 m on coach's instructions

DAY 8   Warm-up only or relay practice

DAY 9   Warm-up only; omit strengthening exercises in
                    both sessions

DAY 10   Race; omit strengthening exercises in both sessions

13	800 m/1500 m	CLUB	CONDITIONING

Target time: 1.56/4.00 min

SESSION 1   daily

10 min easy running
10 min loosening and stretching exercises [A] [B]
10 min steady running

SESSION 2   at least 4 h after session 1

Daily warm-up	20 min including stretching exercises
MONDAY	6–8 × 150–200 m (10% slope) with walk-back recovery 6–8 × 60 m (12% slope) with walk-back recovery
TUESDAY	10 km (6 miles) run (increasing to 3.30 min/km; 5.30 min/mile) 30 min circuit training in gym
WEDNESDAY	10 × 200 m (30–31 s); 45 s recovery 5 min slow jogging 10 × 200 m (30–31 s); 45 s recovery
THURSDAY	On the road, 5 min hard effort – 5 min jog 2 × (3 min hard – 3 min jog – 2 min hard – 2 min jog – 1 min hard – 5 min jog)
FRIDAY	30 min circuit training in gym
SATURDAY	3–5 km (2–3 miles) road or cross-country race or time trial
SUNDAY	Omit session 1 13–16 km (8–10 miles) starting slowly, increasing to 3.45 min/km (6.00 min/mile)

| 14 | 800 m/1500 m | CLUB | PRE-COMPETITION |

Target time: 1.56/4.00 min

SESSION 1   daily

10 min easy running
10 min loosening and stretching exercises [A] [B]
10 min steady running

SESSION 2   at least 4 h after session 1

Daily warm-up   20 min including stretching exercises

MONDAY   4–5 × 800 m on grass; 5 min jog recovery

TUESDAY   6 × 50 m bounding; 400 m jog
6 × 50 m high-knee stepping; 400 m jog
6 × 150 m stride – sprint – stride
30 min steady running

WEDNESDAY   4 × 400 m (65 s); 200 m jog recovery (90–120 s)
4 × 400 m (63 s); 200 m jog recovery (90–120 s)
1½ km (1 mile) steady run
or   2 × (400+200 m) (56 s/400 m) with 60 s walk between 400 m and 200 m and 4 min jog after each set
2 × 300 m (42 s); 2 min jog recovery

THURSDAY   8–10 km (5–6 miles) steady run (3.35 min/km; 5.40 min/mile)

FRIDAY   Rest or 30 min easy run

SATURDAY   Time trials, e.g. 2 × 800 m (100% effort); 10 min rest between
or   Speed training, e.g. 6 × 300 m at top speed; 4 min rest between

SUNDAY   Omit session 1
10–13 km (6–8 miles) starting slowly, increasing to 3.45 min/km (6.00 min/mile)

15	800 m/1500 m	CLUB	COMPETITION

Target time: 1.56/4.00 min

SESSION 1   daily

10 min easy running
10 min loosening and stretching exercises [A] [B]
10 min steady running

SESSION 2   Daily at same time of day as next competition

Daily warm-up
1600 m easy running
5 min stretching exercises [B]
800 m steady running including 4 × 80 m striding, accelerating to top speed

MONDAY
2 × 600 m; 2 × 400 m; 2 × 300 m (63–64 s/400 m); 2 min jog recovery (no additional recovery between sets)
2–3 km (1–2 miles) warm-down

TUESDAY
6 × 50 m bounding
6 × 50 m high-knee stepping
3 km (2 miles) brisk run (3.20 min/km; 5.20 min/mile)
2 × 6 × 50 m sprint drills
2–3 km (1–2 miles) warm-down

WEDNESDAY
4 × 300 m (42–43 s); 2 min jog recovery
2 × 400 m tactical practice, striding at 66 s pace and sprinting in response to coach's signal

THURSDAY
6 km (4 miles) on grass (3.50 min/km; 6.00 min/mile)

FRIDAY
5 km (3 miles) jog

SATURDAY
Race

SUNDAY
Extend session 1 to 8 km (5 miles)
5–6 km (3–4 miles) fartlek

16	800 m/1500 m	ÉLITE	CONDITIONING

Target time: 1.42/3.30 min

SESSION 1   daily (7.00 a.m. approx.)

5–10 min slow jog
10 min loosening and stretching exercises [A] [B]
10 min steady running (3.45 min/km; 6.00 min/mile)

SESSION 2   daily (12.00 noon approx.)

Daily warm-up	10–20 min depending on type of session but including 10 min stretching
MONDAY	10 km (6 miles) steady run (3.45 min/km; 6.00 min/mile) 20 min loosening exercise [A]
TUESDAY	6 km (4 miles) brisk run (3.25 min/km; 5.30 min/mile) 1½ km (1 mile) slow run
WEDNESDAY	10 km (6 miles) steady run (3.45 min/km; 6.00 min/milc)
THURSDAY	6 km (4 miles) steady run (3.45 min/km; 6.00 min/mile) 3 × 5 × 60 m sprint drills
FRIDAY	Rest
SATURDAY	Omit session 1 8 km (5 miles) slow run
SUNDAY	Omit session 1 16 km (10 miles) slow run

SESSION 3   daily, at least 5 h after session 2

Daily warm-up	20 min, including 10 min stretching
MONDAY	8 × 200 m (30 s); 60 s recovery 1½ km (1 mile) jog 8 × 150 m (13–14 s/100 m) 1½ km (1 mile) jog 8 × 60 m (12 s/100 m) 3 km (2 miles) slow run
TUESDAY	30 min weight/gym training for all main muscle groups 6 km (4 miles) slow run
WEDNESDAY	2 × 800 m (2.16 min); 2 min recovery 2 × 400 m (62–66 s); 1 min recovery 1½ km (1 mile) jog 4 × 300 m (44 s); 90 s recovery 1½ km (1 mile) jog
THURSDAY	4 × 2 min hill-training (10% slope) 1½ km (1 mile) jog 8 × 45 s hill-training (12½%) 1½ km (1 mile) jog 4 × 20 s hill-training (15%) all at maximum effort 3 km (2 miles) slow run
FRIDAY	40 min weight/gym training for all main muscle groups 6 km (4 miles) slow run
SATURDAY *or*	Cross-country or road race up to 8 km (5 miles) 1 × 10 min plus 2 × 5 min sustained fast run (below 3.07 min/km; 5.00 min/mile)
SUNDAY	3 km (2 miles) slow run 4 × 5 × 50 m sprint drills, including 5 × 50 m bounding 3 km (2 miles) slow run

| 17 | 800 m/1500 m | ÉLITE | PRE-COMPETITION |

Target time: 1.42/3.30 min

SESSION 1   daily (7.00 a.m. approx.)

5–10 min slow jog
10 min loosening and stretching exercises [A] [B]
15–20 min steady running (3.45 min/km; 6.00 min/mile)

SESSION 2   daily, at least 4 h after session 1

10-day programme:

| **Daily warm-up** | 20 min jogging, stretching and easy striding
5 min strengthening exercises
6 × 30 m sprint drills, e.g. high-knee stepping |
| **DAY 1** | 3 × 1000 m off track (timed); 3 min jog recovery
1½ km (1 mile) warm-down |
| **DAY 2** | 8 km (5 miles) run (3.25 min/km; 5.30 min/mile) |
| **DAY 3** | 6 × 60 m bounding
20–30 min light weight-training, chiefly for legs, e.g. step-ups, squat-jumps, heel-raising, skipping, jumping
3 km (2 miles) warm-down |
| **DAY 4** | 11 km (7 miles) fartlek, with several hard bursts of 200–400 m (not more than 90% effort) |
| **DAY 5** | 2 × 5 × 60 m sprint drills
800 m jog
2 × 300 m (38–39 s); 5 min recovery
5 × 60 m bounding
1½ km (1 mile) warm-down |
| **DAY 6** | 11 km (7 miles) (3.45 min/km; 6.00 min/mile) |
| **DAY 7** | 8 km (5 miles) in 29 min approx.
8 × 150 m striding |
| **DAY 8** | 10 km (6 miles) easy run |

DAY 9   6 km (4 miles) (3.25 min/km; 5.30 min/mile)
                    4 × 200 m (28 s); 60 s recovery
                    1½ km (1 mile) warm-down

DAY 10   13 km (8 miles) cross-country (3.45 min/km; 6.00
                    min/mile)

SESSION 3   daily, at least 5 h after session 2

Daily warm-up   20 min jogging, stretching and easy striding

DAY 1   8 × 100 m downhill (13 s approx.); walk-back
                    recovery
                    8 × 150 m stride – sprint – stride; 200 m jog
                    recovery
                    3 km (2 miles) warm-down

DAY 2   3 × 4 × 400 m (57–59 s); 60 s recovery between
                    fast runs, 5 min recovery between sets
                    1½ km (1 mile) warm-down

DAY 3   11 km (7 miles) (3.25 min/km; 5.30 min/mile)

DAY 4   8 × 100 m uphill (13 s); 30 s recovery
                    1½ km (1 mile) easy run
                    12 × 200 m (28 s); 30 s recovery
                    1½ km (1 mile) easy run
                    8 × 150 m (28 s/200 m); 30 s recovery
                    1½ km (1 mile) easy run

DAY 5   4 × 600 m (87–89 s); 2 min recovery
                    3 km (2 miles) warm-down

DAY 6   8 km (5 miles) run in approx. 26 min

DAY 7   1000 m (2.30 min); 60 s rest
                    200 m (25 s); 3 min rest
                    800 m (2.00 min); 60 s rest
                    200 m (25 s); 3 min rest
                    600 m (1.30 min); 60 s rest
                    200 m (25 s); 3 min rest
                    Warm-down

DAY 8   5 km (3 miles) (3.25 min/km; 5.30 min/mile)
                    400 m (57–58 s); 1600 m (5 min approx.); 400 m
                    (56–57 s)
                    3 km (2 miles) warm-down

DAY 9 400 m (50 s approx.); 4 min rest
300 m (37 s); 3 min rest
200 m (24 s)
1½ km (1 mile) jog
Repeat fast 400 m, 300 m and 200 m
Warm-down

DAY 10 6 × 60 m bounding
20–30 min light weight-training, chiefly for legs,
e.g. step-ups, squat-jumps, heel-raising, skipping, jumping
3 km (2 miles) warm-down

| 18 | 800 m/1500 m | ÉLITE | COMPETITION |

Target time: 1.42/3.30 min

SESSION 1   daily
___

10-day programme:

Daily warm-up   20–25 min warm-up, including 10 min stretching and mobility exercises

DAY 1   50–60 min very slow running

DAY 2   5 km (3 miles) brisk run (3.07 min/km; 5.00 min/mile)

DAY 3   6 km (4 miles) steady run (3.45 min/km; 6.00 min/miles)

DAY 4   10 km (6 miles) steady run (3.45 min/km; 6.00 min/mile)

DAY 5   5 × 1 min hard hill run on grass (10% slope)
5 × 200 m fast downhill (25 s)

DAY 6   6 km (4 miles) steady run (3.45 min/km; 6.00 min/mile)
3 × 5 × 50 m sprint drills

DAY 7   3 km (2 miles) slow run
2 × 300 m (41–42 s)
1½ km (1 mile) slow run

DAY 8   30 min slow run

DAY 9   20 min slow run

DAY 10   20 min slow run

SESSION 2   daily, at least 5 h after session 1

Daily warm-up   20–25 min warm-up, including 10 min stretching and mobility exercises

DAY 1   3 km (2 miles) steady run (3.45 min/km; 6.00 min/mile

8 × 200 m, on grass (26–30 s); 1–2 min recovery

3 km (2 miles) steady run (3.45 min/km; 6.00 min/mile

DAY 2   3 × 500 m (71–72 s); 3 min recovery

DAY 3   2 × 1 mile fast sustained run (4.20 s); 7 min recovery

5 km (3 miles) steady run (3.45 min/km; 6.00 min/mile)

DAY 4   4 × (2 × 400 m) (56–57 s); 40 s recovery between the two and 5 min recovery between sets

DAY 5   Rest

DAY 6   8 km (5 miles) run (3.25 min/km; 5.30 min/mile)

DAY 7   6 × 300/400 m tactical runs at race pace, accelerating in response to coach's signals; 2 min recovery

DAY 8   20 min steady run (3.45 min/km; 6.00 min/mile)

DAY 9   3 × 200/300 m at race pace

1½ km (1 mile) slow run

DAY 10   Race

| 19 | 3000 m/5000 m | CLUB | CONDITIONING |

Target time: 8.10/14.15 min

SESSION 1   daily

10 min steady running
5–10 min loosening and stretching exercises [A] [B]
10 min steady running

SESSION 2   at least 4 h after session 1

Daily warm-up	800 m jog
	5 min stretching exercises
	5 min trunk-strengthening exercises
	5 min steady running

MONDAY (a) 10 km fartlek on hilly course, with hard bursts
   or (b) 8–12 × 150–200 m hill run (10% slope) with jog
down recovery

TUESDAY   10 km (6 miles) steady run, starting at 3.45 min/
km (6.00 min/mile) and increasing speed in the
second half

WEDNESDAY   8 × 300 m; 60–90 s recovery
10 min jog
8 × 300 m; 60–90 s recovery

THURSDAY   3 km (2 miles) fast run (3.05 min/km; <5.00 min/
mile)
10 min easy run
3 km (2 miles) fast run (3.05 min/km; <5.00 min/
mile)
10 min easy run

FRIDAY   Rest or 30 min easy run

SATURDAY   Cross-country race
   or 3 × 1600 m fast run; 5 min rest after each
3000 m warm-down

SUNDAY   16 km (10 miles) steady run (60 min)

| 20 | 3000 m/5000 m | CLUB | PRE-COMPETITION |

Target time: 8.10/14.15 min

SESSION 1   daily (except Sunday)

10 min slow running
5–10 min loosening and stretching exercises [A] [B]
10 min steady running

SESSION 2   at least 4 h after session 1

Daily warm-up   800 m jog
5 min stretching exercises
5 min trunk-strengthening exercises
5 min steady running

MONDAY   (a)   2 × 8 × 200 m (30–31 s); 40 s recovery between
runs and 5 min jog between sets
or (b)   15–20 × 100 m fast hill run (10% slope); jog down
recovery

TUESDAY   10 km (6 miles) steady run (3.35 min/km; 5.35 min/
mile)
5 × 50 m high-knee stepping
5 × 50 m bounding

WEDNESDAY(a)   6 × 1000 m (2.50 min); jog recovery
or (b)   2 × 800 m (65–66 s/400 m); 2.30 min jog recovery
2 × 600 m (65–66 s/400 m); 2.00 min jog recovery
2 × 400 m (65–66 s); 1.30 min jog recovery
2 × 200 m (100% effort); 1.00 min jog recovery

THURSDAY   8 km (5 miles) steady run

FRIDAY   Rest or 30 min easy running

SATURDAY   2–3 km time trial; 10 min rest
2 × 400 m (100% effort); 3 min rest between
2–3 km (1–2 miles) warm-down

SUNDAY   [Omit first session]
13–16 km (8–10 miles) run (3.45 min/km; 6.00
min/mile) with 6 × 80 m acceleration runs at the
end

| 21 | 3000 m/5000 m | ÉLITE | COMPETITION |

Target time: 8.10/14.15 min

SESSION 1   daily (except Sunday when replaced by 8 km (5 miles) run

10 min easy running
10 min loosening and stretching exercises [A] [B]
10 min steady running

SESSION 2   at least 4 h after session 1

Daily warm-up	800 m jog 10 min loosening and stretching exercises [A] [B] 800 m steady run 800 m with 4 × 80 m acceleration runs
MONDAY	5 × 600 m (90–94 s); 5 min recovery 2–3 km (1–2 miles) warm-down
TUESDAY	6 × 50 m high-knee stepping 15 min steady run 4 × 400 m tactical practice, striding (68 s) and sprinting in response to coach's signal 15 min steady run
WEDNESDAY	6 × 400 m (65 s); 60 s jog recovery 4 × 300 m (44 s); 2 min jog recovery 2–3 km (1–2 miles) warm-down
THURSDAY	8 km (5 miles) run on grass (3.35 min/km; 5.45 min/mile) 4 × 100 m acceleration runs
FRIDAY	30 min steady run
SATURDAY	Race
SUNDAY	8–10 km (5–6 miles) fartlek

| 22 | 5000 m/10 000 m | ÉLITE | CONDITIONING |

Target time: 13.00/27.00 min

SESSION 1   daily (except Sunday), 7.00 a.m. approx.

5–10 min slow jog
10 min loosening and stretching exercises [A] [B]
15 min steady run (3.45 min/km; 6.00 min/mile)

SESSION 2   12.00 noon approx.

Daily warm-up	10 min stretching exercises [B]
MONDAY	30 min flexibility exercises 8 km (5 miles) steady run (3.45 min/km; 6.00 min/mile)
TUESDAY	13 km (8 miles) steady run (3.45 min/km; 6.00 min/mile)
WEDNESDAY	10 km (6 miles) steady run (3.45 min/km; 6.00 min/mile)
THURSDAY	13 km (8 miles) steady run (3.45 min/km; 6.00 min/mile)
FRIDAY	8 km (5 miles) steady run (3.45 min/km; 6.00 min/mile)
SATURDAY	Rest
SUNDAY	18–24 km (12–15 miles) run (3.4–4.3 min/km; 6–7 min/mile)

SESSION 3	at least 5 h after session 2

Daily warm-up	20 min including 10 min stretching exercises
MONDAY	5 km (3 miles) steady run (3.45 min/km; 6.00 min/mile) 10 × 200 m (33 s); 20 s recovery 1½ km (1 mile) jog 8 × 150 m (15 s/100 m); 20 s recovery 1½ km (1 mile) jog 6 × 60 m sprint; 20 s recovery 8 km (5 miles) steady run (3.45 min/km; 6.00 min/mile)
TUESDAY	8 km (5 miles) steady run (3.35 min/km; 5.45 min/mile) 20 min weights/gym training for back, abdominal and upper body muscles
WEDNESDAY *or*	High-volume interval training e.g. 8 × 800 m (70 s/400 m); 2 min recovery 8 × 400 m (70 s); 1 min recovery Timed fast runs with equal duration recovery e.g. 1, 2, 3, 4, 3, 2, 1, 3, 2, 1, 3, 2, 1 min
THURSDAY	8 × 2 min hill run (10% slope) 3 km (2 miles) jog 12 × 45 s hill run (12% slope) 3–5 km (2–3 miles) slow run (4.0 min/km; 7.00 min/mile)
FRIDAY	5 km (3 miles) fast run (3.25 min/km; 5.30 min/mile)
SATURDAY *or*	8–16 km (5–10 miles) race Sustained fast running (<3.05 min/km; 5.00 min/mile) for 10, 5 and 5 min; 5 min recovery between each
SUNDAY	5 km (3 miles) run on grass, including 6 × 150 m easy strides

| 23 | 5000 m/10 000 m | ÉLITE | PRE-COMPETITION |

Target time: 13.00/27.00 min

SESSION 1   daily, 7.00 a.m. approx.

5–10 min slow jog
10 min loosening and stretching exercises [A] [B]
15 min steady run (3.45 min/km; 6.00 min/mile)

SESSION 2   at least 4 h after session 1

10-day programme:

Daily warm-up	20 min warm-up of jogging, stretching and easy striding
DAY 1	3 × (12 × 200 m) intervals (30 s); 20 s recovery; 5 min between sets
DAY 2	10 km (6 miles) run (3.25 min/km; 5.30 min/mile)
DAY 3	Off-track but timed runs of 1600 m – 1200 m – 1600 m – 1200 m at 95% effort
DAY 4	8 km (5 miles) run (3.25 min/km; 5.30 min/mile)
DAY 5	4 × 800 m (2.06–2.08 min); 2 min recovery 5 min jog 4 × 400 m (62–64 s); 1 min recovery
DAY 6	10 km (6 miles) run (3.25 min/km; 5.30 min/mile)
DAY 7	Extra 10 min warm-up 3000 m time-trial (with blood lactate or maximum oxygen uptake test)
DAY 8	13 km (8 miles) run (3.25 min/km; 5.30 min/mile)
DAY 9	600 m – 500 m – 400 m (100% effort); 5 min recovery after each 3 km (2 miles) warm-down
DAY 10	13–16 km (8–10 miles) steady run (3.45 min/km; 6.00 min/mile)

SESSION 3   at least 5 h after session 2

Daily warm-up	20 min warm-up of jogging, stretching and easy striding
DAY 1	8 km (5 miles) run (26 min approx.) 2 × 5 × 50 m sprint drills 5 × 200 m (27–28 s); 90 s recovery 1½ km (1 mile) warm-down
DAY 2	13 km (8 miles) fast run (3.15 min/km; 5.15 min/mile)
DAY 3	10 km (6 miles) steady run (3.25 min/km; 5.30 min/mile) 6 × 60 m bounding
DAY 4	11 km (7 miles) fast run (3.15 min/km; 5.15 min/mile)
DAY 5	5 × 600 m (89 s); 4 min recovery
DAY 6	15 min extra flexibility exercises 8 km (5 miles) in approx. 25 min
DAY 7	5 km (3 miles) easy pace 6 × 150 m stride – sprint – stride
DAY 8	8 km (5 miles) run (3.15 min/km; 5.15 min/mile)
DAY 9	3 × 1000 m (2.42–2.45 min) with 1600 m (5.20 min) between each
DAY 10	5 km (3 miles) steady run (3.25 min/km; 5.30 min/mile) 5 × 300 m (45 s); 2 min jog recovery

24	5000 m/10 000 m	COMPETITION

Target time: 13.00/27.00 min
14-day programme:

SESSION 1   daily, a.m.

Daily warm-up	20–25 min, including 10 min stretching and mobility
Mon. 1	3 × 12 × 200 m (30 s); 20 s recovery; 5 min between sets
Tues. 1	13 km (8 miles) steady run (3.25 min/km; 5.30 min/mile)
Wed. 1	10 km (6 miles) steady run (3.25 min/km; 5.30 min/mile)
Thur. 1	13 km (8 miles) slow run
Fri. 1	6 km (4 miles) fast run (3.15 min/km; 5.15 min/mile)
Sat. 1	5 km (3 miles) slow run
Sun. 1	19 km (12 miles) slow run
Mon. 2	10 km (6 miles) steady run (3.25 min/km; 5.30 min/mile)
Tues. 2	5 km (3 miles) slow run
Wed. 2	8 km (5 miles) steady run (3.45 min/km; 6.00 min/mile)
Thur. 2	5 km (3 miles) slow run
Fri. 2	5 km (3 miles) slow run
Sat. 2	5 km (3 miles) slow run
Sun. 2	8 km (5 miles) very easy

SESSION 2   daily, p.m., at least 5 h after session 1

Daily warm-up	20–25 min, including 10 min stretching and mobility
Mon. 1	4 × [(800 m (2.10 min); 90 s recovery; 400 m (60 s); 2 min recovery)]
Tues. 1	8 km (5 miles) slow run, including 10 × 80 m acceleration runs
Wed. 1	1200 m (3.04 min); 5 min recovery 800 m (2.00 min); 5 min recovery 600 m (<90 s); 5 min recovery 2 × 400 m (55–56 s); 3 min recovery 3 km (2 miles) slow run
Thur. 1	4 × 60 m sprint drills 8 km (5 miles) steady run (3.25 min/km; 5.30 min/mile)
Fri. 1	10 km (6 miles) steady run (3.25 min/km; 5.30 min/mile), including 6 × 300 m (42–45 s)
Sat. 1 *either*	5 × 1000 m; 3 min recovery
or, before 5000 m race	3 × (400 m; 30 s jog recovery; 800 m; 60 s jog recovery; 400 m; 3 min jog recovery) (at 5000 m race speed)
or, before 10 000 m race	3 × (800 m; 90 s jog recovery; 1200 m; 2 min jog recovery; 800 m; 3 min jog recovery) (at 10 000 m race speed
Sun. 1	6 km (4 miles) steady run (3.45 min/km; 6.00 min/mile)
Mon. 2	8 km (5 miles) steady run (3.45 min/km; 6.00 min/mile), including 8 × 200 m (27–28 s)
Tues. 2	5 × 600 m (91–93 s with fast bursts in response to signals from coach); 2 min recovery

Wed. 2	6 km (4 miles) slow run
Thur. 2 *either before 5000 m race*	4 × 400 m; 45 s jog recovery
or, before 10 000 m race	4 × 800 m; 90 s jog recovery
plus	3 km (2 miles) slow run
Fri. 2	6 km (4 miles) steady run (3.45 min/km; 6.00 min/mile)
Sat. 2	Race
Sun. 2	16 km (10 miles) steady pace (3.45 min/km; 6.00 min/mile)

25	MARATHON	CLUB	CONDITIONING

Target time: sub 2 h 25 min

SESSION 1   daily (except Sunday)

10 min slow running
5 min loosening and stretching exercises [A] [B]
20 min steady run (3.45 min/km; 6.00 min/mile)

SESSION 2   at least 5 h after session 1

Daily warm-up
10 min slow running
5 min stretching exercises [B]
5 min striding

MONDAY
10 × 200 m hill run (10% slope); jog recovery
2–3 km (1–2 miles) warm-down

TUESDAY
5 × 2000 m approx. repetition running (3.05 min/km; 5.00 min/mile); 5 min jog recovery

WEDNESDAY
11–16 km (7–10 miles), starting at 3.45 min/km (6.00 min/mile) and increasing pace in later stages

THURSDAY
20 × 200 m (33 s); 45 s jog recovery
1½ km (1 mile) warm-down

FRIDAY
Omit session 2

SATURDAY
Race (10–16 km) or time-trial (100% effort), e.g. 1 × 8 km or 2 × 3 km with 10 min recovery

SUNDAY
Omit session 1
21–29 km (13–18 miles) easy pace

26	MARATHON	CLUB	PRE-RACE

Target time: sub 2 h 25 min

SESSION 1   daily (except Sunday)

10 min slow running
5 min loosening and stretching exercises [A] [B]
20 min steady run (3.45 min/km; 6.00 min/mile)

SESSION 2   at least 5 h after session 1

Daily warm-up   10 min slow running
5 min stretching exercises [B]
5 min striding

MONDAY   10 km (6 miles) easy running

TUESDAY   12–15 × 400 m (75 s approx.); 200 m jog recovery in 1 min

WEDNESDAY   3 km (2 miles) fast run (3.10 min/km; 5.05 min/mile)
8 km (5 miles) steady run (3.40 min/km; 5.50 min/mile)
1½ km (1 mile) fast run (3.10 min/km; 5.05 min/mile)
6–8 km (4–5 miles) steady run (3.40 min/km; 5.50 min/mile)

THURSDAY   11–13 km (7–8 miles) fartlek, starting slowly then steady pace with several bursts of 100 m and 200 m both uphill and downhill

FRIDAY   Omit session 2

SATURDAY   10–21 km race or fast run (6–13 miles)

SUNDAY   Long run at slower than 3.45 min/km (6.00 min/mile), 24–32 km (15–20 miles) if Saturday's run short; 19–24km (12–15 miles) if Saturday's run long

| 27 | MARATHON | ÉLITE | CONDITIONING |

Target time: sub 2 h 12 min

SESSION 1   daily

10 min slow running
5 min loosening and stretching exercises [A] [B]
30–40 min steady run (3.30 min/km; 5.30 min/mile)

SESSION 2   at least 5 h after session 1

Daily warm-up	10 min slow running 5 min stretching exercises [B] 5–10 min jogging and striding
MONDAY	13–16 km (8–10 miles) fartlek on hilly course (sub 3.45 min/km; 6.00 min/mile), with bursts on hills
TUESDAY	1 × 4 km; 1 × 3 km; 1 × 2 km; 1 × 1600 m (all at sub 3.00 min/km; 4.50 min/mile); 5 min jog recovery between each
WEDNESDAY	16 km (10 miles) in approx. 52 min
THURSDAY	4 × 400 m (66–67 s); 60 s jog recovery 3 km (2 miles) steady run (3.30 min/km; 5.35 min/mile) 4 × 400 m (66–67 s); 60 s jog recovery 3 km (2 miles) steady run (3.30 min/km; 5.35 min/mile)
FRIDAY	8 km (5 miles) easy run
SATURDAY	Race (10–20 km) or time trial (100% effort), e.g. 1 × 10 km or 2 × 5 km with 10 min recovery
SUNDAY	2 h continuous running at 3.45 min/km (6.00 min/mile) pace with some sections slightly faster

28	MARATHON	ÉLITE	PRE-RACE

Target time: sub 2 h 12 min

SESSION 1   daily

10 min slow running
5 min loosening and stretching exercises [A] [B]
30–40 min steady run (3.30 min/km; 5.30 min/mile)

SESSION 2   at least 5 h after session 1

Daily warm-up   10 min slow running
5 min stretching exercises [B]
5–10 min jogging and striding

MONDAY   10–13 km (6–8 miles) easy fartlek, starting slowly, then at 3.45 min/km (6.00 min/mile) with several bursts over 200 m

TUESDAY   10 × 800 m (2.16 min approx.); 200 m jog recovery in 90 s

WEDNESDAY   1 mile (4.45 min); 2 min recovery
6 km (4 miles) 3.10 min/km; 5.05 min/mile); 3.5 min recovery
1 mile (4.45 min); 2 min recovery
6 km (4 miles) 3.10 min/km; 5.05 min/mile)

THURSDAY   10–13 km (6–8 miles) fartlek, starting slowly then steady pace with several bursts of 100 m and 200 m both uphill and downhill

FRIDAY   8 km (5 miles) easy run

SATURDAY   16 km (10 miles) race or 10 km (6 miles) time-trial (100% effort)

SUNDAY   2½ h steady run (faster than 3.45 min/km; 6.00 min/mile), with some sections at 3.30 min/km (5.30 min/mile)

DETAILS OF EXERCISES

[A] Loosening Exercises

Typical loosening, or mobility, exercises are trunk rotation, arm swinging, ankle rotation and leg swinging. A standard routine, which should only be carried out when the body is warm, would include six to eight of these exercises, each performed for no more than 20 s.

[B] Stretching Exercises

A typical stretching exercise is the 'sitting stretch', in which the athlete sits on the ground with the legs extended forwards. He or she then leans forwards, bending from the hips and stretching towards the toes with head raised. This position is held for 30 s, with the stretch gradually increasing. For runners it is most important that the flexors, at the back of the leg, be stretched regularly to allow the stride to remain maximal. Stretching exercises can be usefully performed after exercise as well as before since the range of muscle movement may become restricted after many repeated contractions. These exercises must always be carried out slowly, to avoid triggering the stretch reflex, and on warm muscles.

[C] Strengthening Exercises

These are carried out to increase the strength and endurance of the general musculature but should not form part of the warm-up routine carried out prior to racing. They are normally employed in the form of a circuit of six to twelve exercises involving all major muscle groups, including legs, arms, trunk and shoulders, with 10–20 repetitions of each. Some, such as 'sit-ups', 'press-ups', 'pull-ups' and 'squat-thrusts', are performed without weights, using the body to provide resistance. Others require weights, either free or fixed. 'Light weights' implies no more than half of the maximum weight that can be managed by the athlete.

[D] Resistance Running

A form of running in which the action is made harder by running through sand, mud or water, or by carrying extra weight. The latter can be achieved by wearing leg weights, weighted boots or a weighted jacket, or by pulling against a belt held by another athlete.

[E] Weight-training

As [C] but using full weights.

[F] Recuperation Running

A warm-down exercise carried out very slowly, between 4 min/km (6.30 min/mile) and 6 min/km (10 min/mile)) to facilitate blood flow after heavy exercise for the removal of waste products.

[G] Differentials

A running exercise in which the two halves of a set distance, typically 400 m, are run at different speeds. A middle-distance runner might run the first 200 m at normal 1500 m pace and the second at 800 m pace, giving times of, say, 31 s and 28 s.

Differentials for endurance runner could be 10 miles with the first and last 2 miles easy and the middle six hard.

Advice for Women Runners

CLOTHING

There is no shortage of recommendations on the clothing which should be worn by the male runner and, although this information is increasingly available for the experienced female runner, the following advice is intended for women who are beginning their running careers.

Underwear

Both pants and bras should be unfussy and preferably cotton to prevent chafing of the skin. A good supporting bra is essential:

- *Marks & Spencer* sell two sports bras. These are good for the beginner but have joins and straps that will undoubtedly chafe the long-distance runner.
- *Minimal-bounce bras* are available in most good sports shops or can be obtained by mail order. It is advisable to get a size that is supportive but that, at the same time, does not restrict chest movement by being too tight.
- Slip-over lycra bras often have few seams and are very good for long-distance running or for those who do not have too full a figure. Such bras are fairly 'fashionable' and so are available in most shops that sell underwear.

Shorts

Often when women (and many men) start running or jogging their legs rub together. If this is the case, cycling shorts rather than 'short' shorts can prevent chafing.

Overdressing

Be careful not to overdress. This is particularly important for the novice runner, who may wear a tracksuit on a warm day, merely because she is self-conscious. More experienced runners learn what to wear according to the conditions. Confidence in running will grow as time goes by to bring the confidence in appearance that will allow the runner to dress according to what is right for the particular day, and not what is right for the other runners or the neighbours to see!

Overheating is a serious problem, so look at the weather before setting out and listen to your body. If you find it takes you a while to warm up, either warm up by stretching and exercising lightly before you leave the house or wear a top that can be easily removed and tied round your waist, leaving a lighter top underneath.

MENSTRUATION

Running does not have to stop at this time of the month. Indeed, running can often alleviate some of the symptoms of pre-menstrual tension (headache, mood swings, etc.) and also some of the pain of menstruation itself (see pp. 170–171). Pain-killers such as paracetamol are necessary for some women at this time of the month but they should not interfere with the running schedule if they are taken an hour before the run.

Although running sometimes temporarily slows the menstrual flow, wearing a sanitary-towel is still a necessity. A 'bum-bag' containing a change of sanitary-towel, taken on a run, especially a long training run, is probably a better idea than wearing too bulky a towel that might chafe the skin.

PREGNANCY

For those who wish to exercise or to continue running during their pregnancy, guidelines have been put forward by the American College of Obstetricians (1985) and more information can be obtained from the book *Exercise in Pregnancy* (Artal and Wiswell, 1985):

- Consult your doctor. Ask if there are any medical reasons why exercising during your *particular* pregnancy should be hazardous. You may be warned against running in certain circumstances, such as a history of miscarriage, an incompetent cervix, blood spotting, abdominal pain or palpitations on running.

- Run when you feel like it, but do not ignore feelings of tiredness or strain.
- Pay particular attention to warming up and cooling down. Warming up and cooling down are important aspects of training at any time, but they are particularly important during the second half of pregnancy, when the body releases relaxin—a hormone which 'loosens' the joints and the connective tissue, especially in the pelvic region, in preparation for delivery. These changes increase the risk of injury to joints, and this risk persists for a few weeks after delivery. And remember that towards the end of pregnancy the body weight has increased by about 20 kg, putting more stress on ankle and knee joints. Also the centre of gravity changes, which can also place more strain on joints.
- Consider changing to a more 'comfortable' form of exercise later in pregnancy; swimming and walking are good alternatives to running.
- Do *not* race or use speedwork in your training: do *not* run for long periods. A decrease in blood flow to the uterus can damage the fetus. Try not to exercise above 70% of your maximum heart rate (the latter is calculated by subtracting your age from 220). Thus, even for a 20-year-old, the maximum should be 140 beats/min. Pregnancy itself increases the heart rate and also the stroke volume, so that the cardiac output (pp. 142–143) is already increased even at rest. Hence there is less capacity to use during exercise.
- Do *not* allow yourself to become overheated—an elevated body temperature of the mother can cause malformation of the foetus and endanger its life. Drink plenty before, during and after running.
- Do *not* start a running programme during pregnancy if you did not run before conception.
- Do *not* design a rigid training programme at the beginning of pregnancy for the coming months. Adapt the training programme, perhaps weekly or even daily, to your changing body shape and feelings.
- In pregnancy it is necessary to consume adequate amounts of vitamins, minerals and energy. Research has shown that, for most women, the extra energy required for pregnancy (estimated to be about 1000 kJ per day) is accommodated by less energy expenditure due to a more sedentary lifestyle. However, for those who continue to train it is important that the extra energy used in the exercise is consumed in the daily food, so that the foetus is not starved:

hypoglycaemia in the mother may be a particular problem for the foetus.

- Exercise while lying on the back (supine exercise) may not be the best way of exercising for the pregnant woman since it can cause a marked lowering of the blood pressure (supine hypotension) which could reduce blood flow to the foetus.
- Once the baby is born, running can be quickly resumed. Some mothers have been running within a few days of giving birth. The problem of 'looser' joints remains for about 4 weeks but, apart from ensuring an *adequate* energy intake if the mother is breastfeeding, there are no other problems.

Psychological Self-Assessment and Training

SPORTS EMOTIONAL-REACTION PROFILE

The Sports Emotional-Reaction Profile (SERP) was devised by Thomas Tutko to help athletes become more aware of psychological 'problems' that might interfere with their performance. The approach is discussed in detail in the book *Sports Psyching* by Thomas Tutko and Umberto Tosi (J.P. Tarcher Inc., Los Angeles, 1978). In the test, the athlete is asked to respond to statements using the responses:

- Almost always (about 90% of the time).
- Often (about 75% of the time).
- Sometimes (about 50% of the time).
- Seldom (about 25% of the time).
- Almost never (about 10% of the time).

On the basis of these responses a score is determined for each of seven psychological traits (Table C.1). By comparing these with

Table C.1. Psychological traits featured in SERP profiles

Desire
Assertiveness
Sensitivity
Tension control
Confidence
Personal accountability
Self-discipline

'normal' values, the athlete is made aware of possible problem areas which might be tackled using appropriate psychological training techniques.

DETERMINE YOUR SERP

The first step it to respond to the 42 items in Table C.2 with one of the five responses listed above. You may find it helpful to use Table C.3 for your answers. The questions for the various traits are listed randomly in Table C2, so each trait must now be scored by circling your response to each item in Table C.4. For instance, if for Question 1 you ticked 'Seldom', that response is worth 2 points in the trait 'Desire'. If for Question 41 you ticked 'Seldom', that response is worth 4 points in the trait 'Personal accountability'. There are six entries for each psychological trait; now for each trait add up the six scores you have circled, then enter the total score.

For each of the seven psychological areas the total score can be as low as 5 or as high as 30. One way of visualising these results is to plot a profile on Figure C.1. Either a high score (25–30) or a low score (5–10) for a particular trait could indicate a potential problem and its size. Advice on how to intrepret your scores is given below.

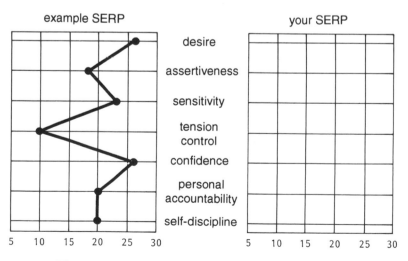

Figure C.1. Your Sports Emotional-Reaction Profile

Table C.2. Statements for determination of SERP

1. I do not consider my running worthwhile unless I am performing near my best.
2. I am intimidated by other aggressive athletes.
3. Little annoyances can affect my running.
4. I am able to remain calm prior to and during a race.
5. I have faith in my ability.
6. I apologize to others when I make a mistake or run poorly.
7. I organize my strategy before running.
8. I run primarily for fun.
9. I speak out whenever I have something to say in an athletic contest.
10. I have nerves of steel during competition.
11. I make more mistakes during competition compared to training.
12. I lack confidence during competition.
13. I avoid looking at what I have done wrong.
14. I run spontaneously rather than having a planned strategy.
15. I want to be the best runner in the event.
16. I laugh things off rather than get angry about them.
17. I am influenced by what others think about my athletic performances.
18. I can control my nervousness prior to and during a race.
19. I usually enter a race expecting to win.
20. My mistakes make me feel bad for days.
21. I have a routine that I adhere to when I train for a race.
22. I prefer to train with people who do not make running a 'contest'.
23. I am a 'take-charge' type of runner.
24. I am 'emotionally numb' during a race.
25. My nervousness interferes with my racing.
26. I think about losing a race even before it begins.
27. I think about the errors my opponent may make rather than running my own race.
28. I jump from one thing to another trying to improve my running performance.
29. I don't feel like running unless I have a challenge.
30. When my opponents show anger, I try to ignore them.
31. An offhand comment by someone can ruin my race.
32. I enjoy the pressure of competition because it stimulates me to do well.
33. I like to challenge the tougher opponents.
34. I worry about my failures more than I enjoy my successes.
35. I try to find ways to be more efficient during training and racing.
36. I can enjoy racing even though I might make a lot of mistakes.
37. I am assertive on the athletic field.
38. I try to blank everything out of my mind during competition.
39. I worry about getting into difficult situations long before they occur.
40. I worry that my opponents will humiliate me.
41. I try to avoid thinking about my mistakes.
42. I do not know what I am going to do until a race gets underway.

Table C.3. SERP responses

	Almost always	Often	Sometimes	Seldom	Almost never
1.					
2.					
3.					
4.					
5.					
6.					
7.					
8.					
9.					
10.					
11.					
12.					
13.					
14.					
15.					
16.					
17.					
18.					
19.					
20.					
21.					
22.					
23.					
24.					
25.					
26.					
27.					
28.					
29.					
30.					
31.					
32.					
33.					
34.					
35.					
36.					
37.					
38.					
39.					
40.					
41.					
42.					

Table C.4. Scoring table for SERP

DESIRE

Item no.	Almost always	Often	Sometimes	Seldom	Almost never
1	5	4	3	2	1
15	5	4	3	2	1
29	5	4	3	2	1
8	1	2	3	4	5
22	1	2	3	4	5
36	1	2	3	4	5

Total score for Desire: ____

ASSERTIVENESS

Item no.	Almost always	Often	Sometimes	Seldom	Almost never
9	5	4	3	2	1
23	5	4	3	2	1
37	5	4	3	2	1
2	1	2	3	4	5
16	1	2	3	4	5
30	1	2	3	4	5

Total score for Assertiveness: ____

SENSITIVITY

Item no.	Almost always	Often	Sometimes	Seldom	Almost never
3	5	4	3	2	1
17	5	4	3	2	1
31	5	4	3	2	1
10	1	2	3	4	5
24	1	2	3	4	5
38	1	2	3	4	5

Total score for Sensitivity: ____

Table C.4. (*continued*)

TENSION CONTROL

Item no.	Almost always	Often	Sometimes	Seldom	Almost never
4	5	4	3	2	1
18	5	4	3	2	1
32	5	4	3	2	1
11	1	2	3	4	5
25	1	2	3	4	5
39	1	2	3	4	5

Total score for Tension control: ____

SELF-DISCIPLINE

Item no.	Almost always	Often	Sometimes	Seldom	Almost never
7	5	4	3	2	1
21	5	4	3	2	1
35	5	4	3	2	1
14	1	2	3	4	5
28	1	2	3	4	5
42	1	2	3	4	5

Total score for Self-discipline: ____

CONFIDENCE

Item no.	Almost always	Often	Sometimes	Seldom	Almost never
5	5	4	3	2	1
19	5	4	3	2	1
33	5	4	3	2	1
12	1	2	3	4	5
26	1	2	3	4	5
40	1	2	3	4	5

Total score for Confidence: ____

Table C.4. (*continued*)

PERSONAL ACCOUNTABILITY

Item no.	Almost always	Often	Sometimes	Seldom	Almost never
6	5	4	3	2	1
20	5	4	3	2	1
34	5	4	3	2	1
13	1	2	3	4	5
27	1	2	3	4	5
41	1	2	3	4	5

Total score for Personal accountability: ____

- *Desire*. An indication of the personal goals of the athlete. A high score is satisfactory provided it does not promote anxiety through trying to achieve too much. The athlete needs to be able to accept limitations if they are real. Emil Zatopek appreciated the importance of setting realistic goals: 'When you set your aim too high and don't fulfil it, then your enthusiasm turns to bitterness. Try for a goal that is reasonable and then gradually raise it. That's the only way to get to the top.'
- *Assertiveness*. A measure of self-confidence—the determination to take oneself to the limit. An athlete with a low score will be easily intimidated and will be 'beaten even before the race starts'. Assertiveness can be increased by planning assertive actions and responses to situations and then putting them into practice. A high assertiveness score may be beneficial for a track athlete but can lead to poor strategy in races since the athlete will want to 'lead from the front'—a characteristic of the athlete who breaks records but does not win gold medals. In 1973, Dave Bedford ran the 10 000 m in the then world record time of 27 min 30.8 s but did not win any gold medals. Noakes (1992) writes: 'I think unquestionably, like Clayton, Bedford tried too hard and trained too much.' Assertiveness can lead to aggression, and those with a high score in this area must learn not to waste energy through aggression in training before the race but to channel their aggression into the competition itself and particularly the final stages of the race. Was Liz McColgan's poor performance in the 10 000 m event in the Barcelona Olympic Games caused by overtraining? Assertive athletes are more prone to overtraining (see Chapter 12).

- *Sensitivity*. An index of how much pleasure and elation are gained from success. A high scorer can too easily become discouraged by mistakes or failure. This is an area where a sympathetic coach can help a great deal. A low sensitivity score is rarely a problem since it suggests emotional resilience.
- *Tension control*. The ability to cope with anxiety. In an athlete with poor tension control, emotions interfere with performance in a way that has already been described. Poor performance increases anxiety, which causes more anxiety and the athlete spirals downwards according to the catastrophe theory. The problem, as explained above, is the long road back to peak performance. A high score here is only a problem if it is accompanied by a lack of desire, in which case there will be little incentive to train hard.
- *Confidence*. Belief in one's own ability, which must be based on a full understanding of this ability. Low confidence can be boosted by a coach who is aware of the problem. But confidence can also be too high and may occur, for example, in someone with considerable natural ability who in their earlier days won medals without much training. Subsequently they find the discipline and hard work of training impossible to accept. Noakes (1992) points out that none of the following outstanding marathon runners—Emil Zatopek, Jim Peters, Frank Shorter, Steve Jones or Carlos Lopes—were outstanding schoolboy athletes. Coaches should be aware, however, that apparent over-confidence may be a cover-up for a lack of confidence or ability.
- *Personal accountability*. The ability to deal realistically with failures and mistakes. A low score may mean that the athlete blames others for mistakes; a high score may mean that the athlete is too hard on himself or herself and becomes angry or even depressed at the slightest error. This, too, readily leads to overtraining.
- *Self-discipline*. The ability to stick at a task and not give up. A low score can mean that the athlete does not train enough, may fail to heed the coach's advice and fails to learn from others and from their own mistakes. A high score is good unless it leads to an inflexible attitude.

LEARN TO RELAX

If you scored poorly in 'Tension control' you may benefit from relaxation techniques which help you to learn not only how to relax your body but how to do it so well that it becomes almost a reflex action. This is important not only during intensive peak training, but especially before important competitions.

The technique described was developed by Jacobson (1929) to induce muscular relaxation in individuals who have difficulty falling asleep. It involves the athlete contracting and then relaxing groups of muscles and, in so doing, learning the difference between high levels of muscle tension and relaxation. The repetitive contraction/relaxation sequence, repeated every day, provides a learning process for the athlete, so when tension and anxiety build up he or she can cause the muscles to relax.

Preparation is important. Find a quiet comfortable room without distractions such as television, radio or cassette player. Change into a tracksuit and light shoes and begin by warming up—as important for relaxation exercises as it is for training on the track. The warm-up involves lying on your back (on a bed or on the floor) with a pillow beneath your head. Your feet should be 30–45 cm apart and your arms by your sides. Allow your body to go as limp as possible, shake your arms and legs gently and roll your head from side to side. Now you are ready for the relaxation exercises themselves, which will take about 20 min a day.

- *Leg muscles*. Flex the muscles of your left leg by raising it 10–18 cm above the floor. Point your toes slightly back toward your head.

  Hold this position of tension for as long as you can—about 10 s or so—until you begin to feel the muscles start to tremble. Then relax the muscles, i.e. let the leg drop.

  Let the leg rest for another 10 s, noting the feeling of relaxation in those muscles. Repeat the procedure for the same leg. Associating the relaxation with a word or a phrase—*easy, relax, be calm*—each time a muscle group is relaxed this phrase may be useful as a verbal cue for initiating relaxation at other times.

  The same procedure should now be done for the right leg.
- *Buttocks and thighs*. Tighten your buttock and thigh muscles, keeping them as tight as possible for as long as possible. Then relax while saying out loud the association-relaxation word. Once again, for about 10 s, focus on the relaxed feeling in the muscles. Repeat the procedure.
- *Stomach*. Do the same procedure twice for your abdominal muscles.
- *Arms and shoulders*. Imagine that there is a bar above you and that you want to use it to pull yourself up. Raise your hands, palms upward, above your chest. Grab the imaginary bar and clench your

fists around it as hard as you can, flexing the muscles in your arms and shoulders. Hunch your shoulders as tightly as possible, hold for as long as you can and then relax again for about 10 s.

- Similar procedures can be followed for the *back* and *neck, jaw* and *face* muscles.
- Finally relax your *entire body*. Close your eyes and try to relax all the muscle groups in the body at the same time. Keeping your eyes closed, stay in this relaxed state for the rest of the 10 min session.

Think of a very pleasant, peaceful place—floating in a small boat on a peaceful lake with a soft breeze gently rocking you back and forth, back and forth; or relaxing on a quiet beach, with sunlight, warm breeze and the sound of sea on the beach. Note the pleasant, calm feelings. Associate this state with the word or phrase you have chosen to initiate relaxation.

Another means of achieving relaxation is to breathe slowly and deeply, holding your breath both after inhaling and after exhaling. This should be done for 5–10 min and can be repeated several times a day.

IMPROVE YOUR CONCENTRATION

To increase arousal and to focus it effectively, try the following each day. This time, instead of lying down, sit at a desk or table, and put an object in front of you as the focus of attention for the concentration exercises. The object should be something familiar and of interest, described by a simple word, such as book, ball, mug or pen.

Repeat the total relaxation exercises, but in the less elaborate way of *thinking* through the sequence of tension–relaxation of the muscles. Finally, relax your whole body by association with relaxing thoughts, as described above and by using the cue-word to initiate the deeply relaxed state. Breathe slowly and deeply.

In this state you can begin the concentration exercises. Let us assume you are using a book as the concentration object.

- *Say the word 'book'.* Look at the book and repeat the word to yourself, to prevent the mind from wandering.
- *Examine the object of concentration.* Now begin to examine the book visually in great detail attempting to ignore all other features in the room.

- *Feel the object.* Pick up the book. Turn it around and look at it from various angles. This aids the focus of concentration.
- *Imagine the object.* Put the book down and focus your mind and eyes on it. See the book as fully as you can so that its smallest detail will stand out in your mind, but do not try to 'overpower' the book. As you relax and keep your eye on the book, you will find that the object will seem to 'come to you'. It should be possible to concentrate on the subject quite naturally; the process cannot be forced. Eventually you should be able to 'switch on' this ability to concentrate quite naturally and when you do you will find that this seemingly mysterious process blots out all other influences except that of the book.

The first time you try to focus attention on the book you will find that your mind will wander; a wide variety of unrelated outside thoughts enter the mind, and you will become aware of other objects, noises from the street or the next room. This is quite normal and simply demonstrates the difficulty of concentration for any period of time without training. Bring your mind back to the book and keep repeating the word. As your training improves, your mind will stay with the object for longer and longer periods, so that your power of concentration develops in a similar manner to the way that aerobic capacity responds to repetitive intervals!

Practise the above technique for 20 min every day. At the end of a week, you will be able to concentrate for a longer period than when you started—not perhaps for 2 min at a time, not even for one, unless you are very good at this, but longer than before the training.

This training will be of great value for competition; to be able to focus total attention on the upcoming race and to remove all distractions from the mind, including other competitors, the importance of the event, the crowd, the coach, and the relatives, is of enormous importance for performance in the event.

The Runner's Diet

Mention the word diet and images of fat people trying to become thin, or ill people striving to recover, come to mind. But our diet is simply what we eat and by eating the right things we can almost certainly enhance athletic performance.

Since athletes are people, a good balanced diet, such as that recommended by the UK National Advisory Committee on Nutritional Education (NACNE), should provide the basis for deciding what athletes ought to eat. Athletes, however, are special people and that means that they have some special dietary needs. These have been elaborated in Chapter 11 and can be summarized:

- Total energy requirements are high.
- At least 60% of this energy should come from carbohydrate.
- This can include a larger amount of sugar than is recommended for the general public.
- Intake of essential fatty acids must be maintained and, since total fat intake is reduced, this means substitution of unsaturated fats for saturated ones whenever possible.
- Protein intake must be kept fairly high.
- Certain vitamins and minerals are required in larger amounts, and supplementation of the diet may well be required.
- Foods must be easy and quick to prepare—athletes are busy people but, unfortunately, almost all so-called convenience or fast foods are rich in fat.

KEEPING UP THE CARBOHYDRATES

No fuel: no run. Both carbohydrate and fat provide fuel and the body's fat stores are enormous, so what is the problem? Quite simply, they are stored and used in different ways. What the runner undergoing

Table D.1. Foods containing sufficient carbohydrate to be of use to the intensively training athlete

---

1. **Complex carbohydrate**
   Grains and cereals
   Bread
   Oats
   Pasta
   Rice

   Vegetables
   Potatoes
   Sweetcorn
   Beans
   Peas
   Lentils
   Chick-peas
   Broccoli

2. **Simple sugars**
   Table sugar
   Fizzy drinks
   Sweets
   Fruit (especially dried)

Box D.1   The fast food factor

Imagine you are a 50 kg middle-distance athlete engaged in intensive pre-competition training. You don't have much time to cook so you attempt to satisfy your daily requirement for 500 g of carbohydrate by eating hamburgers at the local fast-food establishment. You consult their thoughtfully provided nutritional data and discover that each large hamburger in a bun contains 40 g of carbohydrate. That means you will have to eat 12½ large hamburgers each day. If you could manage this feat you would be consuming a staggering 26 600 kJ— far in excess of the 13 000 kJ you probably need (Table D.2). You would get fatter, not faster.

If you do find yourself in a fast-food establishment, try the milk-shake. With 72.2% of its energy in carbohydrate and only 17.5% in fat it is almost good news!

intensive training needs is to refill his or her muscle *carbohydrate* stores as quickly as possible after exercise, and that is only achieved on a high-carbohydrate diet—not on a fat-rich diet. Table D.1 lists some of the foods rich in carbohydrate.

Complex carbohydrates must be digested to sugars before they can enter the blood for transport to the muscles and this takes time. Sugars are absorbed much more rapidly, so ingestion of substantial quantities of simple sugars may be essential if the athlete is to replenish muscle glycogen reserves fast enough. This would not be good advice for the non-athlete.

THE PROBLEM WITH FAT

The athlete's dietary difficulties lie here, in the fact that it is difficult to accommodate this need for carbohydrate when most meals contain considerable amounts of fat. As a nation, 46% of our energy comes from carbohydrate—less than the NACNE recommendation of 55–60% and far less than the 60–70% recommended for athletes. Some 42% of the

Table D.2. Recommended daily energy and carbohydrate intakes for athletes undertaking heavy training

Body mass (kg)	Energy intake[a,b] (kJ/day)	Carbohydrate intake (g/day[c])
40	10 400	400
45	11 700	450
50	13 000	500
55	14 300	550
60	15 600	600
65	16 900	650
70	18 200	700

[a]Female athletes will require slightly less because of their lower *lean* body mass.

[b]It should be noted that the basic (resting) energy expenditure varies quite considerably between individuals, so that this value is only a guide. If the energy intakes does not satisfy the energy expenditure, body weight will fall and the intake must be increased.

[c]On the basis of 65% energy provided by carbohydrate.

Data from W. M. Sherman and G. S. Wimer (1991). Insufficient dietary carbohydrate during training: does it impair athletic performance? *Int. J. Sport Nutr.*, **1**, 28–44.

energy in the British diet is provided by fat. Why is this bad and why is it so high?

First, many people overeat, consuming more energy than they use, and fat contains more energy than the same weight of carbohydrate (pp. 74–75). The two important variable factors that influence the amount of energy required by a person are body mass and the level of activity. Table D.2 provides a guide for those undergoing intense training.

Secondly, much of the fat consumed is of animal origin, which means that it is likely to be saturated (see p. 230) and associated with cholesterol. There is a strong possibility that, at least in some people, these factors increase the likelihood of a heart attack.

Thirdly, for the intensively training athlete on a diet which produces no increase in body weight, a high proportion of fat must mean a low proportion, and therefore a low quantity, of carbohydrate.

Where does all this fat come from? Because fat is so energy rich, it 'sneaks up' on us. Take a lean steak, the traditional body-building food (but note that traditional is not synonymous with beneficial): a 250 g (8 oz) steak provides about 80 g of protein (1350 kJ of energy) but also about 60 g of fat, which provides almost 2250 kJ of energy (there is more than 100 g of water in the steak). Therefore, *just* the fat in this single food item provides over 20% of a whole day's energy-intake of 10 000 kJ for the average person.

Carbohydrate is not only much less energy rich than fat but it comes, especially when cooked, much more 'diluted'. A tablespoon of butter (25 g) contains approximately the same energy (760 kJ) as 150 g of cooked pasta. However, it is the pasta, not the butter, which replaces the glycogen in the muscle. Since the body somehow measures the amount of energy consumed in the meal and suppresses appetite when sufficient energy has been consumed, the presence of fat will produce a feeling of satiety long before enough carbohydrate has been consumed to replenish glycogen stores.

OUR MENUS

Athletes have long been brought up to 'think protein'; now they have to re-educate themselves to 'think carbohydrate'. The essence of planning a diet is to adjust quantities over a period, most usefully a day, so that, for example, a slightly fat-rich breakfast can be compensated for by a lunch richer in carbohydrate. The sample menus that we have

Table D.3. A week of high-carbohydrate menus

Recipes for items marked [R] will be found at the end of this section.

DAY 1

Menu	Portion size	Weight (g) of			Energy (%) from			Total energy (kJ)
		Carbo.	Prot.	Fat	Carbo.	Prot.	Fat	
Coffee/tea with semi-skimmed milk	25 ml milk	2	0.8	0.2	60	26	14	53
BREAKFAST								
Muesli	150 g	110	20	10	73	13	14	2 647
	100 ml milk							
Orange juice	100 ml	10	0.8	0.1				
LUNCH								
Wholewheat spaghetti with tomato sauce [R]	See recipe	80	15	3				
Wholemeal roll	50 g	21	4.7	3	74	16	10	3 125
+ low-fat margarine	1 tsp. (5 g)							
Cardamom custard [R]	See recipe	42	9	2				
Coffee/tea	25 ml milk	2	0.8	0.2				
DINNER								
Mackerel risotto [R] with side salad	See recipe	93	43.5	24.5				
Lemon curd tart [R]	See recipe	46	10	7	53	21	26	4 476
Orange juice	100 ml	10	0.8	0.1				
TOTAL		416	105.4	50.1	65	17	18	10 301

Table D.3. (*continued*)

DAY 2

Menu	Portion size	Weight (g) of Carbo.	Prot.	Fat	Energy (%) from Carbo.	Prot.	Fat	Total energy (kJ)
Coffee/tea with semi-skimmed milk	25 ml milk	2	0.8	0.2	60	26	14	53
BREAKFAST								
Cereal (cornflakes)	100 g	106	15	3	83	12	5	2 239
+ skimmed milk	200 ml							
+ sugar	1 dsp. (15g)							
Orange juice	100 ml	10	0.8	0.1				
LUNCH								
Thick pasta and bean soup [R]	See recipe	65	20	6	73	15	12	3 409
Oriental-style nan bread	150 g	72	9	5				
+ low-fat margarine	1 tsp. (5 g)							
Pear	150 g	16	0.5	–				
Coffee/tea	25 ml milk	2	0.8	0.2				
DINNER								
Chicken noodle casserole [R]	See recipe	72	48	7	58	24	18	4 551
+ green beans	100 g cooked	3	1	–				
+ tomatoes	100 g	3	1	–				
Wholemeal roll	50 g	21	4.7	1				
+ low-fat margarine	1 tsp. (5 g)	0.1	0.3	2				
Rich chocolate mousse [R]	See recipe	57	7.5	12				
+ banana + sponge fingers								
Orange juice	100 ml	10	0.8	0.1				
TOTAL		439.1	110.2	36.6	69	18	13	10 252

DAY 3

Menu	Portion size	Weight (g) of			Energy (%) from			Total energy (kJ)
		Carbo.	Prot.	Fat	Carbo.	Prot.	Fat	
Coffee/tea with semi-skimmed milk	25 ml milk	2	0.8	0.2	60	26	14	53
BREAKFAST								
Muscavado porridge: porridge oats	30 g							
+ semi-skimmed milk	240 ml	67	16.5	7				
+ topping of wheatgerm	15 g							
+ muscavado sugar	25 g				71	14	15	2 876
Wholemeal toast	2 slices	50	6	5				
+ low-fat margarine	10 g							
+ honey	20 g							
Orange juice	100 ml	10	0.8	0.1				
LUNCH								
Jacket potato	250 g	70	33.5	10				
+ low-fat cottage cheese	220 g							
+ pineapple chunks	125 g							
Large banana	160 g	30	1	0.6	63	18	19	3 836
Banana cake (slice) [R]	See recipe	48	5	9.5				
Coffee/tea with semi-skimmed milk	25 ml milk	2	0.8	0.2				
DINNER								
Seafood lasagne [R]	See recipe	84.5	46.5	20.5				
+ broccoli	100 g cooked	5	3	0.3	56	24	20	4 190
Almond-flavour rice pudding [R]	See recipe	48	7.5	2				
Orange juice	100 ml	10	0.8	0.1				
TOTAL		426.5	121.3	55.5	62	19	19	10 955

Table D.3. (continued)

DAY 4

Menu	Portion size	Weight (g) of Carbo.	Prot.	Fat	Energy (%) from Carbo.	Prot.	Fat	Total energy (kJ)
Coffee/tea with semi-skimmed milk	25 ml milk	2	0.8	0.2	60	26	14	53
BREAKFAST								
Cereal (e.g. Crunchy Nut Cornflakes)	100 g	123	15	6.5				
+ semi-skimmed milk	200 ml				81	10	9	2 641
+ large banana	160 g							
Orange juice	100 ml	10	0.8	0.1				
LUNCH								
Tuna and sweetcorn sandwiches incl. wholemeal bread	4 slices (200 g)	100	42	10				
Tuna	100 g							
+ drained sweetcorn	150 g				61	23	16	3 902
Lemon curd tart [R]	See recipe	46	10	7				
Coffee/tea with semi-skimmed milk	25 ml milk	2	0.8	0.2				
DINNER								
Sausage and bean bake [R]	See recipe	107	36	26				
Honey fruit cake [R]	See recipe	64.5	4	4	62	15	23	4 711
Orange juice	100 ml	10	0.8	0.1				
TOTAL		464.5	110.2	54.1	66	16	18	11 307

DAY 5

Menu	Portion size	Weight (g) of			Energy (%) from			Total energy (kJ)
		Carbo.	Prot.	Fat.	Carbo.	Prot.	Fat.	
Coffee/tea with semi-skimmed milk	25 ml milk	2	0.8	0.2	60	26	14	53
BREAKFAST								
Pancakes	2 × 20 cm diam.							
inc. plain flour	75–100 g	90	15	18	63	11	26	2 538
maple-flavoured syrup	30–40 g							
Orange juice	10C ml	10	0.8	0.1				
LUNCH								
Turkey and apricot oatie rolls								
incl. oat-covered rolls	2 (150 g)	85.5	40	17	55	20	25	3 934
+ low-fat margarine	10 g							
+ roast turkey breast	85 g							
+ apricot chutney	25 g							
Banana cake [R]	See recipe	48	5	9.5				
Coffee/tea with semi-skimmed milk	25 ml milk	2	0.8	0.2				
DINNER								
Tuna tagliatelle [R]	See recipe	88	35	9	70	16	14	5 046
Lettuce, tomato + cucumber salad	250 g	6	2.5	0.5				
Nan bread	150 g	72	9	3				
Chocolate fudge delight [R]	See recipe	44	2	6				
Orange juice	100 ml	10	0.8	0.1				
TOTAL		457.5	111.7	63.6	63	17	20	11 571

Table D.3. (*continued*)

DAY 6

Menu	Portion size	Weight (g) of Carbo.	Prot.	Fat.	Energy (%) from Carbo.	Prot.	Fat	Total energy (kJ)
Coffee/tea with semi-skimmed milk	25 ml milk	2	0.8	0.2	60	26	14	53
BREAKFAST								
Spaghetti on toast incl. tin spaghetti (approx. ¾ tin)	300 g	88.5	15	7	75	13	12	2 107
+ wholemeal toast	3 rounds (150 g)							
+ low-fat margarine	10 g							
Orange juice	100 ml	10	0.8	0.1				
LUNCH								
Oriental-style rice with chick-peas								
½ tin chick-peas	200 g (cooked)	96	16	6	82	10	8	3 079.5
Bachelors pilau rice (100 g uncooked)	250 g uncooked							
+ green pepper	½							
1 fresh fruit (e.g. banana)	145 g	27	1	0.5				
1 dried fruit (e.g. dates)	50 g	32	1	–				
Coffee/tea with semi-skimmed milk	25 ml milk	2	0.8	0.2				
DINNER								
Pizza ½	190–200 g							
+ baked beans (½ tin)	220 g	105	36	19.5	64	18	18	4 105
+ chopped beef tomatoes	100 g							
Ice cream (low fat)	250 ml	49	5.5	1				
Orange juice	100 ml	10	0.8	0.1				
TOTAL		421.5	77.7	34.6	72	14	14	9 344.5

DAY 7

Menu	Portion size	Weight (g) of			Energy (%) from			Total energy (kJ)
		Carbo.	Prot.	Fat.	Carbo.	Prot.	Fat.	
Coffee/tea with semi-skimmed milk	25 ml milk	2	0.8	0.2	60	26	14	53
BREAKFAST								
Sweet-crisp rolls	4 (8 halves)							
+ low-fat margarine	10 g							
+ honey	25 g	80	15.5	20	59	11	30	2 461
+ low-fat cream cheese	50 g							
Orange juice	100 ml	10	0.8	0.1				
LUNCH								
Pasta (100 g uncooked)	250–300g cooked	99	16	8				
+ ragu sauce*	220 g							
Dried figs	100 g	53	3.5	–	79	11	10	3 112
Coffee/tea with semi-skimmed milk	25 ml milk	2	0.8	0.2				
DINNER								
Cod steamed in butter sauce (Birds Eye)	170 g							
New potatoes (cooked)	400 g	101	25	7				
Carrots (cooked)	100 g							
Parsnips	100 g							
Fruit salad (incl. melon, mango and banana)	200 g / 100 g / 125 g	48	3	–	77	15	8	3 296
Orange juice	100 ml	10	0.8	0.1				
TOTAL		405	66.2	35.6	73	12	15	8 922

*Or any other tomato based pasta sauce

Table D.4.   Some information to help you plan your own diet

Energy units

  1 kilojoule (kJ) = 1000 joules (J)
  1 megajoule (MJ) = 1000 kilojoules (kJ)

Energy used to be, and sometimes still is, measured in calories. For dietary purposes the most useful form of this unit is the kilocalorie (kcal), which is alternatively written as the Calorie (Cal).

  1 Calorie = 4.2 kilojoules

Conversion factors

  CARBOHYDRATE   16 kJ/g
  PROTEIN   17 kJ/g
  FAT   37 kJ/g

To calculate the percentage energy contributed by carbohydrate:

(i) establish the number of grams of carbohydrate, protein and fat in the food;
(ii) multiply each of these by the appropriate conversion factor to get the energy contributed by each;
(iii) add the three figures together to get total energy;
(iv) % energy contributed by carbohydrate =

$$\frac{\text{energy contributed by carbohydrate}}{\text{total energy}} \times 100.$$

Weights
  1 oz = 28.4 g (recommended nearest conversion 1 oz = 25 g)
  100 g = 3.52 oz (recommended nearest conversion 4 oz = 125 g)
  1 lb = 454 g
  1 kg = 2.2 lb

devised provide between 9000 and 11 500 kJ per day, with between 62% and 73% of the energy coming from carbohydrates (Table D.3).

Menus for days 1–5 all contain some meat or fish and make use of the specially devised recipes detailed at the end of this section. Menus for days 6 and 7 make use of 'off-the-shelf' items to show that tins, and especially frozen foods (which tend to be low in fat), can also provide the basis for a high-carbohydrate diet. Indeed, these latter menus are somewhat higher in carbohydrate (and lower in total energy) than the preceding five, which makes them suitable for the individual trying to lose weight but not athletic form. Note that the menu for day 6 is vegetarian.

To make use of these menus, the first thing to do is to work out what your own daily energy need is likely to be, using Table D.2 as a guide. Unless you are a small athlete, you will probably need to increase the total energy content of the menus by consuming proportionally larger portions or supplementing with carbohydrate-rich snacks. If, after all this, you *feel* you are eating too little (your weight is decreasing) or too much (your weight is increasing), adjust portions appropriately but in proportion over the whole menu.

Of course, you will want to vary your diet to accommodate your own preferences and opportunities (Box D.2). The information provided in Table D.4 should help you to construct your own diet of specified energy and carbohydrate content, and so plan for your athletic success.

Box D.2 Full of beans

Our parents were right; fruit and vegetables are good for us. They are rich in fibre and are good sources of the water-soluble vitamins, but athletes have a problem. If they eat large quantities, the very bulk consumed prevents them from ingesting sufficiently large amounts of digestible carbohydrate. Athletes have to choose their vegetables carefully, eating most of those which bring them the greatest benefit.

Grains—the seeds of certain grasses—are the staple food of almost everyone on the planet; indeed, without the ability to cultivate such plants it is doubtful whether human populations could have reached the level they have. In much of Europe and the USA, wheat is the most widely grown cereal and, when ground to flour, is a particularly versatile component of our diet. The grinding process can be manipulated to separate the three main parts of the wheat grain (Figure D.1): the endosperm, containing the reserves of starch for the developing plant; the germ, or embryo; and the bran which surrounds the grain. White flour is made from endosperm only, but in brown and wholemeal flours part or all of the germ and the bran is included. Bran is a good source of fibre, and the germ is richer in protein and vitamins than the endosperm, making breads made from these flours more nutritious than white bread. Unfortunately, the inclusion of wheatgerm also reduces the time which flour and bread can be kept in a palatable condition. It is possible to buy bran and wheatgerm separately and to supplement the diet by sprinkling them on to other cereals, yoghurt or fruit.

_____ continued _|

— *continued* —

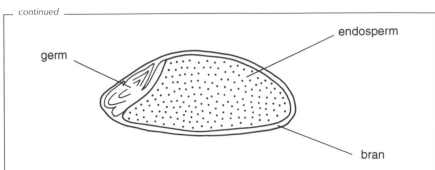

Figure D.1. Section through a wheat grain

A second group of athlete-friendly vegetables are the legumes or pulses—seeds of a large family of plants which gives us kidney beans, haricot beans, white beans, black beans, soya beans, peas, chick-peas, lentils and many other edible products. A characteristic of members of this family is that their roots enter into a mutually advantageous partnership with nitrogen-fixing bacteria so can tap into gaseous nitrogen from the atmosphere as a source of this vital element. In consequence, legumes are much richer in protein than other plants; haricot beans have a higher protein content than steak. The snag is that most are deficient in methionine, an essential sulphur-containing amino acid, but sufficient can be obtained from dairy or wholegrain products. Complex carbohydrate can contribute as much as 75% to the weight of dried pulses, which are also rich in fibre and low in fat.

If green vegetables are not a major part of the athlete's diet then root vegetables should be, for in addition to their carbohydrate content they can provide much-needed vitamins. Potatoes are particularly useful since they are rich in vitamin C and contain twice as much carbohydrate as parsnips and four times as much as carrots. Their failing is their lack of vitamin A but carrots can provide this. An interesting alternative is the sweet potato, which is on a nutritional par with the more familiar kind but with significant amounts of vitamin A and rather less protein.

In the recipes which follow
☐ = protein
▨ = fat
■ = carbohydrate

Wholewheat Spaghetti with a tomato sauce

Proportions of energy supplied

Proportions by weight

No. of servings: 2
Preparation time: 5 min
Cooking time: 12–15 min

Energy per serving: 1680 kJ
Energy from carbohydrates: 1300 kJ

INGREDIENTS

200 g (uncooked) wholewheat spaghetti
400 g (can of) chopped tomatoes
1 tsp. dried basil or 1 tbsp. chopped fresh basil
1 tbsp. (15 ml) Kraft 'Fat Free Dressing' (optional)

PREPARATION

Cook the spaghetti in boiling water, according to the manufacturer's instructions. In a separate pan gently heat the tomatoes. Mix in the herbs. Drain the spaghetti as soon as it is cooked, stir in the 'Fat Free Dressing' if used and divide between two plates or bowls. Pour the tomato sauce into the centre of the spaghetti. Serve at once.

NOTE: Although this meal is high in carbohydrate, its protein content is incomplete. When not using meat or dairy products complete the vegetable proteins by mixing pulses with grains; for example, beans on toast, rice with kidney (or other) beans, hummus with pitta bread. Or, as in our menu suggestion, follow this course with one containing dairy products—here, cardamom custard (p. 398).

Mackerel Risotto

Proportions of
energy supplied

Proportions
by weight

No. of servings: 4
Preparation time: 10 min
Cooking time: 25–45 min

Energy per serving: 3130 kJ
Energy from carbohydrate: 1485 kJ

INGREDIENTS

400 g (uncooked) brown wholegrain rice, or mixed long-grain and wild rice
450 g (1 lb) smoked mackerel fillets (approx. 4)
400 g (or 1 can) cooked red kidney beans, drained and washed
250 g (cooked) peas
1 red pepper, deseeded and chopped
3 spring onions, chopped
2 tbsp. reduced-calorie mayonnaise
2 tbsp. tartar sauce
2 tbsp. chopped fresh parsley
1 lemon (juice and grated rind)

PREPARATION

Cook the rice for between 20 and 40 min in boiling water (according to manufacturer's instructions). Once the rice has boiled, reduce to a medium heat, adding more water if necessary to ensure rice does not stick to pan. While the rice is cooking, skin and flake the fish, removing all bones, and prepare the vegetables. When the rice is cooked (has absorbed enough water to become soft), drain off excess water and return it to a non-stick pan. Add all the other ingredients and mix well with the rice. Cook gently for 5–10 min or until heated through. Serve at once, garnished with sprigs of parsley.

Chicken Noodle Casserole

Proportions of
energy supplied

Proportions
by weight

No. of servings: 4
Preparation time: 10–15 min
Cooking time: 1 h 45 min

Energy per serving: 2230 kJ
Energy from carbohydrate: 1150 kJ

INGREDIENTS

450 g (1 lb) chicken breasts, cubed or left as individual portions (4)
250 g (uncooked) egg noodles
350 g (1 can) sweetcorn, drained
175 g button mushrooms
1 green pepper, deseeded and chopped
575 ml (1 pint) chicken soup (e.g. Bachelors chicken noodle soup) or
    chicken stock
1 tbsp. light soy sauce (or Worcester sauce to taste)
black pepper

GARNISH

coriander leaves
spring onions, chopped into 1-inch pieces

PREPARATION

Pre-heat oven to 200 °C (400 °F, Gas Mark 6). Wash the chicken pieces
and cut into cubes if preferred. Place chicken pieces or cubes in a large
casserole dish. Mix the green pepper and mushrooms into the soup or
stock and then pour over the chicken. Cover and place in the oven.
Reduce oven temperature after 30–45 min to 180 °C (350 °F). Cook
until the chicken is tender. When the chicken is almost cooked put a
pan of water on to boil. Cook the egg noodles according to manufactur-

er's instructions (approximately 6 min). When the noodles are cooked, drain and mix with chicken in casserole pot. Add the sweetcorn, black pepper and soy sauce.

Cook everything for a further 5 min in the oven before serving, garnished with coriander leaves and spring onions.

Sausage and Bean Bake
(for the unashamed fatty meat eater!)

No. of servings: 4
Preparation time: 20 min
Cooking time: 30 min

Proportions of energy supplied   Proportions by weight

Energy per serving: 3300 kJ
Energy from carbohydrate: 1732 kJ

INGREDIENTS

900 g (2 lb) (approx.) potatoes, peeled and sliced
450 g (1 lb) sausages with oats (lower fat), cut into ¾–1-inch pieces
  (14 g of fat per 100 g)
1 small onion chopped finely
440 g (1 can) baked beans
285 ml (½ pint) semi-skimmed milk
40 g wholemeal flour
40 g low-fat cooking margarine ('Gold' see p. 395)
25 g Cheddar cheese, grated

SEASONING

1 tsp. dried basil or 1 tbsp. chopped fresh basil
1 tsp. paprika

PREPARATION

Cook the sliced potatoes in boiling water for 5–10 min (only, since they
need to be firm). While the potatoes are cooking, melt 25 g (1 oz) of
the margarine in a large pan (use a fairly low heat as this lower-fat
margarine will not tolerate high temperatures). Add the sausage slices
and cook for 5 min. Add the onion and cook for a further 5 min. Add
the flour and cook for 1 min, stirring continuously. Gradually add the

milk; continue stirring. Bring to the boil and then simmer for 1–2 min, still stirring until a 'sauce' texture is achieved. Stir in the baked beans and the cheese. Transfer the mixture to an ovenproof dish and arrange the partly cooked potato slices on top. Dot with the remaining margarine and sprinkle with paprika. Cook for 20 min or until the potatoes have browned, in an oven pre-heated to 200 °C (400 °F, Gas mark 6). Sprinkle with fresh chopped basil and serve.

Seafood Lasagne

Proportions of
energy supplied

Proportions
by weight

No. of servings: 4
Preparation time: 25 min
Cooking time: 35–40 min

Energy per serving: 2900 kJ
Energy from carbohydrate: 1355 kJ

INGREDIENTS

450 g (1 lb) smoked haddock
250 g lasagne verdi (ready-to-cook)
330 g (1 can) sweetcorn, drained
200 g (½ can) chopped tomatoes
575 ml (1 pint) fresh seafood soup (now available in good supermarkets) or fish stock
575 ml (1 pint) semi-skimmed milk
50 g low-fat margarine
50 g plain flour
25 g parsley (or 1 tbsp.) finely chopped
1 lemon (juice of)

SEASONING

Sprigs of parsley
Lemon wedges

PREPARATION

Heat the milk gently in a large saucepan and add the fish pieces. Poach
for about 10 min or until the fish begins to flake. Remove the pan from
the heat. Place the fish in a bowl to cool and retain the milk as this
will be used to make the sauce. In another pan melt the margarine.
Once melted add the flour and cook over a gentle to moderate heat for
1 min. Now gradually add the milk (that used to cook the fish), stirring
all the time. Bring the mixture to the boil (turn up heat if necessary)

and then allow to simmer. The mixture should have thickened, but should also be smooth—any lumps can be removed by straining the mixture through a colander. Add the parsley to the sauce, then the sweetcorn and the seafood soup. Stir the mixture.

Flake the haddock now that it is cool enough to touch, and remove all the skin and bones. Place the flaked fish into the sauce and mix, adding the lemon juice. Season. The sauce is now ready.

Pour a layer of sauce into the lasagne dish (or casserole dish) then place a layer of lasagne on top. Repeat the layers until all the sauce and lasagne are used up, ending with a layer of sauce. Take care to cover all the lasagne with sauce as it absorbs the moisture in the sauce during cooking. Pour the chopped tomatoes into the middle of the dish to complete.

Cover dish with aluminium foil and cook in a pre-heated oven (195 °C, 380 °F, Gas mark 5) for 30–40 min or until lasagne is cooked. The foil can be removed for the last 5–10 min to allow the lasagne to brown slightly.

Garnish with sprigs of parsley and lemon wedges.

Thick Pasta and Bean Soup 'Italian Style'

No. of servings: 4–6
Preparation time: 15 min
Cooking time: 20 min

Proportions of
energy supplied

Proportions
by weight

Energy per serving: 1610 kJ
Energy from carbohydrate: 1040 kJ

INGREDIENTS

350 g (uncooked) filled fresh pasta shapes (filled with vegetables or
    ricotta cheese)
430 g (1 can) cannellini beans, drained and washed
430 g (1 can) borlotti beans, drained and washed
1 litre vegetable stock
400 g (1 can) Italian sieved tomatoes
2 tbsps. tomato paste
225 g carrots, chopped
1 small onion, finely chopped
25 g low-fat cooking margarine (e.g. 'Gold', see p. 395)

SEASONING

1 tsp. dried basil or 1 tbsp. chopped fresh basil
1 bay leaf

PREPARATION

Melt the fat over a low heat in a large saucepan. Add the onion and
carrots and cook for 4–5 min until slightly softened. Make up the
vegetable stock and pour over the vegetables in the pan. Turn up the
heat. Add the sieved tomatoes, tomato paste, beans, and filled pasta
shapes and bring to the boil. Add the basil and the bay leaf. Once

boiled reduce heat and simmer for 15 min. When the soup is cooked, remove the bay leaf and serve while piping hot with warm nan bread.

NOTE: Nan bread is an oriental form of bread (like pitta bread). It can be bought in most large supermarkets and is delicious warm as well as having a very high carbohydrate content. Nan bread is thus ideal to have as a tasty snack itself, with a main meal or, as here, with soup.

Tuna Tagliatelle

Proportions of
energy supplied

Proportions
by weight

No. of servings: 4
Preparation time: 10 min
Cooking time: 20 min (approx.)

Energy per serving: 2310 kJ
Energy from carbohydrate: 1408 kJ

INGREDIENTS

500 g (1 lb) fresh wholemeal or spinach tagliatelle (can usually be
   bought fresh in 250 g packs)
365 g (2 small tins or 1 large) tuna, in brine, drained
350 g (1 can) chopped tomatoes
35 g (½) onion, chopped
1 garlic clove, crushed
1 tbsp. olive oil
2 tbsp. red wine
50 g black olives, slivered (optional)
2 tbsp. chopped parsley (fresh)

PREPARATION

Heat the oil in a large saucepan. Add the onion and cook gently until
translucent. Add the garlic and brown slightly. Do not allow garlic to
burn. Add the tuna, tomatoes, red wine and the olives (if using) to the
pan, mix well and bring to the boil. Now reduce the heat and allow the
mixture to simmer gently for 20 min. While the sauce is cooking, the
tagliatelle can be made ready. Put a large pan of water on to boil.
Between 3 and 10 min before the sauce is ready (depending on how
fresh the pasta is; see manufacturer's instructions) place the tagliatelle in the boiling water. Once cooked, drain and divide the tagliatelle between four plates. Leave a space in the middle of each plate
and fill this with the cooked sauce. Sprinkle each serving with chopped
fresh parsley and serve at once.

Rich Chocolate Mousse with Sponge Fingers

Proportions of
energy supplied

Proportions
by weight

No. of servings: 6
Preparation time: 20–25 min
Chilling time: 2 h

Energy per serving: 1500 kJ
Energy from carbohydrate: 912 kJ

INGREDIENTS

175 g Bourneville plain chocolate
3 eggs, separated into yolks and whites
50 g dark brown sugar ⎫ or 65 g dark brown sugar
15 g muscavado sugar ⎭
3 tbsp. water
pinch of salt

TOPPING

1 packet sponge fingers
2 bananas, chopped
(*Note:* Prepare topping when about to serve the dessert.)

PREPARATION

Break the chocolate bar into pieces and melt over hot, but not boiling, water in a suitable bowl. Keep the chocolate melted (do not let it return to its solid state) while preparing the other ingredients. Add the egg yolks, one at a time, to the melted chocolate, beating well after each addition. Keep the bowl containing the chocolate mixture over the hot water if possible to help prevent the mixture from becoming too thick and stiff. Now add 3 tbsp. water to the mixture and whisk until smooth. In a separate bowl combine the egg whites and the salt; whisk the whites until soft peaks form. Gradually add the sugar and whisk until stiff peaks form. Gently fold this mixture into the chocolate mixture. The mousse is now complete but needs to be chilled for at least 2 h before serving. The mousse can be chilled in serving dishes or glasses, but decorate with sponge fingers and chopped bananas just before serving.

NOTE: This is a rich dessert for those who love chocolate. Its taste is not impaired in the least by the fact that it does not contain cream and therefore, although not low in fat, it is lower in fat than most home-made mousses. Serve with sponge fingers and chopped bananas in order to increase the carbohydrate content of this dessert.

Almond Rice Pudding

No. of servings: 2–3
Preparation time: 5 min
Cooking time: 1½–2 h

Energy per serving: 970 kJ
Energy from carbohydrate: 768 kJ

Proportions of
energy supplied

Proportions
by weight

INGREDIENTS

60 g pudding rice (30 g or more per person)
600 ml semi-skimmed milk (300 ml per person)
50 g caster sugar
1–2 tsp. almond essence
1 tsp. vanilla essence

PREPARATION

Mix all the ingredients together in a lightly greased ovenproof dish.
Cover and place in pre-heated oven (150 °C/300 °F, Gas mark 2) and
cook for 1½–2 h. During this time the rice will absorb most of the fluid
and so will be soft when cooked. This dessert can be served on its own,
or with dried or fresh fruit.

Note: Almonds themselves are, like other nuts, high in fat (approximately 80% of their energy value comes from fat). Almond essence is
used in this recipe to improve the taste without the addition of fat.

Lemon 'Curd' Tart

Proportions of
energy supplied

Proportions
by weight

No. of servings: 4
Preparation: 20–30 min
Cooking time: 15–20 min

Energy per serving: 1170 kJ
Energy from carbohydrate: 740 kJ

INGREDIENTS

175 g curd cheese (10% fat)
65 g wholemeal flour
65 g low-fat cooking margarine (e.g. 'Gold', see p. 395)
52 ml (3½ tbsp.) semi-skimmed milk
1 egg, beaten
50 g caster sugar
½ lemon (½ rind grated plus juice of half of lemon)

DECORATION

50 g (2 oz) lemon jellies
or orange+lemon sugar slices

PREPARATION

Place the flour in a bowl and rub in the margarine until the mixture resembles fine breadcrumbs. Mix with 2 tbsp. milk to form a dough. Roll out the dough on a floured work surface. Use this pastry to line an 18 cm (7-inch) flan ring. Blind bake in a pre-heated oven at 200 °C (400 °F, Gas mark 6) for about 15 min.

While the pastry case is cooking in the oven beat the curd cheese with 1½ tbsp. of the remaining milk and ½ tbsp. (7.5 ml) lemon juice (about the juice of ½ lemon). Grate the rind of the lemon and beat this in too.

Whisk the egg and sugar until thick and pale, then gradually beat this mixture into the cheese mixture. Pour into the cooked pastry case and bake at 190 °C (375 °F/Gas mark 5) for 20 min until set.

Decorate with the lemon sweets.

Chocolate Fudge Delights

No. of servings: 16, or 35 (approx.)
   sweet pieces
Preparation time: 15–20 min
Chilling time: At least 2 h but
   preferably overnight

Energy per serving:
cake: 972 kJ
sweet: 445 kJ
Energy from carbohydrate:
cake: 710 kJ
sweet: 325 kJ

Proportions of energy supplied   Proportions by weight

INGREDIENTS

450 g (1 lb) light or dark muscavado sugar
150 ml (¼ pint) semi-skimmed milk
175 g 'crunchy' chocolate spread
125 g porridge oats
125 g 'crunchy' oat cereal (or muesli)
125 g glacé cherries, chopped
15 g margarine
1 tsp. vanilla essence

PREPARATION

Place the milk, brown sugar, margarine and vanilla essence into a large saucepan. Bring this mixture to the boil and then continue to boil for 2 min or until the sugar has dissolved, stirring the mixture continuously. Once the sugar has dissolved remove the pan from the heat and stir in the chocolate spread.

Mix together the oats, crunchy oat cereal (or muesli) and the chopped glacé cherries in a separate bowl. Gradually add this cereal mixture to the chocolate fudge mixture. Add enough cereal to ensure a fairly stiff consistency. Mix well.

If making sweets, take spoonfuls of the mixture and form sweet shapes on a tray covered with baking foil or non-stick baking paper. Place the tray, once filled with sweets, in the fridge to chill.

If making cakes with the mixture, pour (or spread) into a large flan dish (or two 20 cm flan dishes) lined with non-stick baking paper and place this in the fridge.

The mixture sets better if left overnight in the fridge. When set the sweets can be placed in paper sweet cases. Alternatively the flan, once set, can be divided to form 16 slices or triangles.

Wholemeal Banana Cake

Proportions of
energy supplied

Proportions
by weight

No. of servings: 10–12
large slices
Preparation time: 15 min
Cooking time: 40–50 min

Energy per serving: 1210 kJ
Energy from carbohydrate: 765 kJ

INGREDIENTS

900 g (2 lb) ripe medium bananas (6–7) mashed with a fork
265 g wholemeal self-raising flour
125 g low-fat cooking margarine (e.g. 'Gold')
125 g caster sugar
2 medium-sized eggs, beaten
1 tsp. nutmeg

PREPARATION

Cream the margarine with the sugar until the mixture is creamy. Then beat in the (beaten) eggs until thoroughly mixed. Blend in the mashed bananas and again beat until mixed. Blend in sifted flour and nutmeg (wholemeal in flour might get caught in sieve but add this to mixture). Once blended, pour the mixture, with the help of a spoon, into a greased 2 lb loaf tin (or 22 cm diameter cake tin). Place the tin in a pre-heated oven (180°C/350°F/Gas mark 4) and cook for 40–50 min until golden brown and firm to the touch. Serve warm or cold with sweetened fromage frais.

NOTE: Cooking with 'Gold'. 'Gold' cooking margarine can now be bought in most larger supermarkets. It contains 40% less fat than most traditional cooking margarines. Remember most low-fat *spreads* are only suitable for spreading and not for cooking.

Rich Fruit Cake

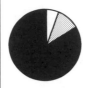

No. of servings: 20 or more pieces.
This is a large cake!
Preparation time: 30 min
Cooking time: 3 h plus

Energy per serving: 1322 kJ
Energy from carbohydrate: 1108 kJ

Proportions of
energy supplied

Proportions
by weight

INGREDIENTS

250 g (ready-to-eat) dried apricots, quartered
250 g sultanas
250 g raisins
250 g glacé cherries, halved
250 g chopped crystallized pineapple
500 ml orange or pineapple juice
100 g (runny) honey
90 g low-fat cooking margarine (e.g. 'Gold', see p. 395)
225 g plain flour
225 g wholemeal self-raising flour
150 ml semi-skimmed milk
(optional: 1 tsp. mixed spice)

PREPARATION

Chop the dried apricots into quarters and the glacé cherries into halves
and place in a large mixing bowl. Add the sultanas, raisins and
crystallized pineapple. Mix together then tip into a large saucepan
with the honey, margarine and the fruit juice. Heat the mixture until
the margarine has melted. Bring the mixture to the boil, then reduce
the heat, cover the pan and simmer for 5 min. Pour the mixture back
into the large mixing bowl. Leave the mixture to cool to about room
temperature. Once the mixture is cool enough, stir in the milk, sifted

flour and spice; do this half at a time. Spread the mixture into a prepared baking tin (line a deep 23 cm square cake pan with 3 layers of greaseproof paper) and then bake in a pre-heated oven (150 °C/ 300 °F/Gas mark 2) for about 3 h. Cool in the tin.

NOTE: If stored in an air-tight container this cake will keep for up to a month. This cake can be made in advance of a special occasion and is perfect for birthdays and even for Christmas. It can be decorated with marzipan and icing; the only difference from a 'normal' Christmas cake or special-occasion cake is the low fat content of this cake, so you can indulge without the heavy stomach and guilty mind! This cake has the highest percentage energy from carbohydrate of all the recipes— as high as cornflakes.

Cardamom Custard

Proportions of   Proportions
energy supplied   by weight

No. of servings: 2
Preparation and cooking time: 10 min

Energy per serving: 900 kJ
Energy from carbohydrate: 672 kJ

INGREDIENTS

25 g (1 sachet Bird's) custard powder
500 ml (1 pint) skimmed milk
40 g castor sugar
10–15 cardamom seeds or whole pods or ⅛ tsp. cardamom powder

PREPARATION

Make the custard as usual but stir in the cardamom powder with the custard powder at the outset. Alternatively, use cardamom seeds or pods (wrapped in muslin, for easy removal before serving) while cooking and stirring the custard in order to bring out their aromatic qualities and bitter-sweet taste; who said custard couldn't be exotic?

Cereal
(Cornflakes or Rice Krispies)

Proportions of   Proportions
energy supplied   by weight

No. of servings: 1
Preparation time: 2 min

Energy per serving: 2100 kJ
Energy from carbohydrate: 1700 kJ

INGREDIENTS

100 g cereal (either cornflakes or Rice Krispies)
200 ml semi-skimmed milk (skimmed milk can be used—as in menu
   on day 2—to reduce fat content still further)
15 g sugar, to sprinkle on top

Tinned Fruit with Yoghurt (or Rice Pudding)

Proportions of energy supplied

Proportions by weight

No. of servings: 1
Preparation time: 3 min

Energy per serving: 1150 kJ
(information provided uses yoghurt, not rice pudding)
Energy from carbohydrate: 1005 kJ

INGREDIENTS

200 g (½ tin) peach slices in syrup
150 g carton sweetened low-fat fruit yoghurt

NOTE: Tinned fruit is a quick way of including extra simple sugars (plus potassium) in the diet. Tinned fruit preserved in syrup contains more carbohydrate (in the form of sugars) than that preserved in fruit juice (about 18 g per 100 g compared with 12 g per 100 g for fruit in natural juice).

Beans on Toast

Proportions of
energy supplied

Proportions
by weight

No. of servings: 1
Preparation time: 5 min

Energy per serving: 1745 kJ
Energy from carbohydrate: 1130 kJ

INGREDIENTS

220 g (½ tin) baked beans
2 thick slices wholemeal toast (50 g per slice)
10 g low-fat margarine for spreading

Mars Bar

No. of servings: 1
Preparation time: as long as it takes
    to remove the wrapper!

Energy per serving: 1830 kJ
Energy from carbohydrate: 1115 kJ

Proportions of
energy supplied

Proportions
by weight

INGREDIENTS

King-size (100 g) Mars bar

NOTE: The percentage of energy from fat!

☐ = protein
▨ = fat
■ = carbohydrate

Appendix: Composition of Recipes

These are more precise values for the percentages by weight and by energy for carbohydrate, protein and fat for the recipes given on the previous pages.

Recipe	% by weight			% energy		
	carbo.	prot.	fat	carbo.	prot.	fat
Almond rice pudding	83	13	4	78	13	9
Banana cake	77	8	15	64	7	29
Beans on toast	72	21	7	65	20	15
Cardamom custard	79	17	4	75	17	8
Cereal	85	12	3	81	12	7
Chicken noodle casserole	57	38	5	51	37	12
Chocolate fudge delight	85	4	11	73	4	23
Chocolate mousse	74	10	16	61	9	30
Lemon curd tart	73	16	11	63	14	23
Mackerel risotto	58	27	15	47	24	29
Mars bar	75	6	19	61	5	34
Pasta and bean soup	71	22	7	65	22	13
Rich fruit cake	89	6	5	84	5	11
Sausage and bean bake	63	21	16	53	18	29
Seafood lasagna	56	31	13	47	27	26
Tinned fruit with yoghurt	82	16	2	79	17	4
Tuna tagliatelle	67	26	7	64	25	11
Wholewheat spaghetti	82	15	3	78	15	7

Noakes' Advice on Injuries and Running Shoes

The information contained in this section is summarized from Dr Tim Noakes' book *Lore of Running* (1992).

INJURIES

A major topic of conversation when runners gather together is their latest injury. As with other aspects of athletics, as much misinformation as information is usually exchanged. For a medically informed common-sense approach to sports injuries it is hard to better the advice of Dr Tim Noakes—a South African doctor, author and runner—which we reproduce here with some of his comments.

1. *Running injuries are not acts of God.* They result from unfortunate interactions between the athlete and the environment, usually as a result of an inherent biomechanical defect in the athlete (e.g. one leg is shorter than the other).

2. *Most running injuries progress through four stages.*
   - Pain occurs only *after*, usually several hours after, cessation of exercise.
   - Discomfort, but not pain, occurs during exercise but is not sufficiently severe to interfere with performance.
   - The pain is great enough to reduce training and interfere with performance.
   - The pain is severe enough to prevent running.

Except in the case of stress fractures and iliotibial band friction syndrome, a stage 1 injury will not *suddenly* become a stage 4 problem, but treatment is needed to prevent progression through the stages.

3. *Virtually all running injuries are curable.* Finding the cure first involves finding the cause, then treating it. Some of the common causes are as follows.
   - *Running surfaces.* Hard surfaces can cause impact damage; road camber can cause over-pronation of the foot on the higher part of the road; grass surfaces are uneven and can lead to damage; uphill running stretches calf muscles and the Achilles tendons; downhill running can cause damage to muscles because of eccentric contraction (working the muscles while they are being stretched); track work involves running around bends and this causes the outer leg to overstride.
   - *Training shoes.* The problems that arise with shoes are discussed in more detail below. Shoes must be replaced when worn out (which may occur well before the shoe has an appearance of 'old age').
   - *Training.* Too much, too rapidly, too often and without sufficient rest explains most injury problems.

4. *X-rays and other sophisticated investigations are seldom necessary for the diagnosis of running injuries.* Most running injuries are soft-tissue injuries, so that X-rays provide no useful information. Sports physicians should use their hands and take a detailed history to make a diagnosis.

5. *Rest is seldom the most appropriate treatment.* Rest may cure the acute symptoms of a running injury but it is the most unacceptable form of treatment for the serious runner. Complete rest is only required in those injuries in which, in any case, running is impossible (e.g. stress fracture). Indeed for many injuries some exercise is beneficial in providing for proper alignment of new fibres in the damaged area and for increasing the strength of the repaired tissue. Running should be permitted but only to the point where discomfort is experienced; it should not be continued when it becomes painful. Treatment should gradually permit longer and faster runs before discomfort occurs. If an injury does not respond to treatment, further investigation into the injury should be performed since it may be unrelated to running.

6. *Never accept as a final opinion the advice of a non-runner (physician or otherwise)*. Runners appreciate the importance of running to the individual and therefore are unlikely to give the advice 'stop running'!

7. *Avoid surgery if at all possible*. Surgery is irreversible. It may not cure the injury but it may seriously affect the athlete's future

Table E.1. Foot injuries

Noakes (1992) has pointed out that different 'types' of foot are prone to different injuries. He advocates the 'bathroom test' to identify foot type. Stand on a flat surface with wet feet and note the pattern left.

Rigid foot	Normal foot	Over-mobile foot

Possible problems
Stress fractures
   (dull ache that persists
   after exercise; mild swelling,
   tenderness)

Iliotibial band friction syndrome
   (tenderness at the outside of
   knee; pain may radiate up the
   outside of thigh)

Ill-defined muscle and joint pain
   particularly after long runs

Possible problems
Achilles tendinitis
   (soreness, tightness and pain
   in Achilles tendon—especially
   when running or walking fast)

Runner's knee
   (aching pain behind or
   around kneecap)

Shinsplints
   (severe discomfort or burning
   pain in shin or calf)

From Noakes, T. (1992). *Lore of Running*. Oxford University Press, Cape Town.

running career. Surgery is only sensible for a few groups of injuries and only when these injuries have reached stages 3 or 4 (see item 2 above).

8. *There is no scientific evidence that running causes osteoarthritis* in runners whose joints were normal when they started running.

These rules are presented as a guide for the consideration of injuries if and when they arise. However, we advise that as soon as an injury occurs, help and advice from the coach, physiotherapist or other experienced runner should be sought as soon as possible. A list of some common injuries is provided in Table E.1.

THE FOOT

The force of landing on the foot during running is enormous. To compensate and to distribute some of this force, the foot slightly changes its structure. As the heel strikes the ground, the arch flattens to absorb some of the energy; the foot then rolls inwards—a movement known as *pronation*. This inward movement unlocks joints in the ankle and midfoot to absorb the shock. To compensate, the knee rotates outwards. For take-off, the foot rolls outwards, and this *supination* locks the ankle and midfoot joints to provide a rigid lever to transmit a powerful force (Figure E.1). Unfortunately, many runners *over-pronate*; the foot rolls too far inwards and puts strain on the muscle and particularly the joints and tendons of the lower leg. This can be caused or worsened by poor shoes. If the shoe is so worn that it tilts inwards even when not being worn, this may well cause over-pronation and hence damage. Over-pronation may also occur when the mecha-

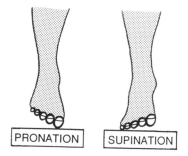

PRONATION   SUPINATION

Figure E.1. Rotations of the right foot. Both supination (during take-off and landing) and pronation (during the first part of the stance phase) are normal movements. Only when these movements are excessive will injury result

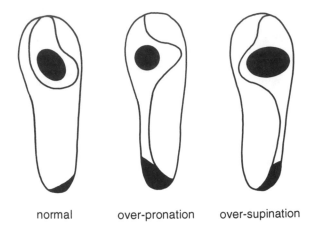

normal   over-pronation   over-supination

Figure E.2. Running-shoe wear (left show) for different foot types. After Noakes, T. (1992). *Lore of Running*. Oxford University Press, Cape Town

nics of what appears to be a normal foot are actually slightly abnormal. This is simply a genetic defect that the runner has to deal with by wearing the correct running shoe for this problem. Alternatively a rigid foot may roll inwards too little, so failing to absorb the impact energy.

A clue to any mechanical problem affecting the feet may be found in the wear pattern of a well-used running shoe (Figure E.2). If there is no problem, wear is greatest at the outer edge of the heel, under the ball of the foot and at the front of the sole. Extreme pronation increases the wear along the inside edge and, conversely, excessive supination causes wear along the outer edge.

Another test can be carried out in the bathroom. Place your naked and wet feet on a dry paper bath mat (even newspaper will do), first sitting and then, after moving your feet, standing. See how the print changes (Table E.1). If the footprint narrows on standing you have a rigid foot; if it broadens you have an over-mobile, or flat, foot.

- *The rigid foot* provides a firm lever and is an ideal foot for sprinting but it is not that good for the long-distance runner. Without properly controlled pronation, shock is not absorbed and may be transmitted to the knee, which is unable to deal with it and in time becomes injured.
- *The over-mobile foot* absorbs impact well but is unstable during the push-off for the next stride. It fails to provide a firm enough lever so the lower limb rotates too far inwards.

THE RUNNING SHOE

Since few runners have ideal foot mechanics, correct choice of running shoe is vital if injuries are to be minimized. Running shoes designed for maximum shock absorption are needed by those with rigid feet, while running shoes with best motion control benefit those with over-mobile feet. Unfortunately some feet combine elements of both weaknesses and cause their owners much distress, since no running shoe can correct both at the same time.

Shoes are generally chosen by trial and error; the runner experiments until a pair is found which causes least injury. This can be an expensive process to find the correct running shoe. The following information might reduce the cost.

There are at least five important features of the running shoe:

- The outer sole.
- The midsole.
- Slip or board lasting.
- Heel counter.
- Straight or curved lasting.

Outer Sole

This is the part of the shoe that comes into direct contact with the ground. Watch for wear, especially on the outer heel edge.

Midsole

The midsole is very important for three reasons:

- It must absorb the shock of landing.
- It must resist excessive pronation of the ankle.
- It must be able to flex about two-thirds from the heel for the 'toe off' in the next stride.

The softer the midsole the greater is its ability to absorb impact force. This can be tested by squeezing the midsole with finger and thumb in the shoe shop. The hardness of the midsole can vary along the length of the shoe to provide impact-absorbing properties in the heel but more stiffness to control pronation in the remainder of the shoe. Those runners with a rigid foot need a soft midsole and those with an over-mobile foot need a firmer midsole.

Slip or Board Lasting

If the upper portion of the shoe is stuck directly to the midsole, this is slip lasting; if another piece of material overlies this connection, the shoe is board lasted. The latter increases the ability of the shoe to withstand pronation. The board may extend from heel to toe or may end at about the back of the foot.

Heel Counter

This is the part of the shoe that supports the heel. For those that pronate excessively a firm heel counter is required. The firmness can be assessed by simply squeezing the heel of the shoe.

Straight or Curved Lasting

Draw a straight line from the middle of the heel to the middle of the toe. If the shoe forms two equal halves (i.e. is symmetrical) it is straight lasted. If the shoe provides more sole inside such a line, this is curved or 'banana' lasting. For those who require pronation control, the straight-lasted shoe is recommended.

Other points which should be taken into account when buying a pair of shoes include the following.

- The running shoe should be slightly larger than the normal shoe, since the foot swells by about half a size on running. Some space should be left between the longest toe and the front end of the shoe upper.
- Despite this, the heel must not slip out of the heel counter at toe-off.
- The running shoe must feel comfortable immediately upon walking.
- The width of the shoe is also important; room should be available to move the toes upwards and there should be room over the bridge of the foot.
- If running shoes are used every day they will last less than 6 months, and a 'hundred-a-week' runner will get through a pair in a matter of weeks.

Medicines to Avoid

In its efforts to control the use of drugs to enhance performance, the International Olympic Committee (IOC) has drawn up a list of substances which, if found in the urine of competing athletes, will lead to their being banned from competition. Many national committees and sports regulatory bodies use the same list. The problem for the athlete is that the list is very long and includes many drugs that have legitimate medical uses, some of which may even be bought over the counter without prescription. As far as sport is concerned, the offence is having a banned substance in the urine; whether it was taken for a medical complaint or indeed how it entered the body is of no consequence. Competitors beware!

DRUG NAMES

An added complication for the athlete is that drugs have three kinds of name. First is their chemical name—precise but rarely used owing to its length. For example, the chemical name for aspirin is ethanoyl-2-oxybenzoic acid. Aspirin itself is the drug's *generic* name—the official name for the active chemical. This is marketed under a variety of *brand* names differing, often very slightly, in formulation or in the inclusion of other active ingredients. Thus aspirin is sold under such names as Aspro, Disprin, Solprin and, combined with other drugs, as Codis, Alka-Seltzer, Solpadeine and many more. Since banned drugs are listed under generic names it is important to read the small print on your medicine.

POINTS TO NOTE

- Caffeine, although on the banned list, is permitted at levels below 12 μg/ml in the urine. This level would only be reached if six to eight cups of coffee were consumed in a single sitting some 2 to 3 h before testing.

- Most decongestants contain sympathomimetic amines which are considered to be stimulant drugs. Many cold 'cures' contain decongestants.
- Herbal teas, such as Ma Huang and ginseng, contain ephedrine—a banned substance.
- Codeine, is permitted for medical use.
- Injection of corticosteroids into joints is permitted but must be declared in writing, with full details.
- Tests for beta-blockers are only likely to be carried out on competitors in sports such as archery, shooting, biathlon, modern pentathlon, diving luge, bobsleigh and ski-jumping.
- All beta-2 agonists are prohibited except salbutamol and terbutaline which may be administered by inhalation provided the IOC Medical Commission is notified in writing by a doctor.

BANNED SUBSTANCES

NOTE: The drugs listed below are examples of prohibited drugs; the list is not exhaustive. In some cases the same drug is listed under more than one name. New drugs and formulations continue to appear on the market and the IOC have banned whole classes of drugs to prevent minor chemical modifications from being used to get round the regulations. For each class of drugs listed below the Commission uses the phrase 'and related substances' to include drugs that are related either by chemical structure or pharmacological action. *ANY ATHLETE TAKING ANY MEDICATION IN THE DAYS BEFORE COMPETITION SHOULD SEEK EXPERT ADVICE ABOUT ITS ACCEPTABILITY BY THE APPROPRIATE GOVERNING BODY.*

Key: AB   Anabolic agents
          BB   Beta-blockers
          DT   Diuretics
          NA   Narcotic analgesics
          PP   Peptide hormones
          SM   Stimulants

acebutolol	BB	diamorphine	NA
acetazolamide	DT	diclofenamide	DT
alphaprodine	NA	diethylpropion	SM
alprenolol	BB	dihydrocodeine	NA
amfepramone	SM	dimetamfetamine	SM
amfetamine	SM	dimetamphetamine	SM
amfetaminil	SM	dipipanone	NA
amineptine	SM	ephedrine	SM
amiphenazole	SM	epitestosterone	AB
amphetamine	SM	erythropoietin	PP
amphetaminil	SM	etacrynic acid	DT
anileridine	NA	etafedrine	SM
atenolol	BB	etamivan	SM
bendroflumethiazide	DT	ethacrynic acid	DT
benzfetamine	SM	ethamivan	SM
benzphetamine	SM	ethoheptazine	NA
benzthiazide	DT	ethylmorphine	NA
bolasterone	AB	etilamfetamine	SM
boldenone	AB	fencamfamin	SM
bumetanide	DT	fenethylline	SM
buprenorphine	NA	fenetylline	SM
caffeine	SM	fenproporex	SM
canrenone	DT	fluoxymesterone	AB
cathine	SM	frusemide	DT
chlordehydromethyl-	AB	furfenorex	SM
testosterone		furosemide	DT
chlormerodrin	DT	growth hormone	PP
chlorphentermine	SM	heroin	NA
chlortalidone	DT	hydrochlorothiazide	DT
chlorthalidone	DT	labetalol	BB
chorionic gonadotrophin	PP	levorphanol	NA
clenbuterol	AB	mefenorex	SM
clobenzorex	SM	mersalyl	DT
clorprenaline	SM	mesocarb	SM
clostebol	AB	mesterolone	AB
cocaine	SM	metandienone	AB
corticotrophin	PP	metenolone	AB
cropropamide	SM	methadone	NA
crotetamide	SM	methamphetamine	SM
crothetamide	SM	methandienone	AB
dextromoramide	NA	methenolone	AB
dextropropoxyphene	NA	methoxyphenamine	SM

methylephedrine	SM	phenazocine	NA
methylphenidate	SM	phendimetrazine	SM
methyltestosterone	AB	phenmetrazine	SM
metoprolol	BB	phentermine	SM
morazone	SM	phenylpropanolamine	SM
morphine	NA	pipradol	SM
nadolol	BB	prolintane	SM
nalbuphine	NA	propranolol	BB
nandrolone	AB	propylhexedrine	SM
nikethamide	SM	pseudoephedrine	SM
norethandrolone	AB	pyrovalerone	SM
norpseudoephedrine	SM	somatotropin	PP
oxandrolone	AB	sotalol	BB
oxprenolol	BB	spironolactone	DT
oxymesterone	AB	stanozolol	AB
oxymetholone	AB	strychnine	SM
pemoline	SM	testosterone	AB
pentazocine	NA	triamterene	DT
pentetrazol	SM	trimeperidine	NA
pethidine	NA	trimeperidinum	NA

Further Reading and Bibliography

SOME GENERAL TEXTBOOKS

Åstrand, P.-O. and Radahl., K. (1986). *Textbook of Work Physiology*. McGraw-Hill, New York.

Brooks, G. A. and Fahey, T. D. (1984). *Exercise Physiology: Human Bioenergetics and Its Applications*. Wiley, New York.

Costill, D. L. (1986). *Inside Running: Basics of Sports Physiology*. Benchmark Press, Indianapolis.

Martin, D. E. and Coe, P. N. (1991). *Training Distance Runners*. Human Kinetic Publishers, Champaign, IL.

McArdle, W. D., Katch, F. I. and Katch, V. L. (1991). *Exercise Physiology: Energy, Nutrition and Human Performance*. Lea and Febiger, Philadelphia/London.

Noakes, T. (1992). *Lore of Running*, 2nd ed. Oxford University Press, Cape Town.

Powers, S. K. and Howley, E. T. (1990). *Exercise Physiology: Theory and Application to Fitness and Performance*. W. C. Brown, Dubuque, IA.

Simmons, R. M. (ed.) (1992). *Muscle Contraction*. Cambridge University Press.

Wootton, S. (1988). *Nutrition for Sport*. Simon & Schuster, London.

Wirhed, R. (1994). *Athletic ability and the Anatomy of Motion*. Wolfe Medical, London.

PART I

Chapter 1

Finley, M. I. and Pleket, H. W. (1976). *The Olympic Games: The First 1000 Years*. Chatto & Windus, London.

Gardiner, E. (1930). *Athletics in the Ancient World*. Oxford University Press, Oxford.

Harris, A. (1972). *Sport in Greece and Rome*. Thames & Hudson, London.

Murrell, J. (1975). *Athletics, Sports and Games*. George, Allen & Unwin, London.
Noel-Baker, P. (1978). In *Physical Activity and Human Well-Being: The International Congress of Physical Activity Sciences* (eds Landry, F. and Orban, W. A. R.) Symposia Specialists Inc., Miami, Florida.

Chapter 2

Alexander, R. McN. (1992). *The Human Machine*. Natural History Museum Publications, London.
Eddington, D. W. and Edgerton, V. R. (1976). *The Biology of Physical Activity*. Houghton-Mifflin, Boston, MA.
Edgerton, V. R., Roy, R. R., Gregor, R. J. *et al.* (1986). Morphological basis of skeletal muscle power output. In *Human Muscle Power*, pp. 43–64 (eds Jones, N. L., McCartney, N. and McComas, A. J.). Human Kinetic Publishers, Champaign, IL.
Goldspink, G. (1977). Design of muscles in relation to locomotion. In *Mechanics and Energetics of Animal Locomotion*, pp. 1–22 (eds Alexander, R. McN. and Goldspink, G.). Chapman & Hall, London.
Komi, P. V. (1986) The stretch-shortening cycle and human power output. In *Human Muscle Power*, pp. 27–39 (eds Jones, N. L., McCartney, N. and McComas, A. J.). Human Kinetic Publishers, Champaign, IL.
Merton, P. A. (1972). How we control the contraction of our muscles. *Sci. Am.*, **226**, *No. 5*, 30–37.
White, D. C. S. (1977). Muscle mechanics. In *Mechanics and Energetics of Animal Locomotion*, pp. 23–56 (eds Alexander, R. McN. and Goldspink, G.). Chapman & Hall, London.
Wilkie, D. R. (1976). *Muscle*. Edward Arnold, London.

Chapter 3

Alexander, R. McN. (1977). Terrestrial locomotion. In *Mechanics and Energetics of Animal Locomotion*, pp. 118–203 (eds Alexander, R. McN. and Goldspink, G.). Chapman & Hall, London.
Alexander, R. McN. (1988). *Elastic Mechanisms in Animal Movement*. Cambridge University Press, Cambridge.
Alexander, R. McN. and Ker, R. F. (1990). Running is priced by the step. *Nature*, **346**, 220–221.
Alexander, R. McN. (1992). *The Human Machine*. Natural History Museum Publications, London.
Durnin, J. G. V. A. and Passmore, R. (1967). *Energy, Work and Leisure*. Heinemann, London.
Gleim, G. W., Stacherfeld, N. S. and Nicholas, J. A. (1990). The influence of flexibility on the economy of walking and jogging. *J. Orthop. Res.*, **8**, 814–823.
Goldspink, G. (1977). Energy cost of locomotion. In *Mechanics and Energetics of Animal Locomotion*, pp. 153–167 (eds Alexander, R. McN. and Goldspink, G.). Chapman & Hall, London.

Kram, R. and Taylor, C. R. (1990). Energetics of running: a new perspective. *Nature*, **346**, 265–267.

Margaria, R. (1976). *Biomechanics and Energetics of Muscular Exercise*. Clarendon Press, Oxford.

Newsholme, E. A. and Leech, A. R. (1983). *Biochemistry for the Medical Sciences*. Wiley, Chichester.

Chapter 4

Costill, D. L. and Fox, E. L. (1969). Energetics of marathon running. *Med. Sci. Sports Exerc.*, **1**, 81–86.

Costill, D. L., Coyle, E., Dalsky, G. *et al.* (1977). Effects of elevated plasma FFA and insulin on muscle glycogen usage during exercise. *J. Appl. Physiol.*, **43**, 695–699.

Henricksson, J. (1992). Metabolism in the contracting skeletal muscle. In *Endurance in Sport*, pp. 226–243 (eds Shephard, R. J. and Astrand, P.-O.). Blackwell Scientific Publications, Oxford.

Henricksson, J. (1992). Cellular metabolism and endurance. In *Endurance in Sport*, pp. 46–60 (eds Shephard, R. J. and Astrand, P.-O.). Blackwell Scientific Publications, Oxford.

Hultman, E., Greenhaff, P. L., Ren, J. M. *et al.* (1991). Energy metabolism and fatigue during intense muscle contraction. *Biochem. Soc. Trans.*, **19**, 347–353.

Hultman, E. and Greenhaff, P. L. (1992). Food stores and energy reserves. In *Endurance in Sport*, pp. 127–138 (eds Shephard, R. J. and Astrand, P.-O.). Blackwell Scientific Publications, Oxford.

Wilmore, J. H. (1992). Body composition and body energy stores. In *Endurance in Sport*, pp. 244–255 (eds Shephard, R. J. and Astrand, P.-O.). Blackwell Scientific Publications, Oxford.

Chapter 5

Hultman, E. and Greenhaff, P. L. (1992). Food stores and energy reserves. In *Endurance in Sport*, pp. 127–138 (eds Shephard, R. J. and Astrand, P.-O.). Blackwell Scientific Publications, Oxford.

Newsholme, E. A., Blomstrand, E. and Ekblom, B. (1992). Physical and mental fatigue: metabolic mechanisms and importance of plasma amino acids. *Br. Med. Bull.*, **48**, 477–495.

Chapter 6

Asmussen, E. (1979). Muscle fatigue. *Med. Sci. Sports Exerc.*, **11**, 313–321.

Edwards, R. H. T. (1981). Human muscle function and fatigue. *Ciba Found. Symp.*, **82**, 1–18.

Hermansen, L. (1981). Effect of metabolic changes on force generation in skeletal muscle during maximal exercise. *Ciba Found. Symp.*, **82**, 75–88.

Hultman, E. and Sjoholm, H. (1986). Biochemical causes of fatigue. In *Human*

Muscle Power, pp. 215–238 (eds Jones, N. L., McCartney, N. and McComas, A. J.). Human Kinetic Publishers, Champaign, IL.

Newsholme, E. A., Blomstrand, E. and Ekblom, B. (1992). Physical and mental fatigue: metabolic mechanisms and importance of plasma amino acids. *Br. Med. Bull.*, **48**, 477–495.

Chapter 7

Blix, A. S. (1976). Metabolic consequences of submersion asphyxia in mammals and birds. *Biochem. Soc. Symp.* **41**, 169–178.

Costill, D. L. (1979). *A Scientific Approach to Distance Running*. Track & Field News, Los Altos, CA.

Green, S. and Dawson, B. (1993). Measurement of anaerobic capacities in humans: definitions, limitations and unsolved problems. *Sports Med.*, **15**, 312–327.

Karvonen, J. and Vuorimaa, T. (1988). Heart rate and exercise intensity during sports activities: practical application. *Sports Med.*, **5**, 303–311.

Sjodin, B. and Svedenhag, J. (1985). Applied physiology of marathon running. *Sports Med.*, **2**, 83–99.

Wagner, P. D. (1991). Central and peripheral aspects of oxygen transport and adaptations with exercise. *Sports Med.*, **11**, 133–142.

Chapter 8

American College of Obstetricians and Gynecologists (1985). Women and Exercise. *ACOG Tech. Bull.*, **87**, 1–5.

Artal, R. and Wiswell, R. A. (1985). *Exercise in Pregnancy*. Williams & Wilkins, Baltimore.

Constantine, N. W. and Warren, M. P. (1994). Physical activity, fitness, and reproductive health in women: clinical observations. In: *Physical Activity, Fitness and Health. International Proceedings and Consensus Statement*, pp. 955–966. (eds Bouchard, C., Shepherd, R. J., Stephens, T.). Human Kinetics Publishers, Champaign, Il., U.S.A.

Cummings, D. C. (1988). Reproduction: exercise-related adaptations and the health of women and men. In *Exercise, Fitness and Health*, pp. 677–685 (eds Bouchard, C., Shephard, R. J., Stephens, T., Sutton, J. R. and McPherson, B. D.). Human Kinetic Publishers, Champaign, IL.

De Souza, M. J., Maguire, M. S., Rubin, K. R. *et al.* (1990). Effects of menstrual phase and amenorrhoea on exercise performance in runners. *Med. Sci. Sports Exerc.*, **22**, 575–580.

Fox, J. C. (1990). The fairer sex: how fair the test? *Sports Med. Soft Tissue Trauma*, **2**, 5–6.

Keizer, H. A. (1986). Exercise- and training-induced menstrual cycle irregularities. *Int. J. Sports Med.*, **7**, 38–44.

Kuscsik, N. (1977). The history of women's participation in the marathon. *Ann. NY Acad. Sci.*, **301**, 862–876.

Loucks, A. B. Physical activity, fitness, and female reproductive morbidity (1994). In: *Physical Activity, Fitness, and Health. International Proceedings and Consensus Statement*, pp. 943–954. (eds Bouchard, C., Shepherd, R. J., Stephens, T.) Human Kinetics Publishers, Champaign, Il., U.S.A.

McKenzie, D. C. (1992). Pregnant women and endurance exercise. In *Endurance in Sport*, pp. 385–389 (eds Shephard, R. J. and Astrand, P.-O.). Blackwell Scientific Publications, Oxford.

Moller-Nielson, M. and Hammar, M. (1991). Sports injuries and oral contraceptive use: is there a relationship? *Sports Med.*, **12**, 152–160.

Prior, J. C. (1988). Reproduction: exercise-related adaptions and the health of women and men. In *Exercise, Fitness and Health*, pp. 661–676. (eds Bouchard, C., Shephard, R. J., Stephens, T., Sutton, J. C. and McPherson, B. D.). Human Kinetic Publishers, Champaign, IL.

Vines, G. (1992). Last Olympics for the sex test? *New Scientist*, **135**, 39–42.

Wardle, M. G., Gloss, M. R. and Gloss, D. S. (1987). Response differences. In *Sex Differences in Human Performance* (ed. Baker, M. A.). Wiley, Chichester.

Warren, M. P., Brooks-Gunn, J., Hamilton, L. H. *et al.* (1986). Scoliosis and fractures in young ballet dancers. *N. Engl. J. Med.*, **314**, 1348–1353.

Wells, C. L. (1980). The female athlete: myths and superstitions put to rest. In *Toward an Understanding of Human Performance: Readings in Exercise Physiology for the Coach and Athlete*, pp. 141–1476 (ed Burke, E. J.). Movement Publications, New York.

Whipp, B. J. and Ward, S. A. (1992). Will women soon outrun men? *Nature*, **355**, 25.

Williford, H. N., Scharff-Olson, M. and Blessing, D. L. (1993). Exercise prescription for women. *Sports Med.*, **15**, 299–311.

Wilmore, J. H., Brown, C. H. and Davis, J. A. (1977). Body physique and composition of the female distance runner. *Ann. NY Acad. Sci.*, **301**, 764–776.

Wolfe, L. A., Hall, P., Webb, K. A. *et al.* (1989). Prescription of aerobic exercise during pregnancy. *Sports Med.*, **8**, 273–301.

Chapter 9

Ainsworth, B. E., Montoye, H. J. & Leon, A. S. (1994). Methods of assessing physical activity during leisure and work. In: *Physical Activity, Fitness, and Health*. International Proceedings and Consensus Statement, pp. 146–159. (eds Bouchard, C., Shephard, R. J., Stephens, T.). Human Kinetics Publishers, Champaign, Il., U.S.A.

Anderson, P. (1975). Capillary density in skeletal muscle of man. *Acta Physiol. Scand.*, **95**, 203–205.

Dal-Monte, A. and Lupo, S. (1989). Specific ergometry in the functional assessment of top class sportsman. *J. Sports Med. Phys. Fitness*, **29**, 4–8.

Lucas, J. (1977). A brief history of modern trends in marathon training. *Ann. NY Acad. Sci.*, **301**, 858–861.

Lydiard, A. (1978). *Run the Lydiard Way*. Hodder, London.

Salmons, S. and Jarvis, J. C. (1990). The working capacity of skeletal muscle transformed for use in a cardiac assisted role. In *Tranformed Muscle for Cardiac Assistant Repair*, pp. 89–104 (eds Chin, R. C-J and Bourgeois, I.) Futura, Mount Kisno, NY.

Sargeant, A. J., Davies, C. T. M., Edwards, R. H. T. *et al.* (1977). Functional and structural changes after disuse of human muscle. *Clin. Sci. Mol. Med.*, **52**, 337–342.

Sharp, C. (1988). Fitness and its measurement. *The Practitioner*, **232**, 974–976.

Shephard, R. J. (1978). *The Fit Athlete*. Oxford University Press, Oxford.

Spurway, N. C. (1992). Aerobic exercise, anaerobic exercise and the lactate threshold. *Br. Med. Bull.*, **48**, 569–591.

Viru, A. The mechanism of training effects: a hypothesis (1984). *Int. J. Sports Med.*, **5**, 219–227.

Chapter 10

Bannister, R. G. (1955). *The First Four Minutes*. Putnam, London.

Bannister, R. G. (1956). Muscular Effort. *Br. Med. Bull.*, **12**, 222–225.

Blomstrand, E., Hassmen, P. and Newsholme, E. A. (1991). Effect of branched-chain amino acid supplementation on mental performance. *Acta Physiol. Scand.*, **143**, 225–226.

Hardy, L. (1990). A catastrophe model of performance in sport. In *Stress and Performance in Sport*, pp. 81–106 (ed. Jones, J. G. and Hardy, L.). Wiley, Chichester.

Hardy, L. and Parfitt, G. (1991). A catastrophe model of anxiety and performance. *Br. J. Psychol.*, **82**, 163–178.

Johnson, R. W. and Morgan, W. P. (1981). Personality characteristics of college athletes in different sports. *Scand. J. Sports. Sci.*, **3**, 41–49.

Jones, J. G. and Hardy, L. (1990). The academic study of stress in sport. In *Stress and Performance in Sport*, pp. 3–16 (ed. Jones, J. G. and Hardy, L.). Wiley, Chichester.

Koltyn, K. F., O'Connor, P. J. and Morgan, W. P. (1991). Perception of effort in female and male competitive swimmers. *Int. J. Sports Med.* **12**, 427–429.

Martens, R., Burton, D. and Vealey, R. (1990). *Competitive Anxiety in Sport*. Champaign, Ill: Human Kinetics.

Miller, T. W., Vaughn, M. P. and Miller, J. M. (1990). Clinical issues and treatment strategies in stress-oriented athletes. *Sports Med.*, **9**, 370–379.

Morgan, W. P. (1980). Test of the champions: the iceberg profile. *Psychol. Today*, 6th July, 92–108.

Morgan, W. P., Brown, D. R., Raglin, J. S. *et al.* (1987). Psychological monitoring of overtraining and staleness. *Br. J. Sports Med.*, **21**, 107–114.

Morgan, W. P., O'Connor, P. J., Sparling, P. B. *et al.* (1987). Psychological characterization of the elite female distance runner. *Int. J. Sports Med.*, **8**, 124–131.

Morgan, W. P., Costill, D. L., Flynn, M. G. *et al.* (1988). Mood disturbance following increased training in swimmers. *Med. Sci. Sports Exerc.*, **20** 408–414.

Morgan, W. P., O'Connor, P. J., Ellickson, K. A. *et al.* (1988). Personality structure, mood states, and performance in elite male distance runners. *Int. J. Sport Psychol.*, **19**, 247–263.

Morgan, W. P. (1992). Monitoring and prevention of the staleness syndrome. *Second IOC World Congress on Sport Sciences*, pp. 19–23. COOB, Barcelona.

Neiss, R. (1988). Reconceptualizing arousal: psychobiological states in motor performance. *Psychological Bulletin*, **103**, 345–366.

Newsholme, E. A., Blomstrand, E., Hassmen, P. *et al.* (1991). Physical and mental fatigue: do changes in plasma amino acids play a role? *Biochem. Soc. Trans.*, **19**, 358–362.

Nideffer, R. M. (1985). *An Athlete's Guide to Mental Training.* Human Kinetic Publishers, Champaign, IL.

Nideffer, R. M. (1992). Preparation of individual athletes for Olympic competition. *Second IOC World Congress on Sport Sciences*, pp. 62–67. COOB, Barcelona.

Noakes, T. (1992). *Lore of Running* 2nd edit. Oxford University Press, Cape Town.

O'Connor, P. J., Morgan, W. P. and Raglin, J. S. (1991). Psychobiologic effects of increased training in female and male swimmers. *Med. Sci. Sports Exerc.*, **23**, 1055–1061.

O'Connor, P. J., Morgan, W. P., Koltyn, K. F. *et al.* (1991). Air travel across four time zones in college swimmers. *Am. Physiol. Soc.*, **70**, 756–763.

Raglin, J. S., Morgan, W. P. and Luchsinger, A. E. (1990). Mood and self-motivation in successful and unsuccessful female rowers. *Med. Sci. Sports Exerc.*, **22**, 849–853.

Raglin, J. S., Morgan, W. P. and Wise, K. J. (1990). Pre-competition anxiety and performance in female high school swimmers: a test of optimal function theory. *Int. J. Sports Med.*, **11**, 171–175.

Raglin, J. S., Wise, K. J. and Morgan, W. P. (1990). Predicted and actual pre-competition anxiety in high school girl swimmers. *J. Swimming Res.*, **6**, 6–8.

Rushall, B. S. (1979). *Psyching in Sport: The Psychological Preparation for Serious Competition in Sport.* Pelham Books, London.

Smith, A. M., Scott, S. G. and Wiese, D. M. (1990). The psychological effects of sports injuries: coping. *Sports Med.*, **9**, 352–369.

Tutko, T. and Tosi, U. (1978). *Sports Psyching: Playing Your Best Game All the Time.* Tarcher, Los Angeles.

Yerkes, R. M. and Dodson, J. D. (1908). The relation of strength of stimulus to rapidity of habit formation. *J. Comp. Neurol. Psychol.* **18**, 459–482.

Chapter 11

Alhadeff, L., Gualtieri, T. and Lipton, M. (1984). Toxic effects of water-soluble vitamins. *Nutr. Rev.*, **42**, 33–40.

Anderson, R. A. (1991). New insights on the trace elements, chromium, copper and zinc, and exercise. *Med. Sport Sci*, **32**, 38–58.

Applegate, E. A. (1991). Nutritional considerations for ultra-endurance performance. *Int. J. Sports. Nutr.*, **1**, 118–126.

Barnett, D. W. and Conlee, R. K. (1984). The effects of a commercial dietary supplement on human performance. *Am. J. Clin. Nutr.*, **40**, 586–590.

Belko, A. Z. (1987). Vitamins and exercise: an update. *Med. Sci. Sports Exerc.*, **19**, S191–S196.

Brouns, F., Saris, W. H. and Stroecken, J. (1989). Eating, drinking and cycling: a controlled Tour de France simulation study. *Int. J. Sports Med.*, **10**, S32–S40, S41–S48, S49–S62.

Burke, L. M. and Read, R. S. O. (1987). Diet patterns of elite Australian male triathletes. *Physician Sports Med.*, **15**, 140–155.

Campbell, W. W. and Anderson, R. A. (1987). Effects of aerobic exercise and training on the trace minerals chromium, zinc and copper. *Sports Med.*, **4**, 9–18.

Coggan, A. R. and Coyle, E. F. (1991). Carbohydrate ingestion during prolonged exercise: effects on metabolism and performance. *Exerc. Sport. Sci. Rev.*, **19**, 1–40.

Costill, D. L. (1988). Carbohydrates for exercise: dietary demands for optimal performance. *Int. J. Sports Med.*, **9**, 1–18.

Drinkwater, B. L. Physical activity, fitness, and osteoporosis (1994). In: *Physical Activity, Fitness, and Health. International Proceedings and Consensus Statement*, pp. 724–736. (eds Bouchard, C., Shephard, R. J., Stephens, T.). Human Kinetics Publishers, Champaign, Il., U.S.A.

Ellsworth, N. M., Hewitt, B. F. and Haskell, V. L. (1985). Nutrient intake of elite male and female nordic skiers. *Physician Sports Med.*, **13**, 78–92.

Fogoros, R. N. (1980). Runner's trots: gastrointestinal disturbances in runners. *JAMA*, **243**, 1743–1744.

Friedman, J. E., Neufer, P. D. and Dohm, G. L. (1991). Regulation of glycogen re-synthesis following exercise: dietary considerations. *Sports Med.*, **11**, 232 –243.

Hellemans, I. (1991). Nutrition for the iron man triathlete. *NZ J. Sports Med.*, **19**, 5–7.

Horswill, C. A., Hickner, R. C., Scott, J. R. *et al.* (1990). Weight loss, dietary carbohydrate modifications, and high intensity physical performance. *Med. Sci. Sports Exerc.*, **22**, 470–476.

Horton, E. S. (1986). Metabolic aspects of exercise and weight reduction. *Med. Sci. Sports Exerc.*, **18**, 10–18.

Hunding, A., Jordal, R. and Paulav, P-E. (1981). Runner's anaemia and iron deficiency. *Acta Med. Scand.*, **209**, 315–318.

Kreider, R. B., Miriel, V. and Bertun, E. (1993). Amino acid supplementation and exercise performance: analysis of the proposed ergogenic value. *Sports Med.*, **16**, 190–209.

Kunz, P., Steiner, G. and Wenk, C. (1989). The importance of providing minerals to long distance runners during a 30 km course. *Int. J. Vit. Nutr. Res.*, **59**, 426.

Lawrence, J. D., Bower, R. C., Riehl, W. P. and Smith, J. L. (1975). Effects of α-tocopherol acetate on the swimming endurance of trained swimmers. *Am. J. Clin. Nutr.*, **28**, 205–208.

Lefavi, R. G., Anderson, R. A., Keith, R. E., Wilson, G. D., McMillan, J. L. and Stone, M. H. (1992). Efficacy of chromium supplementation in athletes: emphasis on anabolism. *Intern. J. Sports Nutr.*, **2**, 111–122.

Lemon, P. W. (1987). Protein and exercise: update 1987. *Med. Sci. Sports Exerc.*, **9**, S179–S190.

Lemon, P. W. (1991). Effect of exercise on protein requirements. *J. Sports. Sci.*, **9**, 53–70.

Lemon, P. W. and Proctor, D. N. (1991). Protein intake and athletic performance. *Sports Med.*, **12**, 313–325.

Machlin, L. J. (ed.) (1990). *Handbook of Vitamins: Nutritional, Biochemical and Clinical Aspects*. Marcel Dekker, New York.

Martin, D. E., Vroon, D. H., May, D. F. and Pilbeam, S. P. (1986). Physiological changes in elite male distance runners training. *Physician Sports Med.*, **14**, 152–171.

Maughan, R. J. (1991). Fluid and electrolyte loss and replacement in exercise. *J. Sports Sci.*, **9**, 117–142.

McDonald, R. and Keen, C. L. (1988). Iron, zinc and magnesium nutrition and athletic performance. *Sports Med.*, **5**, 171–184.

Niemann, D. C., Butler, J. V., Pollett, L. M. *et al.* (1989). Nutrient intake of marathon runners. *J. Am. Diet. Assoc.*, **89**, 1273–1278.

Niemann, D. C., Butler, J. V., Pollet, L. M. *et al.*, (1989). Supplementation patterns in marathon runners. *J. Am. Diet. Assoc.*, **89**, 1615–1619.

Saris, W. H. and Brouns, F. (1986). Nutritional concerns for the young athlete. In *Children and Exercise XII*, pp. 11–18 (eds Rutenfranz, J., Mocelin, R. and Klimt, F.). University Park Press, Champaign, IL.

Saris, W. H., van Erp-Baart, M. A., Brouns, F. *et al.* (1989). Study on food intake and energy expenditure during extreme sustained exercise: the Tour de France. *Int. J. Sports Med.*, **10**, S1, S26–S31.

Schofield, W. N. (1985). Predicting basal metabolic rate: new standards and review of previous work. *Hum. Nutr. Clin. Nutr.*, **39**, (Suppl. 1), 5–41.

Sherman, W. M. and Costill, D. L. (1984). The marathon: dietary manipulation to optimize performance. *Am. J. Sports Med.*, **12**, 44–50.

Sherman, W. M. and Wimer, G. S. (1991). Insufficient dietary carbohydrate during training: does it impair athletic performance? *Int. J. Sports Nutr.*, **1**, 28–44.

Simon-Schnass, I. and Pabst, H. (1988). Influence of vitamin E on physical performance. *Int. J. Vit. Nutr. Res.*, **58**, 49–54.

Simonsen, J. C., Sherman, W. M., Lamb, D. R. *et al.* (1991). Dietary carbohydrate, muscle glycogen and power output during rowing training. *J. Appl. Physiol.*, **70**, 1500–1505.

Simopoulos, A. P. (1989). Opening address. Nutrition and fitness from the first Olympiad in 776 B.C. to 393 A.D. and the concept of positive health. *Am. J. Clin. Nutr.*, **49**, 921–926.

Stewart, M. L., McDonalds, J. T., Levy, A. S. *et al.* (1985). Vitamin/mineral supplement use: a telephone survey of adults in the United States. *J. Am. Diet. Assoc.*, **85**, 1585–1590.

van Dam, B. (1978). Vitamins and sports. *Br. J. Sports Med.*, **12**, 74–79.

van der Beek, E. J. (1985). Vitamins and endurance training: food for running or faddish claims? *Sports Med.*, **2**, 175–197.

van Erp-Baart, M. A., Saris, W., Binkhorst, J. A. *et al.* (1989). Nationwide survey on nutrient habits in élite athletes. Energy, carbohydrates, protein and fat intake. *Intern. J. Sports Med.* **10**, 3–10.

Weight, L. M., Myburgh, K. H. and Noakes, T. D. (1988). Vitamin and mineral supplementation: effect on the running performance of trained athletes. *Am. J. Clin. Nutr.*, **47**, 192–195.

Weight, L. M., Noakes, T. D., Labadarios, D., Graves, J., Jacobs, P. and Berman, P. A. (1988). Vitamin and mineral status of trained athletes including the effects of supplementation. *Am. J. Clin. Nutr.*, **47**, 186–191.

Williams, M. H. (1985). *Nutritional Aspects of Human Physical and Athletic Performance*, 2nd edn. Charles C. Thomas, Springfield, IL.

Williams, M. H. (1991). Focus: nutritional ergogenic aids. *Int. J. Sport Nutr.*, **1**, 213.

Wilmore, J. H. (1991). Eating and weight disorders in the female athlete. *Int. J. Sports Nutr.*, **1**, 104–117.

Chapter 12

Dressendorger, R. H., Wade, C. E. and Scaff, J. H. (1985). Increased morning heart rate in runners: a valid sign of overtraining. *Physician Sports Med.*, **13**, 77–86.

Fry, R. W., Morton, A. R. and Keast, D. (1991). Overtraining in athletes: an update. *Sports Med.*, **12**, 32–65.

Grisogono, V. (1984). *Sports Injuries: A Self-help Guide*. John Murray, London.

Hanley, D. F. (1976). Medical care of the U.S. Olympic team. *JAMA*, **236**, 147–148.

Kreider, R. B., Miriel, V. and Bertun, E. (1993). Amino acid supplementation and exercise performance: analysis of the proposed ergogenic value. *Sports Med.*, **16**, 190–209.

Lachmann, S. (1988). *Soft Tissue Injuries in Sport*. Blackwell Scientific, Oxford.

Muckle, D. S. (1982). Injuries in sport. *R. Soc. Health J.*, **102**, 93–94.

Noakes, T. (1992). *Lore of Running*, 2nd edit. Oxford University Press, Cape Town.

Nieman, D. C. Physical activity, fitness, and infection (1994). In: *Physical Activity, Fitness, and Health. International Proceedings and Consensus Statement*, pp. 796–813. (eds Bouchard, C., Shephard, R. J., Stephens, T.). Human Kinetics Publishers, Champaign, Il., U.S.A.

O'Connor, P. J., Morgan, W. P., Koltyn, K. F. *et al.* (1991). Air travel across four time zones in college swimmers. *J. Appl. Physiol.*, **70**, 756–763.

Pagliano, J. W. and Jackson, D. W. (1987). A clinical study of 3,000 long-distance runners. *Ann. Sports Med.*, **3**, 88–91.

Read, M. R. and Wade, P. I. (1984). *Sports Injuries. A Unique Guide to Self Diagnosis and Rehabilitation*. Breshlich & Foss, London.

Roberts, J. A. (1986). Viral illnesses and sports performance. *Sports Med.*, **3**, 296–303.

Vines, G. (1993). Overdosing on exercise. *New Scientist* (Suppl.), 9th October, 13–14.

Chapter 13

Berglund, B. and Ekblom, B. (1991). Effect of recombinant human erythropoietin treatment on blood pressure and some haematological parameters in healthy men. *J. Intern. Med.*, **229**, 125–130.

Bierly, J. R. (1987). Use of anabolic steroids by athletes: do the risks outweigh the benefits? *Postgrad. Med.*, **82**, 67–75.

Burks, T. F. (1991). Drug use in athletics. *Trends Pharmacol. Sci.*, **2**, 66–68.

Chol, P. Y. L., Parrott, A. C. and Cowan, D. (1989). Adverse behavioural effects of anabolic steroids in athletes: a brief review. *Sports. Med.*, **1**, 183–187.

Cowart, V. (1986). Control and treatment of drug abuse have challenged nation and its physicians for much of history. *JAMA*, **256**, 2465–2469.

Cregler, L. L. and Mark, H. (1986). Cardiovascular dangers of cocaine abuse. *Am. J. Cardiol.*, **57**, 1185–1186.

Ekblom, B. and Berglund, B. (1991). Effect of erythropoietin administration on maximal aerobic power. *Scand. J. Med. Sci. Sports*, **1**, 88–93.

Frankle, M. A., Cicero, G. J. and Payne, J. (1984). Use of androgenic anabolic steroids by athletes. *JAMA*, **252**, 482.

Goldman, B., Klatz, R. and Bush, P. (1984). *Death in the Locker Room*. Century Publishing, London.

Hervey, G. R., Knibbs, A. V., Burkinshaw, L. *et al.* (1981). Effects of methandienone on the performance and body composition of men undergoing athletic training. *Clin. Sci.*, **60**, 457–461.

Hickson, R. C., Ball, K. L. and Falduto, M. T. (1989). Adverse effects of anabolic steroids. *Med. Toxicol. Adverse Drug Exp.*, **4**, 254–271.

Lamb, D. R. (1984). Anabolic steroids in athletics: how well do they work and how dangerous are they? *Am. J. Sports Med.*, **12**, 31–38.

Laties, V. G. and Weiss, B. (1981). The amphetamine margin in sports. *Fed. Proc.*, **40**, 2689–2692.

Lombardo, J. A., Longrope, C. and Voy, R. O. (1985). Recognising anabolic steroid abuse. *Patient Care*, **19**, 28–47.

McCaughan, G. W., Bilous, M. J. and Gallagher, N. D. (1985). Long-term survival with tumor regression in androgen-induced tumors. *Cancer*, **56**, 2622–2626.

Mottram, D. R. (ed.) (1988). *Drugs in Sport*. E. & F.N. Spon Ltd, London.

Ryan, A. J. (1981). Anabolic steroids are fools' gold. *Fed. Proc.*, **40**, 2682–2688.

Ryan, A. J. (1984). Causes and remedies for drug misuse and abuse by athletes. *JAMA*, **252**, 517–519.

Sklarek, H. M., Mantovani, R. P., Erens, E. *et al.* (1984). AIDS in a body builder using anabolic steroids. *N. Engl. J. Med.*, **311**, 1701.

Strauss, R. H., Liggett, M. T. and Lanese, R. R. (1985). Anabolic steroid use and perceived effects in ten weight trained women athletes. *JAMA*, **253**, 2871–2873.

Taylor, V. N. (1985). *Hormonal Manipulation*. Jefferson, N. C. McFarland & Co., London.

Tennant, F., Black, D. L. and Voy, R. O. (1988). Anabolic steroid dependence with opioid-type features. *N. Engl. J. Med.*, **319**, 578.

Wade, N. (1972). Anabolic steroids: doctors denounce them, but athletes aren't listening. *Science*, **176**, 1399–1403.

Yesalis, C. E., Wright, J. E. and Bahrke, M. S. (1989). Epidemiological and policy issues in the measurement of the long term health effects of anabolic–androgenic steroids. *Sports Med.*, **8**, 129–138.

PART II

Section B

American College of Obstetricians and Gynecologists (1985). Pregnancy and the post-natal period. *ACOG Home Exercise Programs*, 1–5.

Artal, R. and Wiswell, R. A. (1985). *Exercise in Pregnancy*. Williams & Wilkins, Baltimore.

Carpenter, M. W. Physical activity, fitness, and health of the pregnant mother and fetus (1994). In: *Physical Activity, Fitness, and Health. International Proceedings and Consensus Statement*, pp. 967–989. (eds Bouchard, C.,

Shephard, R. J., Stephens, T.). Human Kinetics Publishers, Champaign, Il., U.S.A.

Section C

Jacobson, E. (1929). *Progressive Relaxation*. University of Chicago Press, Chicago, Ill., U.S.A.
Tutko, T. and Tosi, U. (1978) *Sports Psyching*. J. P. Tarcher, Los Angeles.

Section E

Cook, S. D., Brinker, M. R. and Poche, M. (1990). Running shoes: their relationship to running injuries. *Sports Med.*, **10**, 1–8.

Records*

WORLD RECORDS

Men

100 m	9.85 s	Leroy Burrell (USA)	1994
200 m	19.72 s	Pietro Mennea (ITA)	1979
400 m	43.29 s	Butch Reynolds (USA)	1988
800 m	1 m 41.73 s	Sebastian Coe (GBR)	1981
1500 m	3 m 28.86 s	Noureddine Morceli (ALG)	1992
Mile	3 m 44.39 s	Noureddine Morceli (ALG)	1993
3000 m	7 m 25.11 s	Noureddine Morceli (ALG)	1994
5000 m	12 m 56.96 s	Haile Gebresilasie (ETH)	1994
10 000 m	26 m 52.23 s	William Segei (KEN)	1994
Marathon	2 h 06 m 50s	Belayneh Dinsamo (ETH)	1988
110 m Hurdles	12.91 s	Colin Jackson (GBR)	1993
400 m Hurdles	46.78 s	Kevin Young (USA)	1992
3 km Steeplechase	8 m 02.08 s	Moses Kiptanui (KEN)	1992
4 × 100 m Relay	37.40 s	USA	1992 and 1993
4 × 400 m Relay	2 m 54.29 s	USA	1993
High Jump	2.45 m	Javier Sotomayor (CUB)	1993
Pole Vault	6.14 m	Sergei Bubka (UKR)	1994
Long Jump	8.95 m	Mike Powell (USA)	1991
Triple Jump	17.97 m	Willie Banks (USA)	1985
Shot	23.12 m	Randy Barnes (USA)	1990

WORLD RECORDS

Men continued

Discus	74.08 m	Jurgen Schult (GDR)	1986
Hammer	86.74 m	Yuri Sedykh (URS)	1986
Javelin	95.66 m	Jan Zelezny (Cz Rep)	1993
Decathlon	8891 pts	Dan O'Brien (USA)	1992

Women

100 m	10.49 s	Florence Griffith-Joyner (USA)	1988
200 m	21.34 s	Florence Griffith-Joyner (USA)	1988
400 m	47.60 s	Marita Koch (GDR)	1985
800 m	1 m 53.28 s	Jarmila Kratochvilova (TCH)	1983
1500 m	3 m 50.46 s	Qu Yunxia (CHN)	1993
Mile	4 m 15.61 s	Paula Ivan (ROM)	1989
3000 m	8 m 06.11 s	Wang Junxia (CHN)	1993
5000 m	14 m 37.33 s	Ingrid Kristiansen (NOR)	1986
10 000 m	29 m 31.78 s	Wang Junxia (CHN)	1993
Marathon	2 h 21 m 06 s	Ingrid Kristiansen (NOR)	1985
100 m Hurdles	12.21 s	Yordanka Donkova (BUL)	1988
400 m Hurdles	52.74 s	Sally Gunnell (GBR)	1993
4 × 100 m Relay	41.37 s	GDR	1985
4 × 400 m Relay	3 m 15.17 s	USSR	1988
High Jump	2.09 m	Stefka Kostadinova (BUL)	1987
Pole Vault	4.11 m	Sun Caiyun (CHN)	1993
Long Jump	7.52 m	Galina Chistiakova (URS)	1988
Triple Jump	15.09 m	Ana Biryukova (RUS)	1993
Shot	22.63 m	Natalya Lisovskaya (URS)	1987
Discus	76.80 m	Gabriele Reinisch (GDR)	1988
Hammer	66.84 m	Olga Kuzenkova (RUS)	1994
Javelin	80.00 m	Petra Felke (GDR)	1988
Heptathlon	7291 pts	Jackie Joyner-Kersee (USA)	1988

BRITISH RECORDS

Men

100 m	9.87 s	Linford Christie	1993
200 m	19.87 s	John Regis	1994
400 m	44.47 s	David Grindley	1992
800 m	1 m 41.73 s	Sebastian Coe	1981
1500 m	3 m 29.67 s	Steve Cram	1985
Mile	3 m 46.32 s	Steve Cram	1985
3000 m	7 m 32.79 s	David Moorcroft	1982
5000 m	13 m 00.41 s	David Moorcroft	1982
10 000 m	27 m 23.06 s	Eamonn Martin	1988
Marathon	2 h 07 m 13 s	Steve Jones	1985
110 m Hurdles	12.91 s	Colin Jackson	1993
400 m Hurdles	47.82 s	Kriss Akabusi	1992
3 km Steeplechase	8 m 07.96 s	Mark Rowland	1988
4 × 100 m Relay	37.77 s	(Great Britain)	1993
4 × 400 m Relay	2 m 57.53 s	(Great Britain)	1991
High Jump	2.37 m	Steve Smith	1992 and 1993
Pole Vault	5.65 m	Keith Stock	1981
Long Jump	8.23 m	Lynn Davies	1968
Triple Jump	17.57 m	Keith Connor	1982
Shot	21.68 m	Geoff Capes	1980
Discus	64.32 m	Bill Tancred	1974
Hammer	77.54 m	Martin Girvan	1984
Javelin	91.46 m	Steve Backley	1992
Decathlon	8847 pts	Daley Thompson	1984

BRITISH RECORDS

Women

100 m	11.10 s	Kathy Cook	1981
200 m	22.10 s	Kathy Cook	1984
400 m	49.43 s	Kathy Cook	1984
800 m	1 m 57.42 s	Kirsty Wade	1985
1500 m	3 m 59.96 s	Zola Budd	1985
Mile	4 m 17.57 s	Zola Budd	1985
3000 m	8 m 28.83 s	Zola Budd	1985
5000 m	14 m 48.07 s	Zola Budd	1985
10 000 m	30 m 57.07 s	Liz McColgan	1991
Marathon	2 h 25 m 56 s	Veronique Marot	1989
100 m Hurdles	12.82 s	Sally Gunnell	1988
400 m Hurdles	52.74 s	Sally Gunnell	1993
4 × 100 m Relay	42.43 s	(Great Britain)	1980
4 × 400 m Relay	3 m 22.01 s	(Great Britain)	1991
High Jump	1.95 m	Diana Davies	1982
Pole Vault	3.65 m	Kate Staples	1994
Long Jump	6.90 m	Bev Kinch	1983
Triple Jump	14.09 m	Ashia Hansen	1994
Shot	19.36 m	Judy Oakes	1988
Discus	67.48 m	Meg Ritchie	1981
Hammer	59.92 m	Lorraine Shaw	1994
Javelin	77.44 m	Fatima Whitbread	1986
Heptathlon	6623 pts	Judy Simpson	1986

USA RECORDS

Men

100 m	9.85 s	Leroy Burrell	1994
200 m	19.73 s	Mike Marsh	1992
400 m	43.29 s	Butch Reynolds	1988
800 m	1 m 42.60 s	Johnny Grey	1985
1500 m	3 m 29.77 s	Sydney Maree	1985
3000 m	7 m 33.37 s	Sydney Maree	1982
5000 m	13 m 01.15 s	Sydney Maree	1985
10 000 m	27 m 20.56 s	Mark Nenow	1986
Marathon	2 h 08m 52 s	Alberto Salazar	1982
3 km Steeplechase	8 m 09.17 s	Henry Marsh	1985
110 m Hurdles	12.92 s	Roger Kingdom	1989
400 m Hurdles	46.78 s	Kevin Young	1992
High Jump	2.40 m	Charles Austin	1991
Pole Vault	5.97 m	Scott Huffman	1994
Long Jump	8.95 m	Mike Powell	1991
Triple Jump	17.97 m	Willie Banks	1985
Shot	23.12 m	Randy Barnes	1990
Discus	71.32 m	Ben Plucknet	1983
Hammer	82.50 m	Lance Deal	1994
Javelin	85.70 m	Tom Pukstys	1993
Decathlon	8891 pts	Dan O'Brien	1992

USA RECORDS

Women

100 m	10.49 s	Florence Griffith-Joyner	1988
200 m	21.34 s	Florence Griffith-Joyner	1988
400 m	48.83 s	Valerie Brisco	1984
800 m	1 m 56.90 s	Mary Slaney	1985
1500 m	3 m 57.12 s	Mary Slaney	1993
3000 m	8 m 25.83 s	Mary Slaney	1985
5000 m	14 m 56.07 s	Annette Peters	1993
10 000 m	31 m 19.89 s	Lynn Jennings	1992
Marathon	2 h 21 m 21 s	Joan Benoit	1985
110 m Hurdles	12.40 s	Gail Devers	1993
400 m Hurdles	52.79 s	Sandra Farmer-Patrick	1993
High Jump	2.03 m	Louise Ritter	1988
Long Jump	7.49 m	Jackie Joyner-Kersee	1987
Triple Jump	14.23 m	Sheila Hudson	1992
Shot	20.18 m	Ramona Pagel	1988
Discus	66.10 m	Carol Cady	1986
Javelin	69.32 m	Kate Schmidt	1977
Heptathlon	7291 pts	Jackie Joyner-Kersee	1988

Index

Compiled by Annette Musker